THERAPEUTIC APPROACHES IN MENTAL HEALTH/PSYCHIATRIC NURSING

THERAPEUTIC APPROACHES IN MENTAL HEALTH/PSYCHIATRIC NURSING

Edition 4

David S. Bailey, EdD, FAClinP
Affiliated Psychological and Medical Consultants, Gainesville,
Georgia; Affiliate Medical Staff, Northeast Georgia Medical Center
and Laurelwood Psychiatric and Substance Abuse Hospital,
Gainesville, Georgia; and Consultant, Department of Human
Resources and Department of Family and Children's Services,
State of Georgia

Deborah Robinson Bailey, RN, BSN, BS, MSN
Director of Administrative Projects, Legislative Liaison,
and Healthcare Lobbyist, Northeast Georgia Health Systems;
and Wharton Fellow

 F. A. DAVIS COMPANY · Philadelphia

F. A. Davis Company
1915 Arch Street
Philadelphia, PA 19103

Printed in the United States of America

Last digit indicates print number: 10 9 8 7 6 5 4 3 2 1

Publisher, Nursing: Robert G. Martone
Nursing Editor: Alan Sorkowitz
Production Editor: Stephen D. Johnson
Cover Designer: Louis J. Forgione

As new scientific information becomes available through basic and clinical research, recommended treatments and drug therapies undergo changes. The authors and publisher have done everything possible to make this book accurate, up to date, and in accord with accepted standards at the time of publication. The authors, editors, and publisher are not responsible for errors or omissions or for consequences from application of the book, and make no warranty, expressed or implied, in regard to the contents of the book. Any practice described in this book should be applied by the reader in accordance with professional standards of care used in regard to the unique circumstances that may apply in each situation. The reader is advised always to check product information (package inserts) for changes and new information regarding dose and contraindictions before administering any drug. Caution is especially urged when using new or infrequently ordered drugs.

Library of Congress Cataloging in Publication Data

Bailey, David S.
    Therapeutic approaches in mental health/psychiatric nursing / David S. Bailey, Deborah Robinson Bailey.—Ed. 4.
        p.   cm.
    Rev. ed. of: Therapeutic approaches to the care of the mentally ill / David S. Bailey, Deborah R. Bailey. Ed. 3. c1993.
    Includes bibliographical references and index.
    ISBN 0-8036-0213-8 (pbk.)
    1. Psychiatric nursing.   I. Bailey, Deborah R.   II. Bailey, David D.   Therapeutic approaches to the care of the mentally ill.   III. Title.
    [DNLM: 1. Mental Disorders—therapy.   2. Mental Disorders—prevention & control.   WM 400 B154t 1997]
    RC440.B245   1997
    616.89'1—dc21
DNLM/DLC
for Library of Congress   96-40370
                                                              CIP

This book is dedicated to my wife, *Deborah Bailey*, who is also my coauthor. I am sure that most every man believes he is married to the perfect woman, but I consider myself to be the luckiest of the lucky. Deborah is a kind and loving person, and every day of my life, since we were married 20 years ago, I have looked forward to going home to her. While most everyone is struck by her physical beauty, by her intelligence, and by her skill as a nurse and healthcare executive, our daughter, Kelley, and I have had the private pleasure of appreciating her as supermom and lifemate. She has contributed immeasurably to our enjoyment of life and has been a kindred spirit in our adventurous exploration of the world. Since her diagnosis with breast cancer 2½ years ago, I have come to appreciate her uncommon courage. It was she who sought to comfort us when her doctors gave us the bad news. Fortunately, being a good nurse always, she found the problem early. We believe that saved her life. And if, on the basis of a kind heart and good deeds, persons are spared, she will be at the top of the list. I wish all of you could know her as I do. Your life would be enriched.

DSB

Listen

When I ask you to listen to me
  and you start giving advice
  you have not done what I asked.

When I ask you to listen to me
  and you begin to tell me why I shouldn't feel that way,
  you are trampling on my *feelings*.

When I ask you to listen to me
  and you feel you have to *do* something to solve my problem,
  you have failed me, strange as that may seem.

Listen! All I asked, was that you listen.
  not talk or do—just hear me.
Advise is cheap: 10 cents will get you both Dear Abby and
  Billy Graham in the same newspaper.
And I can do for myself; I'm not helpless.
  Maybe discouraged and faltering, but not helpless.

When you do something for me *that I can and need to do
  for myself,* you contribute to my fear and weakness.

But, when you accept as a simple fact that I do feel what I feel,
  no matter how irrational, then I can quit trying to convince
  you and can get about the business of understanding what's
  behind this irrational feeling.
  And when that's clear, the answers are obvious and I
  don't need advice.
Irrational feelings make sense when we understand what's
  behind them.

Perhaps that's why prayer works, sometimes, for some people
  because God is mute, and he doesn't give advice or
  try to fix things. "They" just listen and let you
  work it out for yourself.

So, please listen and just hear me. And, if you want to
  talk, wait a minute for your turn; and I'll listen to you.

Anonymous

▽ Preface

In the 20 years since the first edition of this book was published, we have moved from hospitalizing thousands of mentally ill persons in large state hospitals, to decentralized mental health care through the use of community programs, to almost no hospital care (thanks to "managed care"). It seems that economic "realities" have spawned a managed care industry that serves no one but itself, yet professes to "manage" on behalf of the payer and, implicitly, at the expense of the patient, the hospital, and doctor and nurse providers.

Lest we sound too cynical, let us acknowledge that there were providers who abused the previous system and who contributed to the current unhappy state of health care in the United States. In the end, patients lose, providers lose, and the payer still pays—and, in the eyes of many, the system is approaching shambles. But we will find a way out of this—we Americans always do.

In the midst of all this chaos you, as a student, are asked to carry on, to provide the care, the human touch, that heals in a way that medicine, electroshock treatment, and surgery cannot. You are asked to rise above the turmoil, to be therapeutic despite the frustrations and to sacrifice in order to preserve the profession. And you will—we have faith because that is what we have come to know about the tens of thousands of you who have used our books over the last 20 years. You will preserve on behalf of people like our neighbor whose house burned as this was being written. He lost every material treasure that he and his wife of 47 years had accumulated, and along with it, the evidence of their history of half a century of life together. They lost a history they can never touch again—and with it lost their sense of invulnerability that allowed them, and us, to take for granted a history that can never be relived but only dimly remembered. It is for them, and for others in pain, that our profession endures.

Thus, it is with our heartfelt thanks to those who carry on that we offer this fourth edition. We have updated all the chapters, altered the diagnostic chapters to conform to the *DSM-IV* nomenclature, and have added a chapter on therapeutic tools of the nurse as a person. We are grateful for the significant numbers of you who have expressed support and appreciation for the practical nature of the book and for our willingness to make specific verbal and behavioral suggestions and recommendations. We know we risk the wrath of those who would handle such situations differently and stress that we offer our suggestions as *one* way to approach problems and not as the *only* way to handle those problems.

So what of the future of mental health? The dawn of the third millennium lies quietly before us, a sleeping enigma that will, before its end, redefine what it means to be human. A thousand years from now interstellar travel will be as commonplace as going to the beach and mental health "adjustments" will mean accessing a transneural interface device that will download neuronal sequences to stabilize aberrant homeostatic brain mechanisms.

However, we will not go that far with the fourth edition of this book. While this edition marks the 20th year that we have been adding our modest efforts to the battle against "aberrant neuronal sequences," it seems that a concerted effort continues in some corners to have mental illness reduced to just such a biologic manifestation. The authors continue to believe that at least some part of such neuronal sequences reflects the efforts of wholly functioning human beings to adapt to their environment. Which came first? The aberrant neuronal sequence or a stressor that set into motion an adaptation to that stressor which altered a previously "normally" functioning neuronal sequence? This is a question whose time has come—and it is at the interface between the mind and body that answers will be found. Hopefully we will know the answer or answers soon because many of us believe that in those answers may lie solutions to many biologic conditions such as heart disease and cancer.

David S. Bailey
Deborah Robinson Bailey

Contents

Introduction to Mental Healthcare Settings

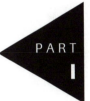

PART

I

Introduction to Working with the Mentally Ill

OBJECTIVES: Student will be able to:

1. Evaluate own feelings and attitudes about mental illness.
2. Compare personal views with those commonly held by practitioners in the mental health field.
3. Understand the importance of the relationship between the mental health worker and patient.
4. Increase awareness of own anxieties related to caring for the mentally ill.

▼ Attitude Inventory Exercise*

Before you begin to use this book, take a few minutes to examine your own feelings and attitudes about mental illness. React to the following statements and decide whether you believe them to be true or false. Let your feelings be your guide. Circle your choice: True or False.

T	F	1. People who enjoy working with mentally ill patients are somewhat mentally unstable themselves.
T	F	2. Most people who are emotionally disturbed are overly active.
T	F	3. Mental illness may develop suddenly.
T	F	4. Mentally ill people are also mentally deficient.
T	F	5. People who have been mentally ill may recover from their illness and live normal lives again.

---

* Slightly modified from Dreyer, S., Bailey, D., and Doucet, W.: *A Guide to Nursing Management of Psychiatric Patients*. St. Louis: Mosby, 1975, with permission.

T F   6. People who have mental illness should not marry or have children.

T F   7. Heavy consumption of alcohol may be a symptom of mental illness.

T F   8. People who work with mentally ill patients soon realize that their own emotional problems are insignificant.

T F   9. Most mentally ill patients are dangerous and may kill others.

T F   10. People who are wealthy rarely become mentally ill.

T F   11. Most people doubt their own sanity at one time or another.

T F   12. Most people who are mentally ill have a certain look that identifies them as being disturbed.

T F   13. The largest number of mentally ill people come from underprivileged families.

T F   14. The actions and speech of most mental patients are revolting and disgusting to others.

T F   15. The main reason that people are committed for psychiatric treatment is to protect the community.

T F   16. It is usually necessary to put emotionally ill patients in seclusion rooms.

T F   17. Hereditary factors determine whether a person becomes mentally ill.

T F   18. Physical disease may influence emotional balance.

T F   19. People who are mentally ill are often very sensitive to the happenings in their environment.

T F   20. Working with mentally ill patients may often cause a person to become mentally ill.

T F   21. Learning about mental disease, psychiatry, and the functions of the mind is harmful to well-adjusted, normal people.

T F   22. Unfortunately, not much can be done for mental patients aside from administering to their physical needs and hoping that they will get well.

T F   23. Mentally ill patients have no sense of humor.

T F   24. To convince a patient to behave in a socially acceptable manner, it is necessary to use punishment.

T F   25. Mentally ill patients often have feelings and emotions similar to those of normal people.

T   F   26. People who are mentally ill can be dangerous to themselves.

T   F   27. Working long hours causes mental illness.

T   F   28. Withdrawal from normal activities may be a sign of mental illness.

T   F   29. A person may handle anxiety by becoming mentally ill.

T   F   30. Mentally ill persons develop strong sexual urges and are unable to control their behavior.

T   F   31. Mentally ill patients who are doing well and seem capable of assuming responsibility for their behavior should not be allowed to do so because they may suddenly become ill again.

T   F   32. It is easy to identify the needs of the mentally ill.

T   F   33. Symptoms of mental illness may be very deeply hidden within a person.

T   F   34. Children should be protected from all frustrating situations.

T   F   35. Experiencing feelings of inferiority is a sign of mental illness.

T   F   36. Early recognition and treatment do not affect the course of mental illness.

T   F   37. Today mentally ill people have no problem being accepted by other members of society.

T   F   38. People readily admit that they need help for emotional disturbances.

T   F   39. Members of the medical and nursing profession accept and have an understanding attitude toward mental illness, just as they do about other types of illness.

T   F   40. People whose behavior is deeply disturbed are best treated on the back wards of state hospitals.

T   F   41. Attitudes and feelings about mental illness learned previously may affect a person's ability to deal effectively with mentally disturbed patients.

Using the mental health attitude inventory that you have just completed, compare your views with those commonly held by practitioners in the mental health field. (The answers are given in the Appendix.) If your responses differ significantly from the views held by mental health practitioners, you should not feel too uncomfortable. Even in this day of organ transplants, interplanetary exploration, rescues of wayward satellites, and laser beam surgery, a large part of our population still attaches a great deal of fear and shame to mental illness.

Although some unhealthy attitudes toward mental illness still exist, during the last hundred years or so considerable gains have been made in treating persons afflicted with mental disorders. Society no longer considers them to be under spells or curses or to be possessed by demons. For the most part, mental illness is now viewed as a sickness that may be caused by a wide variety of factors.

Although pinpointing a specific reason for a given person's becoming mentally ill at a particular time is difficult, factors such as physical illness, work, family crises, broken love relationships, repeated disappointments, and prolonged frustration are frequently associated with loss of a person's ability to cope with the demands of day-to-day living. Many authorities believe that a person cannot inherit a specific mental illness but can inherit a predisposition to certain types of mental problems. It is also clear that biologic factors play a major role in certain types of mental illness. Whether people develop an illness to which they are predisposed depends largely upon personal life experiences and the environment in which they live. The question of why a particular person becomes mentally ill under certain conditions whereas another person exposed to the same conditions manages to continue to function is a puzzling one.

The most reasonable explanation probably lies in the fact that different personal experiences cause a difference in what a person perceives as stressful and how much stress a person can tolerate. Some people are afraid of all snakes, some are afraid of only poisonous snakes, and some do not fear snakes at all. Some people fear heights; some do not. The way an individual views a situation determines her or his response. The mentally ill patient often has learned many inappropriate behaviors that must be unlearned or replaced with more acceptable behaviors. Such relearning frequently takes a great deal of time, and hospitalization or prolonged outpatient treatment may be required. There is also a significant question as to the role biologic factors play in determining a person's sensitivity to environmental events. A further question involves whether environmental events *cause* biologic or biochemical abnormalities or whether biologic or biochemical abnormalities *shape* a person's response to environmental events.

Thanks to recent medical advances leading to the development of more effective drugs and improved treatment methods, many hospitalized psychiatric patients are able to return home to their families in a matter of days or weeks. Others do not require hospitalization at all but are treated as outpatients or in day care programs. Some continue to perform their jobs and receive therapy in evening programs. No longer is it necessary to send mentally ill patients to large institutions far from their homes and families to receive treatment.

With treatment, many patients are able to make a complete recovery, and some are better adjusted than before their symptoms appeared. Others are helped to function more effectively but may need to remain on medication for prolonged periods and avoid certain stressful situations that might cause their symptoms to reappear.

Most people, however, are still extremely concerned about what their friends, relatives, boss, and neighbors would think if they were hospitalized for mental illness. Because of these fears, many people who need help do not seek it, and those who are hospitalized are extremely concerned about confidentiality of information. Until they develop a trusting relationship with staff members, they may be very reluctant to disclose any information about themselves. Trusting relationships are not built quickly. Mentally ill patients are very sensitive to how other people feel and react toward them. Perhaps this acute sensitivity is one of the reasons they have become ill, for in society it is extremely important to be accepted, well liked, and a member of the group.

Because mental illness affects all races, ages, and socioeconomic groups, any of us, if subjected to enough stress, may suffer an emotional crisis. In fact, new workers in the mental health field often worry about their own "wellness" in that they see many similarities between their patients and themselves. At one time or another, everyone has minor mood swings, gets depressed, or feels anger, anxiety, or fear. All people occasionally mistrust others. Most people have said, at one time or another, "I'm going to go crazy" or "Are you off your rocker?" The difference between being mentally healthy and mentally ill lies in the frequency and intensity of inappropriate behavior and often in the public's tolerance of such behavior.

New mental health workers often experience considerable anxiety because they feel they do not know what to do for their patients. Physical health team members work in a more structured environment. They have tests to run, medicines to give, patients to be bathed, diagnostic and treatment procedures to do, and patients who are generally cooperative. Of course, they, too, must listen to their patients, but mental health workers must realize that often their primary contribution to a patient may be simply that they are there and available to listen if the patient wishes to talk. In their book, *Psychiatric Nursing in the Hospital and the Community* (Prentice-Hall, 1973), Burgess and Lazare state: "It takes some time to realize that listening to that which aches in the heart of the patient may touch him more profoundly than a back rub."

Finally, as has been pointed out by Erbs-Palmer and Anthony (1995), mental health workers in psychiatric settings are significantly influenced "by myths about the illness, diagnosis, prognosis, and the success rates for treatment." They go on to say, "Whenever nurses try to predict the future based on diagnosis and current symptoms, we are constantly surprised by the progress and success of individuals diagnosed with psychiatric disabilities." In keeping with those thoughts, consider making it your priority to focus on the person for whom you are caring and do not be discouraged by myths and other factors that suggest an inability to succeed. After all, Columbus did not, as was feared by most people of his time, fall off the edge of the world when he set sail for the horizon.

This brief overview of selected general factors related to mental health was intended to provide the mental health worker with a framework for viewing mental illness as it is seen by people currently active in this field. Keep these points in mind as you study the other chapters in this book.

Annotated Bibliography

Agostinelli, B., Demers, K., Garrigan, D., and Waszynski, C.: Targeted interventions: Use of the mini-mental state exam. *Journal of Gerontology Nursing,* 1994, 20(8):15–23.

Authors favor the MMSE for a global cognitive assessment as well as for clues to patients' abilities and disabilities with daily living skills.

Erbs-Palmer, V. K., and Anthony, W.: Incorporating psychiatric rehabilitation principles into mental health nursing. *Journal of Psychosocial Nursing,* 1995, 8(3):36–44.

Dispels myths about mental illness. Discusses the negative impact of severe mental illness. Explores the differences between the rehabilitation and treatment approaches to mental illness.

Fabrega, H.: Psychiatric stigma in the classical and medieval period: A review of the literature. *Comprehensive Psychiatry,* 1990, 31(4):289–306.

Explores how mental illness was viewed in the classical and medieval periods and how these perspectives have affected the view and therefore the treatment of mental illness today.

Jost, K. E.: Psychosocial care: Document it. *American Journal of Nursing,* July 1995, 46–49.

Discusses ways to document psychosocial care with chart example entries and intervention terms.

Lowery, B. J.: Psychiatric nursing in the 1990s and beyond. *Journal of Psychosocial Nursing,* 1992, 30(1):7–13.

Discusses the major advances in the mental health field and the rapid changes in psychiatric nursing due to these advances.

Reinhard, S. C.: Living with mental illness: Effects of professional support and personal control on care giving. *Research in Nursing & Health,* 1994, 17:79–88.

Explores the burdens on caregivers for the mentally ill.

Riley, J. A.: Dual diagnosis: Comorbid substance abuse or dependency and mental illness. *Nursing Clinics of North America,* 1995, 29(1):29–33.

Discusses the importance of proper assessment with dual diagnosis and how these patients do not fit into the traditional 12-step programs that use confrontation and self-management principles.

Robin, R., Vaicunas, J., and Akers, J.: Abnormal behavior: Yesterday and today. In Bootzin, R. R., Acocella, J. R., and Alloy, L. B. (eds.): *Abnormal Psychology: Current Perspectives* (6th ed.). New York: McGraw-Hill, 1993.

Discusses deviations from cultural norms as determinants of abnormal behavior.

References

Burgess, A. W., and Lazare, A.: *Psychiatric Nursing in the Hospital and the Community.* Englewood Cliffs, N.J.: Prentice-Hall, 1973.

Erbs-Palmer, V. K., and Anthony, W.: Incorporating psychiatric rehabilitation principles into mental health nursing. *Journal of Psychosocial Nursing,* 1995, 8(3):37.

Post-Test

True or False. Circle your choice.

T   F   1. A person may inherit a predisposition to certain types of mental illness.

T   F   2. Mentally ill patients are usually very sensitive to how other people feel toward them.

T   F   3. The treatment of mental illness is usually a very clear-cut process.

T   F   4. Any person, if subjected to enough stress, may have a "mental breakdown."

T   F   5. Minor mood swings are signs of mental illness.

T   F   6. People do not inherit mental disorders but may inherit a predisposition to certain types of mental problems.

T   F   7. Trusting relationships are easily established with the mentally ill.

T   F   8. If you feel you have said the wrong thing to a patient and feel it has caused the patient harm, continue to apologize until the apology is accepted.

T   F   9. It is not normal for a mental health worker to be disappointed or angry with a patient.

T   F   10. It is usually quite simple to pinpoint why a person has become mentally ill at a particular time.

Post-Test

(continued)

Fill in the Blanks. From the group of terms listed on the right, select the letter of the most appropriate term(s) to complete the following sentences.

1. The difference between being mentally healthy and mentally ill lies in the _____ and _____ of inappropriate behavior.

2. Mentally ill patients are very _____ to how people feel and react toward them.

3. It is the way people view a situation that determines their _____.

4. New drugs have helped to _____ the length of hospitalization of the mentally ill.

5. Mental health workers must realize that often their primary contribution to a patient may be simply that they are _____.

A. decrease

B. increase

C. response

D. intensity

E. sensitive

F. frequency

G. available to listen

H. insensitive

I. confused

J. aware of the problem

Multiple Choice. Circle the number or letter you think represents the best answer.

1. As a member of the community, the mental health worker can help reduce the loss to society that often occurs when someone becomes mentally ill by:
   a. Increasing the public's knowledge of the mental health services available in the community.
   b. Remembering that the mentally ill are permanently disabled.
   c. Having a personal attitude of acceptance in regard to mentally ill persons.

Post-Test

(continued)

    d. Alerting the public to the early signs of mental illness through education.
       (1) a and c.
       (2) b and d.
       (3) a, c, and d.
       (4) All of the above.

2. To be an effective mental health worker, an individual must:
    a. Understand the basic dynamics of human behavior.
    b. Be willing to explore his or her own feelings and reactions.
    c. Be able to give patients sound advice.
    d. Be able to work effectively with other members of the psychiatric team.
       (1) a and c.
       (2) a, b, and d.
       (3) a, c, and d.
       (4) All of the above.

3. Which of the following statements are true about community mental health centers, day care programs, and halfway houses?
    a. Offer care to patients without removing them from their community or family for long periods.
    b. Prevent regression and dependency of patients, which often occur during long-term hospitalization.
    c. Are rapidly growing approaches to care of the mentally ill.
    d. Probably help patients learn to cope with the environment in which they became ill.
       (1) a and b.
       (2) b and d.
       (3) a, b, and c.
       (4) All of the above.

Post-Test

(continued)

4. In working with emotionally or mentally compromised patients, effective measures include:
   a. Acceptance of the patient as a unique and worthwhile individual.
   b. Support and understanding of the patient's feelings.
   c. Recognition and reinforcement of the patient's strengths.
   d. Prevention of regression on the part of the patient.
      (1) a and d.
      (2) b and c.
      (3) a, b, and c.
      (4) All of the above.

5. The aim of psychiatric treatment is to:
   a. Relieve the patient of symptoms.
   b. Return the patient to home and family.
   c. Help the patient become a better adjusted individual.
   d. Prevent the patient from becoming psychotic.

Personality Development

OBJECTIVES: Student will be able to:

1. Recognize the stages of personality development.
2. Identify the developmental tasks related to the stages of development.
3. Define *id, ego,* and *superego.*
4. Enumerate and explain Erikson's eight-stage theory of personality development.

To understand abnormal behavior, it is essential to have a basic understanding of how a human being learns to behave in a normal (socially acceptable) manner. Because an individual's personality and perception of self are key factors in determining the type of behavior the individual exhibits, this chapter presents a basic overview of personality development, principally Sigmund Freud's theoretical formulations of the id, ego, and superego and Erik Erikson's eight-stage theory of psychosocial development. Freud's theories spurred much research and led the field of mental health out of a period of hopelessness in treating mental illness. Although many of his ideas are considered inaccurate in present-day theoretical formulations, others are still used to explain how people go about defending themselves against emotional distress (see Chapter 3).

Whereas Freud emphasized psycho*sexual* development, Erik Erikson, initially a follower of freudian principles, broke with Freud and emphasized psycho*social* development. Freud considered that the personality was essentially well established by the age of 5 or 6, but Erikson believed that personality development extends from birth to death.

Despite Erikson's belief that events occurring throughout life may affect emotional adjustment, many mental health experts believe that a person's experiences during the first 20 years have the most significant impact on the development of the personality. The freudians, usually referred to as *psychoanalytic* theorists, say that the first 6 years of life are the most crucial. Regardless of which opinion is correct, all agree that an individual's early life experiences directly influence mental health.

For the sake of discussion, the stages of personality development are usually divided in the following manner: infancy (birth to age 1½), toddler period (age 1½ to 3), preschool period (age 3 to 6), school age (age 6 to puberty, which usually occurs between ages 11 and 13), adolescence (puberty to age 18 or 20), and adulthood (from age 18 or 20 on). Each developmental stage serves as a building block in the foundation of personality. If a stage is completed successfully, the foundation remains firm; if there are serious problems during any of the stages, the personality structure is weakened.

Individuals develop at their own rate, and no two human beings are exactly alike; however, each stage has certain tasks that most people accomplish during that stage. For example, one of the developmental tasks of the toddler is to learn to walk, and most children learn the basics of walking between the ages of 1 and 3. Nevertheless, most of these same children are still refining their ability to walk after they have entered the preschool stage and are busy conquering the tasks of that period.

INFANCY

Most authorities believe that normal newborns possess all the basic ingredients (genetic inheritance) to become biologically functioning human beings; however, their ability to utilize their inherited potential depends on their life experiences. For example, if a child has the genetic potential to become a great pianist but is born into a poor family, never hears a piano, and never has a chance to take piano lessons, this great genetic potential is likely to go unrecognized and unused. Another child who has the finest music lessons and the best piano that money can buy but no genetic potential or musical talent can develop, at best, into an average piano player.

A new computer is mechanically ready to function and solve all sorts of complicated problems, yet it cannot begin to function until it is fed, by a human being, a massive dose of raw information, facts, and formulas (programming). A human infant functions in much the same manner. A 5- or 6-year-old child has great difficulty learning to read unless someone, usually the child's parents, has spent 5 or so years programming the child's "computer" (the brain). They prepare the child by saying over and over that a chair is a chair, that a cow is a cow and not a moo, and that a burner on a stove is hot, and by providing the child with a large variety of learning experiences such as trips to the zoo, the store, and the fire department.

Newborn children also have no concept of morality. They are gradually taught right and wrong over the first few years of life according to what their parents consider right and wrong. Sigmund Freud considered the newborn to be a "bundle of id." Simply stated, *id* was Freud's term for that part of the personality that is unconscious and contains all of the "wants" of an individual (e.g., to eat, to sleep, to be comfortable, to have fun, and to do pleasurable things). In other words, infants want their basic needs (food, diapers changed, sleep, attention) met at the exact moment they want them, regardless of whom they inconvenience (usually Mom and Dad at 2 A.M.). Gradually, throughout the first year of life, infants learn that there are others in the world and that, despite a mother's best efforts, warming a bottle or changing a diaper takes a few minutes.

When 3- or 4-month-old infants demand a feeding, most cry, indicating their hunger need, but become quiet when someone takes the bottle out of the refrigerator and begins to warm it. Children begin to trust their parents to follow through in meeting their needs and thus begin to develop feelings that the world is a good place to live and grow. By contrast, infants who are allowed to cry for hours before being fed or who are constantly abused and neglected begin to mistrust people and to feel that the world is not a very likable place. If deprivation and neglect are severe enough, infants and young children withdraw from the world of reality into a world of fantasy that feels less threatening. Therefore, in the first year of life, infants need as little frustration as possible in order to learn to trust their environment and to feel good about themselves and their world. It is not surprising, then, that Erikson named this first stage of development "basic trust versus mistrust."

An unfortunate characteristic of children is that they tend to blame themselves for their parents' failures and thus develop feelings of inadequacy that may affect them all their lives. For example, when parents divorce, young children often blame themselves, plead with the parents to stay together, and promise never to be bad again. This sense of being able to make all sorts of things happen is apparently a carryover from early infancy when young infants, unable to see well enough to distinguish themselves from others, feel that they themselves meet their own needs. Of course, by the time they are 4 to 6 months old, infants can recognize their mothers and see them as the source of relief for all their tension; therefore, they transfer their feelings of omnipotence to their mothers and expect them to cure all ills. For example, a young child may ask his mother to make the rain go away or ask her father to make an injured finger stop hurting.

Although parents are not omnipotent, the role of a mother (or mother substitute) is extremely important in the life of an infant. Infants need the psychological satisfaction that comes from being held close to another human being while being caressed and talked to in a gentle, caring way. The mother figure is the first love object for all humankind. An infant is completely dependent on her, and thus the mother-child relationship is perhaps more intense than any other relationship in one's life. In the more serious psychological illnesses, one of the causative factors is frequently a flaw in the mother-child relationship. Often to their dismay, children soon realize that neither they nor their mothers are omnipotent. In favorable circumstances, this realization occurs gradually as children master more of the skills of daily living and feel more in control of their environment and thus less insecure and dependent.

TODDLER PERIOD

Between the ages of 1 and 2½ or 3, children begin to develop a sense of autonomy. In other words, they begin to view themselves as individuals in their own right, apart from their parents, although still dependent on them. Children now have minds of their own and want to try to deal with reality in their own way. Parents tend to remember this stage of development well, for all of a sudden the quiet, cuddly, agreeable, helpless, dependent, clinging little infant seems to become a tyrant who states over and over, "No, no, no," while refusing all offers of help and scurrying around as if in training for the Olympics.

Unfortunately, many parents fail to recognize and accept this stage for what it is: the child's first attempts at establishing independence and self-reliance. They feel threatened. A ridiculous battle may ensue, and an insecure parent may be heard yelling, "No 2-year-old is going to say 'no' to me!" What parents may fail to realize is that the world is a frustrating place for toddlers. They are quite interested in their world and want to do a great many things; however, they are too short to see much of what is going on, cannot walk or climb well enough to get them where they want to go, cannot dress themselves, and, most of all, are constantly being told what to do by someone four or five times their size.

The world is also frustrating for adults who have children, especially when they are faced with the delicate task of toilet training. It is hard for most adults to believe that they once thought freedom constituted being able to mess in their pants whenever they wanted or that they once felt that fecal material was something special they had created. This, however, is apparently the way many toddlers view the situation. Toddlers are unable to look ahead and realize that when they are toilet trained their parents will take them more places. They must also be taught by their parents that their feces are not artistic creations, that they smell bad, and that they belong in only one place, the toilet.

In other areas of muscle and motor development, this conflict of interest does not exist because the child and the parents agree about their goals. Parents are delighted when their children learn to walk and encourage and reward them for doing so. With toilet training, children want to please their mothers and fathers and at the same time want to retain their freedom and therefore experience conflict. However, in the end, the desire to please the parents usually wins out, and the adult attitude about fecal material is adopted.

This stage of development progresses much more smoothly when parents do not attempt toilet training until the child is physically and psychologically receptive to the idea. Voluntary control of the anal sphincter muscle does not develop until a child is 18 to 24 months old, and by that time the child is usually beginning to show signs of disgust at having "accidents." Serious psychological problems may occur if a parent tries to toilet train a child too early, is excessively preoccupied with neatness or cleanliness, or is overly permissive and enjoys rearing a child with no shame, guilt, or need to conform to the norms of the society in which they live. Humans do not live in isolation and, therefore, must conform to some extent to societal norms. This socialization process takes place in infancy and childhood, and when parents fail to assume their responsibility for making sure that socialization does indeed occur, the individual usually has a great deal of difficulty adjusting as an adult. For example, people who are considered antisocial or sociopathic because they function as a "bundle of id," wanting what they want, when they want it, regardless of whom it inconveniences or hurts, frequently had overly permissive parents. Society does not tolerate such behavior well, and sociopaths often spend their lives on the fringes of society or in and out of jail or mental institutions.

Erikson calls this toddler stage of psychosocial development "autonomy versus shame and doubt." In this stage (or developmental crisis, as Erikson calls his stages), children either develop an enhanced sense of independence and competence (autonomy) or learn to doubt themselves and to subvert their own will to that of their parents and others. The crucial element in this stage is one of balancing the need for developing an appropriate level of autonomy with an appreciation for observing reasonable social and personal limitations.

PRESCHOOL PERIOD

By the end of the toddler or muscle training period, children have greatly increased motor and intellectual skills. Three-year-olds have fairly good vocabularies that enable them to tell about their experiences, and they can ride tricycles, run with only a few falls, dress themselves if the buttons are big and in the front, and can generally stay dry through the night. These accomplishments boost their self-esteem and help children feel good about themselves. They are then ready to learn more about the world outside their families. During this period (age 3 to 6), the ego and superego begin to function. The superego is the conscience part of the personality. It is composed of all the "controls," the shoulds and should nots learned from parents, churches, schools, and teachers. Its structure depends largely on the type, quality, and severity of discipline.

Parents frequently do not realize how critically they behave toward their children and how little room they allow for mistakes. A child who mispronounces a word may be ridiculed, and parents may try to force the child to say the word correctly. Later, they wonder why the child is so quiet and seldom talks. Parents tend to forget the words they mispronounce or the times they stutter. A child who spills a glass of milk may be called clumsy and be punished by parents who react to the inconvenience of cleaning up without realizing that they caused the problem by not understanding that a 3-year-old child's hand cannot reach around a large milk glass. Events such as these chip away at feelings of self-worth, especially when parents tell children over and over that they are bad or should be ashamed of themselves. Parents do better to identify only a child's *behavior* as bad or unacceptable, rather than calling the child bad or good. It is the behavior that is unacceptable, not the child.

By the time children are 5 or 6 years old, parents no longer have to be physically present to enforce discipline. The children have incorporated their parents' scolding into their own minds, and, before they do something, they hear that still, small voice (the superego or conscience) saying, "You better watch out. You know how clumsy you are, and if you break that toy you're going to be a bad kid."

Of course, children need discipline, but discipline needs to be given consistently, in small doses, and only when absolutely needed. Proper environmental structure tends to reduce the need for excessive discipline because the child knows what is expected. A child needs to learn to respond to reasonable limits. If there is no discipline, children fail to develop a sense of right and wrong and lack respect for other people and their belongings. Then again, if discipline is too severe, the child becomes afraid to try anything new or different, experiences extreme guilt and shame, and, in effect, becomes a maladapted person who is afraid of the world. Erikson labeled this third stage of development "initiative versus guilt." Individuals need well-balanced personalities. They need consciences, superegos that allow them to make changes and mistakes and to be successful in give-and-take situations with other people, yet they must be able to accept blame when they are wrong and change their behavior when necessary without becoming so guilt-ridden that continued functioning is impossible. This balance is where the ego plays its major role.

The ego is conscious and functions as the "manager" of the personality. It deals with reality, manages the impulses or demands of the unconscious id and superego, and finds acceptable ways to meet the demands of the id and superego in the conscious world of reality. Of course, the ego must have help in its managerial role. It gets that help from the psychological defense mechanisms, which are discussed in the next chapter.

The preschool period has been called the *family triangle* (e.g., mother, father, and child) period. It is the first time that boys and girls encounter different conflicts and achievements. By age 3, the baby no longer exists, and the child looks like either a little boy or a little girl. Both sexes are acutely aware of their own bodies and the physical changes that are occurring. The genital area is now the body region of emotional significance, and both boys and girls seek a sexual type of pleasure through manipulation of their external genitals. This behavior occurs in nearly all normal children and is even seen in infants, though more randomly and less purposefully.

Unfortunately, many parents react negatively when they find their child masturbating and may resort to various threats and punishments to stop the behavior. Some parents verbally instruct the child to stop and tell them that masturbation is not nice or may be harmful. Other parents may resort to threats of cutting off a boy's penis or suggest retaliation from supernatural beings because the parents feel masturbation is a sin. Most children stop masturbating or continue with it less frequently and with greater discrimination because of fear or because of their desire to please their parents. In either case, a great deal of guilt is produced that must be handled by the child. The guilt is often handled by repression, an unconscious forgetting of threatening events. Unfortunately, the individual does not really forget the event. Instead, it becomes part of the individual's unconscious where, although not remembered, it may motivate future behavior.

SCHOOL AGE

Psychologically, the early school years are quiet and peaceful ones for the child. Some authorities have even gone so far as to describe the span of time between ages 6 and 10 as the "golden era of childhood." At this point in a child's development, sexual frustrations and problems of the family period have usually been at least partially resolved. Most children have given up masturbation in return for parental approval and are actively attempting to become more like the parent of the same sex, instead of trying to possess the parent of the opposite sex. Children, therefore, have more energy to devote to other areas of interest and thus make great social and intellectual strides in this period. During this stage, children are extremely interested in learning, and sexual curiosity has been replaced by intellectual curiosity. Instead of day-dreaming about sexual achievement, the child seeks success in real-life social interactions. Erikson referred to this period as the stage of "industry versus inferiority." The major "crisis" to be resolved is whether young people can obtain sufficient recognition and praise to encourage them to work and achieve or whether they will feel rejected, put down, or ignored. If the latter is the case, then Erikson believed the children come to see themselves as inferior and poorly equipped to cope with the stresses of academic performance and the sense of personal failure.

Finally, school-age children identify with their parents of the same sex and also begin to identify with other children of the same sex. Boys greatly prefer the company of other boys, and girls enjoy being with other girls. Individual friendships are extremely important, but school-age children begin to become interested in group activities and membership as well.

ADOLESCENCE

The onset of puberty (10 to 14 years) is actually the beginning of adolescence, although Erikson's fifth stage extends from age 12 to 18. He called this stage "identity versus role confusion." He saw the major developmental task to be dealing with the rather extreme physiological changes and developing a personal identity or sense of "Who am I?"

Sexual development once again becomes of prime importance. Masturbation is usually resumed or increased if it was never discontinued. Girls begin their menstrual periods, and boys experience nocturnal emissions (wet dreams). Both sexes begin to have romantic fantasies involving sexual contacts with members of the opposite sex. Instead of the parent of the opposite sex who captured their interest during the family triangle period, their partners in these sexual fantasies are often classmates, older friends, movie stars, or other idolized individuals.

During puberty the parent-child relationship must be a good one. Ideally, all children should have adequate sex education, especially in this day of AIDS and other sexually transmitted diseases, before the onset of puberty. As new and drastic body changes begin, children need to be able to discuss their feelings with their parents. They have questions that need to be answered and fears that need to be expressed and understood.

Because actions often speak louder than words, the way parents relate to each other and their acceptance of their own gender greatly influence adolescents' acceptance of their own developing sexuality. For example, the way a young girl accepts the onset of her menstrual period is influenced by the way her mother has accepted her own sexual and reproductive functions. Fears, inhibitions, and tension related to menstruation are often passed on to daughters and surface in physical complaints such as severe cramps and headaches, moodiness, and incapacitation during a portion of the menstrual period.

Adolescence is a stormy period for both teenagers and their parents; both have ambivalent feelings about the changes that are taking place. Parents are not sure they want to give up control of the adolescent and allow greater independence, and adolescents are not always sure they want to assume the responsibility that goes with more independence. Adolescents sometimes find a great deal of security in allowing parents to make the decisions and be responsible for their care. One of the major problems between parents and adolescents occurs when the adolescent wants the independence without the responsibility. Such dependence-independence conflicts probably account for much of the adolescents' often erratic behavior. One moment the adolescent is the most responsible, mature creature possible and, the next moment, childish and irresponsible.

Although most adolescents are not emotionally capable of engaging in a mature and responsible sexual relationship, they are capable of developing emotionally satisfying relationships that provide companionship and the opportunity for experiences and affection with members of the opposite sex.

Because adolescents are still deeply involved in trying to establish their own feelings of self-worth and are working through feelings of inadequacies and dependence at a time when they also long to be independent and self-sufficient, "love" relationships are likely to be based on what the loved person does to strengthen the adolescent's own self-esteem. A young man may brag to his fraternity brothers about his date with one of the college cheerleaders, or a 16-year-old girl may brag to her friend about the guy she is dating who just happens to drive an expensive sports car.

Peer approval is extremely important to the adolescent. A girl often wants to be asked out on lots of dates in order to appear popular, which increases her status in the eyes of her girlfriends. A boy may accomplish the same status by bragging about his sexual accomplishments to his male friends.

"Falling in love" usually begins around age 16 and is likely to happen a number of times before young adults experience the type of relationship in which their wish to receive is overcome by their wish to give. These fleeting relationships are important, however, because they help adolescents develop the ability to form close relationships based on give-and-take situations and ultimately lead to the establishment of a lasting relationship.

When adolescents establish mature relationships, they at long last have conquered the possessive feelings of early childhood and changed the love object from a parent to a person in their own peer group. With this initial act, they prepare for the transition from adolescence to adulthood and go out to face the world carrying with them all that they have learned to be, a small fear of being alone, and hope for the future. Erikson argued that those who find a secure, positive identity do well and those who flounder in role confusion and a negative identity need more time to resolve this crisis before moving on to the next stage.

Many developmental theories end at adulthood, but Erikson continued to his sixth stage, that of "intimacy versus isolation" (young adulthood). In this stage young adults learn about sharing emotions and emotional contact with others. Strong friendships with both sexes may develop, and "special" relationships also develop. Adults who have not resolved their fifth stage (identity versus role confusion) are limited in their ability to share emotional intimacy and develop close relationships that require a coherent sense of the world and how the individual fits into it. Perhaps failure at this sixth stage accounts in part for the large number of divorces in this age group.

Erikson's seventh stage covers middle adulthood and is called "generativity versus stagnation." By *generativity,* Erikson meant the ability to look beyond a person's own needs and to consider the needs of society and of generations to come. *Stagnation* refers to a state in which the individual cannot get past personal needs and is absorbed with getting those personal needs met. Concerns focused on the environment, involvement in community service, or participation in aiding the welfare of others are examples of generativity.

Erikson's eighth and final stage is "integrity versus despair," which occurs during the time generally referred to as old age. At this point people begin to realize that time is running out and that life will soon end. In looking back, aged people may feel a sense of accomplishment, a sense of having lived life well, and satisfaction with the things and people who will remain after their death. Alternatively, they may feel sorrow for a life misspent, for goals not reached, for friendships not cultivated, and for things not done and places not visited. Old age is a time of contemplation and evaluation—and of designing an emotional chariot to carry a person across the threshold from life to death. Table 2–1 summarizes Erikson's eight stages of development.

Table 2–1. **Erikson's Eight Stages of Development**

Stage	Age Range	Nature of Developmental Crisis
Basic trust versus mistrust	First year of life	Developmental crisis involves the child's attempts to get needs met. If met, the child learns to trust and finds the world a comfortable place.
Autonomy versus shame and doubt	1 through 3	Developmental crisis centers around whether the child's sense of independence and competence is supported or if the child learns to doubt and becomes overly compliant.
Initiative versus guilt	4 through 5	Core developmental crisis relates to whether the child's efforts at "trying out" new ways of doing things results in support and encouragement. Learns that exceeding limits risks personal and social failure, for which one punishes oneself with guilt.
Industry versus inferiority	6 through 11	Developmental crisis centers around learning to be skillful at age-appropriate tasks and winning recognition for achievements. Problems may occur if child overvalues work, becomes overly competitive, or feels inferior and learns to avoid tasks because of perceived incompetence.
Ego identity versus role confusion	Adolescence (12–20)	Developmental crisis is "Who am I and what shall I become?" Adolescents are curious about how others see them. If confused or ambivalent about self and direction, adolescent may enter the "counterculture" or overidentify with "heroes" in music and drugs until an identity emerges.
Intimacy versus isolation	20–40	Developmental crisis is related to the person's ability to form close and warm relationships with others, to learn to love and have compassion for others. Failure results in social withdrawal.

continued

Table 2–1. **Erikson's Eight Stages of Development** *continued*

Stage	Age Range	Nature of Developmental Crisis
Generativity versus stagnation	40–60	Concern for future generations rather than fixation on self-indulgences. Accepts responsibility for contributing to humanity.
Ego integrity versus despair	60 to death	Crisis involves evaluating one's life, developing acceptance of what one has accomplished, and dealing with impending death.

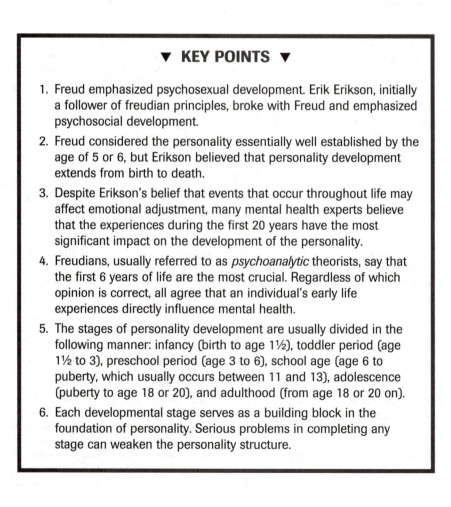

▼ KEY POINTS ▼

1. Freud emphasized psychosexual development. Erik Erikson, initially a follower of freudian principles, broke with Freud and emphasized psychosocial development.

2. Freud considered the personality essentially well established by the age of 5 or 6, but Erikson believed that personality development extends from birth to death.

3. Despite Erikson's belief that events that occur throughout life may affect emotional adjustment, many mental health experts believe that the experiences during the first 20 years have the most significant impact on the development of the personality.

4. Freudians, usually referred to as *psychoanalytic* theorists, say that the first 6 years of life are the most crucial. Regardless of which opinion is correct, all agree that an individual's early life experiences directly influence mental health.

5. The stages of personality development are usually divided in the following manner: infancy (birth to age 1½), toddler period (age 1½ to 3), preschool period (age 3 to 6), school age (age 6 to puberty, which usually occurs between 11 and 13), adolescence (puberty to age 18 or 20), and adulthood (from age 18 or 20 on).

6. Each developmental stage serves as a building block in the foundation of personality. Serious problems in completing any stage can weaken the personality structure.

Key Points continued

7. Individuals develop at their own rate, and no two human beings are exactly alike; however, each stage has certain tasks that most people accomplish during that stage.

8. Most authorities believe that normal newborns possess all the basic ingredients (genetic inheritance) to become biologically functioning human beings; however, the newborn's ability to utilize this inherited potential depends on life experiences.

9. A new computer is mechanically ready to function and solve all sorts of complicated problems, yet it cannot begin to function until it is fed, by a human being, a massive dose of raw information, facts, and formulas (programming). A human infant functions in much the same manner.

10. Newborn children also have no concept of morality. They are gradually taught right and wrong over the first few years of life according to what their parents consider right and wrong.

11. Sigmund Freud considered the newborn to be a "bundle of id." *Id* was Freud's term for that part of a personality that is unconscious and contains all of the "wants" of an individual (e.g., to eat, to sleep, to be comfortable, to have fun, and to do pleasurable things).

12. Infants want their basic needs (food, clean diapers, sleep, attention) met at the exact moment they want them, regardless of whom it inconveniences. Gradually, infants learn that there are others in the world and that it takes a few minutes to warm a bottle or change a diaper.

13. If an infant's needs are met, the child begins to trust the world as a good place. If the infant's needs are not met, the child begins to mistrust people and feel that the world is not a very likable place.

14. In the first year of life, infants need as little frustration as possible to learn to trust their environment and the world in which they live. Erikson named this first stage of development "basic trust versus mistrust."

15. The mother figure is the first love object for all humankind.

16. Between the ages of 1 and 2½, children begin to develop a sense of autonomy.

17. In regard to toilet training, children want to please their parents and at the same time want to retain their freedom. Thus, they

continued on page 28

Key Points continued

experience conflict. Parents do better when they wait until a child is physically and psychologically ready for toilet training.

18. Humans do not live in isolation and therefore, during childhood, must learn to conform reasonably to societal norms.

19. When parents fail to assume their responsibility for making sure socialization does indeed occur, their child usually has a great deal of difficulty adjusting as an adult.

20. People who are considered antisocial, or sociopathic, because they function as a "bundle of id," frequently had overly permissive parents.

21. Erikson calls the toddler stage of psychosocial development "autonomy versus shame and doubt."

22. The crucial element in the toddler stage is balancing the need for developing an appropriate level of autonomy with an appreciation for observing reasonable social and personal limitations.

23. By the end of the toddler or muscle-training period, children have greatly increased motor and intellectual skills.

24. During the preschool period (age 3 to 6) the ego and superego begin to function.

25. The superego is that part of the personality called the *conscience.* It includes all the "controls," the shoulds and should nots, and its structure depends largely on the type, quality, and severity of discipline.

26. Without discipline, children fail to develop a sense of right and wrong and lack respect for other people and their belongings. If discipline is too severe, children become afraid to try anything new or different, experience extreme guilt and shame, and, in effect, become maladapted and afraid of the world.

27. Erikson labeled this third stage of development "initiative versus guilt."

28. The ego is conscious and functions as the "manager" of the personality. It deals with reality and must manage the impulses or demands of the unconscious id and superego.

29. Guilt is often handled by repression, an unconscious forgetting of threatening events. The individual does not really forget the event, but it becomes part of the individual's unconscious where, although not remembered, it may motivate future behavior.

Key Points continued

30. Some authorities have described the span of time between ages 6 and 10 (school age) as the "golden era of childhood."

31. Most children desire parental approval and attempt to become more like the parent of the same sex, instead of trying to possess the parent of the opposite sex.

32. The onset of puberty (age 10 to 14) is actually the beginning of adolescence, although Erikson's fifth stage ("identity versus role confusion") extends from age 12 to 20.

33. Erikson sees the developmental task during puberty to be dealing with the rather extreme physiological changes and developing a personal identity or sense of "Who am I?"

34. One major problem between parents and adolescents occurs when the adolescent wants to exercise independence without responsibility. Such dependence-independence conflicts probably account for much of the adolescent's often irate and erratic behavior.

35. Many developmental theories end at adulthood, but Erikson continues to his sixth stage, that of "intimacy versus isolation" (young adulthood). In this stage the young adult learns about sharing emotions and emotional contact with others.

36. Those who have not resolved the fifth stage ("identity versus role confusion") are limited in their ability to share emotional intimacy and develop close relationships because doing so requires a coherent sense of the world and how one fits into it.

37. Erikson's seventh stage covers middle adulthood and is called "generativity versus stagnation." Generativity is the ability to look beyond one's own needs and consider the needs of future generations.

38. Erikson's eighth and final stage is "integrity versus despair" and occurs during the time generally referred to as "old age."

Annotated Bibliography

Baker, H. S., and Baker, M. N.: Heinz Kohut's Self psychology: An overview. *The American Journal of Psychiatry,* 1987, 144(1):1–9.

Attributes the development of mental illness to inadequate parenting, parental abuse, and unmet needs in childhood.

Carrey, N. J., and Adams, L.: How to deal with sexual acting-out on the child psychiatric inpatient ward. *Journal of Psychosocial Nursing and Mental Health Services,* 1992, 30(5):19–23.

Discusses the causes and patterns of sexual acting-out and provides interventions for modifying these behaviors.

Florenzano, R.: Chronic mental illness in adolescence: A global overview. *Pediatrician,* 1991, 18:142–149.

Provides information on prevalence and types of chronic mental illness in adolescence and discusses current trends in child psychiatry.

Hayes, F. S.: The McCarthy scales of children's abilities: Their usefulness in developmental assessment. *Pediatric Nursing,* 1981, 7(4):35–37.

Describes the use of the MSCA as a tool in the developmental assessment of children age 2½ to 8½.

Kaufmann, P. M., Sparrow, S. S., and Leckman, J. F.: Children with tics and nonverbal learning disability: Preliminary MRI findings. *The Clinical Neuropsychologist,* 5(3):248.

Discusses the neuropsychologic profile similarities observed in children with tic disorders and children with nonverbal learning disability.

Lefley, H. P.: Culture and chronic mental illness. *Hospital and Community Psychiatry,* 1990, 41(3):277–286.

Discusses the effect of cultural beliefs and practices on the development and long-term prognosis of mental illness.

Pontious, S. L.: Practical Piaget: Helping children understand. *American Journal of Nursing,* 1982, 82(1):114–117.

Describes the differences in the perceptions of a child who is in Piaget's preoperational stage (age 2 to 7) and the child who is in the concrete operational stage (age 7 to 12). Offers insights for dealing with the child in each stage.

Rubio-Stipec, M., Bird, H., Canino, G., Bravo, M., and Alegria, M.: Children of alcoholic parents in the community. *Journal of Studies on Alcohol,* 1991, 52(1):78–87.

Provides information on how alcoholism and adverse family conditions increase the risk of maladjustment in children.

Thomas, A., and Chess, S.: Genesis and evolution of behavioral disorders: From infancy to early adult life. *The American Journal of Psychiatry,* 1984, 141(1):1–9.

A study evaluating the effect of temperamental characteristics and environment on psychologic development from birth through adulthood.

Ullmann, R. K., and Sleator, E. K.: Attention deficit disorder children with or without hyperactivity. *Clinical Pediatrics,* 1985, 24(10):547–551.

Discusses the importance of knowing a child's specific problems when treating them for attention deficit disorder.

Reference

Erikson, E. *Identity, Youth and Crisis.* New York: W. W. Norton & Co. Inc., 1968.

Post-Test

Fill in the Blanks. From the group of terms listed on the right, select the letter of the most appropriate term(s) to complete the following sentences.

1. Some experts say that the first _____ years of life are the most crucial.

2. One's ability to utilize all of one's inherited potential depends on

   _____ .

3. If neglect is severe enough, an infant or young child withdraws from reality into a world of fantasy that feels

   _____ .

4. The _____ relationship is perhaps more intense than any other relationship in one's life.

5. Between the ages of _____ , a child's superego develops rapidly.

a. life experiences

b. 6

c. mother-child

d. less threatening

e. 3 to 6

f. 6 to 10

g. sibling

h. husband-wife

True or False. Circle your choice.

T   F   1. All human beings develop in exactly the same pattern and almost at the same rate.

T   F   2. The mother figure is the first love object for all humankind.

T   F   3. If there is no discipline, children fail to develop a sense of right and wrong.

T   F   4. Adolescence appears to be an easy developmental stage for teenagers and their parents.

T   F   5. Peer approval is of little importance to the adolescent.

T   F   6. Erikson identified seven stages of life.

T   F   7. The stage of "integrity versus despair" occurs during the adolescent period.

Post-Test

(continued)

Multiple Choice. Circle the letter or number you think represents the best answer.

1. What is the outstanding characteristic of growth and development?
   a. It occurs at a uniform rate.
   b. Each individual follows a unique pattern.
   c. It is a simple process.
   d. It rarely influences behavior.

2. What is the most important factor in the home environment of a child?
   a. Assurance of proper nutrition.
   b. Provision for play space.
   c. Atmosphere that lets the child feel secure.
   d. Protection from overstimulation.

3. A basic factor contributing to children's security is:
   a. The knowledge that they are individuals.
   b. The setting of realistic boundaries and limits.
   c. Allowing for dependence on their mothers for their needs.
   d. Allowing them to have what they want.

4. The growth and development of children are influenced by their:
   a. Heredity.
   b. Cultural heritage.
   c. Environment.
   d. Treatment by their parents.
      (1) a only.
      (2) a and c.
      (3) b, c, and d.
      (4) All of the above.

5. The fact that boys fight and generally display greater aggressiveness than girls is probably best explained on the basis of difference in:
   a. Social expectation.
   b. Endocrine balance.
   c. Inherited predisposition.
   d. Hereditary factors.

Post-Test

(continued)

6. The freudian theory of personality development divides the mind into three basic parts. Of the terms listed below, which one is not a basic part?
   a. Ego.
   b. Libido.
   c. Id.
   d. Superego.

7. The ego is that part of the "mind" that:
   a. Helps the individual deal with reality.
   b. Constantly attempts to satisfy its own demands.
   c. Is concerned with morals, values, precepts, and standards.
   d. Represses painful thoughts from the conscious.

8. A 2-year-old child is frequently negativistic and resistant to adult demands. This behavior is usually regarded as an indication of:
   a. Inconsistent techniques on the part of the parents.
   b. Overindulgence on the part of the parents.
   c. Too much strictness on the part of the parents.
   d. A growing awareness of self on the part of the child.

9. Independent behavior is learned from a mother who:
   a. Is permissive and allows children to do as they desire.
   b. Is fearful of injury or of the child getting dirty.
   c. Permits exploration and experimentation but sets limits.
   d. Rewards accomplishments and avoids restrictions.

10. The best advice to give parents on the subject of toilet training is:
    a. To wait until the child indicates that readiness via behavioral cues.
    b. To begin bladder training around 15 months of age.
    c. To tell parents it is up to their discretion.
    d. To place the child on the potty for 15 minutes at the same time each day.

11. The best way to manage the aggressive behavior of a 2-year-old boy is:
    a. Tell him he is a bad boy and that you won't love him if the behavior continues.
    b. To rechannel his activity into a more acceptable area.

Post-Test

(continued)

   c. Let him vent his aggressive feelings however he wishes.
   d. Provide punishment for any aggressive behavior.

12. A preschool child's questions may become annoying. Adults should understand that:
   a. This is a period of rapid vocabulary growth.
   b. The child's "computer" is being programmed.
   c. Answers provide the child with a concept of adult attitudes and feelings.
   d. The child should always be given an answer.
     (1) a and c.
     (2) b, c, and d.
     (3) a, b, and d.
     (4) a and d.
     (5) All of the above.

13. The typical characteristic of a girl during the preschool stage of development is:
   a. Little curiosity about sex difference.
   b. Strong interest in and attraction to her father.
   c. Intense admiration of her peers.
   d. Interest in "gangs" with girls her age.

14. The so-called "golden years of childhood" are:
   a. 1 to 3.
   b. 3 to 6.
   c. 6 to 10.
   d. 10 through puberty.
   e. 14 to 20.

15. Family relations for the school child are characterized by:
   a. Identification with the parent of the same sex.
   b. Increasing independence.
   c. Individual friendships becoming important.
   d. Resentment of rigid rules.
     (1) a and d.
     (2) b and c.
     (3) a, b, and c.
     (4) b and d.
     (5) All of the above.

Post-Test

(continued)

16. A teacher finds a group of first-graders involved in dramatizing a funeral. Which idea regarding their play is likely to be most justified?
    a. Realistic play of this nature is unusual in children of this age.
    b. This play behavior is likely to be unrelated to the actual experience.
    c. The children should be gently guided to other types of play.
    d. Such play is an attempt to explore the reality of death.

17. The attitudes of a young girl toward menstruation usually reflect those of:
    a. Her best friend.
    b. The person who tells her about it.
    c. Her mother.
    d. Her family.

18. The major adjustments the adolescent has to make are:
    a. Physical adjustment to body changes.
    b. Social adjustment with peers.
    c. Sexual adjustment in boy-girl relationships.
    d. Moral adjustment so the adolescent will have a moral code to live by in the future.
       (1) a only.
       (2) c only.
       (3) b and c.
       (4) All of the above.

19. Usually the strictest behavioral control over the adolescent is exerted by:
    a. Parents.
    b. Church.
    c. Peers.
    d. School.

20. Which of the following statements are true of Erik Erikson's theory?
    a. It represents a modification of some of Freud's psychoanalytic principles.
    b. It is referred to as a psycho*social* theory as opposed to Freud's theory, which is referred to as a psycho*sexual* theory.
    c. It covers human development from birth to death.
    d. It ignores the importance of early childhood experiences.

Basic Concepts of the Mind

OBJECTIVES: Student will be able to:

1. Define *psychopathology.*
2. List three specific behaviors used to evaluate a person's overall mental health.
3. Define the term *defense mechanism;* give two examples.
4. Define *neurosis* and *psychosis.*

THE MENTAL HEALTH CONTINUUM

A person who successfully accomplishes the developmental tasks discussed in the preceding chapter can approach adulthood with the skills necessary to function as a mentally healthy, mature adult. Maturity and mental health are not dependent on the number of years lived but rather on an individual's problem-solving skills, ability to cope with life stresses, and ability to make good choices.

Emotionally healthy people accept themselves and others and have developed the ability to give as well as receive. They have appropriate self-confidence because they have realistically evaluated their own assets and liabilities and have found that they can cope with the challenges of life. They make decisions based on sound judgment and then accept responsibility for their actions.

Of course, even the most emotionally competent and responsible individual sometimes acts in an immature or childish manner. Only when a person's behavior is frequently irresponsible or is significantly at odds with society's expectations does that person begin to experience the maladjustments of psychopathology.

Psychopathology is a term used to indicate that a person is emotionally unable to deal with the stress and strain of everyday life. Such a condition usually comes about when people's defense mechanisms are no longer able to defend them against the anxiety created by stress and strain, when they have not developed defense mechanisms against such forces, or when they use defense mechanisms so excessively that they do not accurately perceive reality. Those whose defenses work adequately and who seem to get along reasonably well in everyday life are said to be "adjusted." Those who do not get along well and are seen as strange or peculiar and those whose behavior is obviously inappropriate are said to be manifesting a significant degree of psychopathology.

To understand the difference between mental health and mental illness, it is helpful to think in terms of specific behaviors. For example, take the rather simple behavior of laughing. People who never laugh are said to be depressed and unable to enjoy themselves. Those who laugh all the time, particularly at inappropriate times, are thought to have something wrong with them. The point is, of course, that somewhere between never laughing and laughing constantly is a range in which the behavior of laughing is both acceptable and expected. This range demonstrates the idea of the mental health continuum. Looking at behaviors in terms of a mental health continuum shows that any given behavior has a socially acceptable range of occurrence and that either the absolute absence of that behavior or its constant presence might be seen as abnormal.

No laughter	Appropriate laughter	Constant laughter
|----------|	-----------------|	--------------|

With the idea, then, that most behaviors have an appropriate range that is both acceptable and expected, consider some of the specific things that may be used to judge a person's overall mental health.

1. Thinking well of oneself; being fairly free of feelings of inadequacy and inferiority; being able to express or to communicate one's emotions.

2. The ability to trust oneself to make decisions and to act on those decisions after careful consideration of the consequences of one's actions.

3. A genuine feeling of well-being and a realistic degree of optimism (the expectation that things will turn out well).

4. Accepting one's real limitations while developing one's assets.

5. Evaluating one's mistakes, determining their causes, and learning not to repeat the same behavior.

6. Being able to delay immediate gratification for future satisfaction, such as putting off marriage until after career preparation.

7. The ability to form close and lasting relationships with persons of both sexes, being relatively satisfied with one's own sex, and having the ability to enjoy an active and satisfactory sex life.

8. An appropriate conscience that prevents the individual from getting into trouble by resisting behavior that is destructive either to the individual or to others; a conscience that also produces guilt about antisocial behavior.

9. The ability to accept authority (obey traffic laws, follow an employer's rules, and so forth) but, in appropriate situations, not to be afraid of authority and to contest authority if necessary.

10. The ability to meet one's needs in a socially acceptable manner while taking into consideration the needs of others.

11. The absence of petty jealousies and of any need to exploit and manipulate others.

12. An ability to maintain a reasonably accurate perception of realities and of one's social and interpersonal interactions.

13. The ability to work alone and to work effectively with others; compromising and sharing when appropriate but being able to compete and be aggressive when necessary; getting organized and systematic in order to get things done; possessing an acceptable degree of cleanliness, promptness, orderliness, and neatness.

14. The ability to function in both dependent and independent roles; to follow or to lead; to take care of others or to be taken care of, depending on the circumstances.

15. Acceptance of the fact that stress and change are part of everyday life; being flexible enough to adapt to these continual changes without a great deal of psychological discomfort.

16. A sense of humor; the ability to laugh at self and others when life situations are absurd.

17. The ability to maintain a balanced or integrated personality so that one can respond adaptively to life experiences.

It is difficult to define these factors accurately, to measure them, and to decide just how much of a behavior is acceptable or unacceptable. Psychologists and psychiatrists attempt to make these decisions and often are asked to do so in court cases and competency hearings. Value judgments relative to these points should be avoided. For example, some societies reward their young men for stealing, and some subcultures in our country give special status to a young man who has been in a juvenile detention center.

In the final analysis, the degree to which a particular behavior is acceptable to individuals in our society is determined by how much of that particular behavior a society is willing to accept. Of course, what is acceptable to society changes from time to time. In 1950, most people would probably have been quite upset to have naked people running around town; however, in the streaking fad of 1974, a great many young people were running around town wearing nothing but tennis shoes and a smile, and they were frequently applauded for their efforts. This particular fad even made its way to Hollywood, where a very daring young man streaked the televised 1974 Academy Awards presentation.

Had these behaviors occurred in 1950, the streakers would likely have been jailed, and there would have been considerable public outrage; however, the permissiveness of the late 1960s and early 1970s made this behavior merely amusing to a great many Americans. Most of the court cases involving streakers were either dismissed or the streakers were given minimal fines; however, even with the permissive attitudes prevalent in 1974, a "dirty old man" in the park wearing nothing but a raincoat who was exposing himself to young girls as they passed by may not have met with a similar fate in court. Depending on the region of the country, he could have received a substantial sentence for indecent public exposure and, at least, been committed for psychiatric treatment. In 1992, rap musicians were jailed, fined, and otherwise harassed for the lyrics they chose. Those opposing them felt harassed by the words they used and felt the music to be disgusting. In general, however, our courts have held that persons have a right to free speech and that poor taste is no excuse to take away constitutional rights.

One further point should be made. Even though most friends and peers see a person as being well adjusted, it is unlikely that anyone is totally adjusted. In fact, it has been said that the only totally adjusted person is a dead one. Every person who is active and who participates in life is continually subjected to conflicts that must be resolved. The female student who meets a handsome young man and wants to go out with him but also has a big exam the following day must confront the conflict and decide whether to go out or study. A healthy response would be to decide to do one or the other. A less healthy response would be to permit the conflict to remain unresolved and not do either.

Return, then, to the question of what happens when an individual becomes unable to manage anxieties and conflicts and thus cannot function in a "well-adjusted" fashion. By and large, there are two major classifications for such maladjustments: neurotic and psychotic. Before types of maladjustments are discussed, however, the psychological defense mechanisms that help people function in highly stressful situations must be outlined. The following section provides an overview of the defense mechanisms, how they work, and how they may be abused.

DEFENSE MECHANISMS

All people have basic images of themselves (self-images) that are important to their general psychological well-being. Basically, the self-image is the collection of ideas a person has about what kind of person he or she is. Sometimes people who have poor self-images try just as hard to maintain that poor self-image as others try to maintain good self-images. Because people frequently react to other people the way they react to themselves, it is easy to see that the way people view themselves is quite an important factor in their relationships with other people.

In this area of the self-image the defense mechanisms work. To maintain a constant way of viewing themselves, people sometimes face situations that are threats to their worth or adequacy or to their cherished way of viewing themselves. Such situations are stressful because they pressure people to change their ways of seeing themselves and thus upset their feelings of "constancy."

The defense mechanisms are sometimes called *adjustment* or *coping mechanisms*. They are usually unconscious, although people sometimes become aware of their presence or, at times, even use them consciously. These mechanisms are used daily by almost everyone. They are neither good nor bad. Whether they are healthy or unhealthy is probably best determined by whether they serve to help or hurt the individual who uses them. If they help people meet their personal and social goals in acceptable ways, they are healthy; if they cause people to distort reality and deceive themselves, they are unhealthy. For example, people who always explain their failures by blaming someone else or always rationalize away their inadequacies may never consider that they might be more successful if they learned to look for the real reasons for failures. A classic example is a student who fails an examination and blames the teacher for not giving a "fair" exam, for making the exam too difficult, or for not asking what the teacher said would be asked on the exam, while ignoring the fact that the student studied only an hour when satisfactory performance on the exam required 4 or 5 hours of work.

To summarize, almost everyone uses defense mechanisms. They are frequently used without conscious awareness, and they are used to help people maintain cherished beliefs about themselves and the world. The rest of this section lists specific defense mechanisms with a brief example to show how they are used and how they might be abused.

Repression

Repression is often considered the most common defense mechanism. People use repression when they "forget" or exclude from conscious thought what they find too painful or anxiety provoking to remember. The repression of anxiety-producing situations is often incomplete and frequently results in vague feelings of worthlessness and insecurity. Sometimes people feel guilty almost constantly and are unable to discover why they have such feelings.

Perhaps the most classic and usual cases associated with repression involve sexual matters. A young female patient seen by one of the authors complained of not being able to "let go" sexually with her husband. She admitted that she wanted to like intercourse because she knew that it would please her husband, yet each time they started to have intercourse she could feel herself "tighten up." The patient even "tightened up" talking about it to the therapist and became quite anxious. After several visits, the patient started to say something about an incident she dimly remembered but could not quite bring herself to discuss. At the next therapy session, she began talking about an incident in which she and her brother, ages 7 and 9, had been playing together and had become interested in how they were different from each other. Her mother discovered them while they were undressed and marveling at their differences. When the screaming, yelling, and whippings were over, the patient was confused, upset, and unaware of what she had done wrong. She was visibly uncomfortable talking about the incident, but, following her recollection and further discussion and supportive therapy, she began to respond to her husband sexually. At last contact, she was feeling much like a woman who had been, in her words, "set free." Of course, not all episodes of repression are so dramatic or have such an impact on a person's behavior. Lesser incidents of repression occur daily. A boy "forgets" to bring his report card home to be signed. He had an F on it. A husband "forgets" his wife's birthday after a big fight. A businesswoman "forgets" the name of a customer whom she really does not like.

In any case, although it may reduce anxiety temporarily, repression uses up valuable psychological energy and may block a person's efforts toward leading a "comfortable" existence. Dealing with the repressed material usually leads to a healthier adjustment.

Rationalization

Rationalization is a favorite for many people. It allows them to do what they want to do when they know that they should not, and it helps them to accept themselves when they fail to live up to their goals or the expectations that they, and others, have for them. It involves thinking up reasons for behavior that are more acceptable than the "real" reason. A good rationalization may contain some elements of truth that make it seem plausible. For example, a woman was about to be jailed for having written bad checks amounting to more than $9000. When asked why she had written the worthless checks, she stated that her husband deserved to have some of the finer things in life and that all of his hard work had not gotten him anything.

Other examples of rationalization are such statements as "If I were only taller, the girls would like me better," "If I just had some new clothes, I would really knock them dead," "If I were captain of the football team, I'd have 10 girlfriends, too," and "If I had his brains, I could make As, too." One final example is "Everyone else cheats, so I have to; if I don't, I won't pass." The most serious consequence of rationalization is self-deception. Although it may be painful at times, people are probably better off accepting the truth about the motives for their behavior. In doing so, they are more likely to benefit from experiences.

Denial of Reality

Denial of reality occurs when someone simply refuses to see what is obvious to everyone else. The husband who refuses to recognize that his wife is "running around" when everyone else knows she is represents the case in point. This mechanism is also frequently found among persons who have physical disabilities or who have lost limbs due to amputation. One young man was injured in an automobile accident and paralyzed from the waist down. He was extremely attractive and bright. When asked what effect he thought the physical disability would have on his social life, he insisted that there would be little, if any, effect. He was denying the facts that he could not walk, that he had to be picked up to move from a wheelchair to a car or from a wheelchair to a bed, and that he had no control over his bowel and bladder functions.

A more common example of denial as a defense mechanism is demonstrated by the insistence of a woman who wears a size 16 dress that she can wear a size 14 or 12 dress, and, in fact, she buys the smaller dress. Someone who is ashamed of his very large feet may wear a pair of shoes one or two sizes too small for him and suffer the pain rather than admit that he has large feet. The old adage that love is blind also demonstrates a popular usage of the denial mechanism.

Of course, the major problem with denial is that a person who is unable to recognize a legitimate problem is unlikely to react in a way that would lead to more adequate personality development and to a higher level of maturity.

Conversion Reactions

In conversion reactions, the individual's emotional stress is unconsciously converted into physical complaints. This mechanism is so prevalent that the fourth revised edition of the American Psychiatric Association's *Diagnostic and Statistical Manual of Mental Disorders (DSM-IV)* lists it as a diagnostic category (conversion disorder). In conversion reactions the individual develops limitations related to physical factors for which no organic basis can be demonstrated. An extreme example is suggested by a young patient who attempted to get out of bed one morning and discovered that he could not walk. After several days of physical examinations, roentgenography, and neurological examinations, no evidence of physical abnormality was found. The patient was referred for psychiatric treatment. In the course of treatment, it was discovered that the patient had a sister who died from a muscular disease that rendered her progressively less able to care for herself. The young man had been ignored during her illness while the parents took care of her. The patient came to resent his sister, and when she died he felt guilty. The patient apparently repressed most of his guilt feelings and seemed well for a while before becoming "paralyzed." Within a matter of 6 weeks, after treatment with behavior modification techniques, the patient was able to walk. There have been no recurrences of his paralysis.

A more common example of this particular defense mechanism occurs when people get uptight, have a hard day, and subsequently develop a headache. Persons who have peptic ulcers also demonstrate the conversion mechanism.

Perhaps the greatest advantage of conversion is that it permits a great many people to blame their tiredness, headaches, and so forth on physical ailments. The disadvantage is that, once such a satisfactory explanation is discovered, people may not try to discern the cause of their stresses and do something to make their lives more acceptable and more livable.

Compensation

Compensation is a mechanism by which people try to cover up an area of weakness by showing a great deal of strength or excellence in another area. An example of this defense mechanism is the boy who is too frail or too small to play football but becomes an excellent student. A more direct example of compensation occurs when an individual loses the use of an arm and then uses the remaining arm to equal or surpass the performance that would have been possible with the lost arm.

Although the mechanism of compensation frequently produces desirable results, it may also produce undesirable results, for example, the youth from the "wrong side of the tracks" who feels that he is socially unacceptable and undertakes to become the meanest fighter on his block. Numerous television programs are built around the compensation theme: A brilliant scientist is offended by his country and subsequently develops weapons of tremendous capability for a competing power simply to "show" the people who rebuffed him. Positive examples of the use of this defense mechanism occur when an individual compensates for a poor figure by dressing in a particularly flattering manner or an overweight person develops an especially winning personality. Compensation mechanisms frequently help people excel in some particular area when otherwise they might not have excelled in anything.

The negative side of compensation may show up when the chosen areas of compensation are antisocial or detrimental to the individual. Perhaps Evel Knievel, the motorcycle exhibitionist, is an outstanding example of this latter point (such exploits are typically a compensation for low self-esteem or a need for recognition).

Projection

Projection is a defense mechanism that enables people to justify their own behavior and feelings by accusing others of having these same feelings and by permitting them to blame their shortcomings on other people or objects. One of the easiest ways to spot this mechanism is to recognize the "blaming" theme that is usually present. An example of this mechanism occurred in a state hospital. A court service worker who sometimes referred patients to the hospital always wrote letters describing the behavior of the referred patients. He never failed to mention the homosexual tendencies of the patients. As a matter of fact, he always found something to indicate the presence of homosexuality. In reality, very few of the patients referred had homosexual tendencies. He was projecting onto other people his fear of his own homosexual impulses and characteristics. Another example of this mechanism is the tennis player who, after completely missing the ball, looks at the tennis racket as if it had a hole in it, in effect saying, "There must be something wrong with this racket. Surely I couldn't have missed the whole dang ball." Frequently people blame many of life's troubles on bad luck, the stars, tarot cards, or the "fickle finger of fate."

The advantage obtained by the individual who uses projection is avoiding responsibility for behavior and some of the feelings of rejection that might come from having socially unacceptable thoughts and feelings. The major disadvantage is that such individuals may become constant "faultfinders" who do little or nothing to straighten out the internal problems that make the use of projection necessary.

Fantasy

Fantasy is a defense mechanism that practically everyone employs. In reasonable amounts, daydreaming can be fun and even productive. At one time or another, most people have daydreams about being a hero. In his daydreams, an adolescent boy may rescue the girl of his dreams from some terrible situation and thus become her hero and lover. A young girl might imagine herself in a dazzling evening gown that causes the teacher upon whom she has a crush to be taken by surprise when he suddenly recognizes how mature and beautiful she really is. Other typical fantasy activity involves a small, skinny child who imagines herself beating up the school bully and thus becoming a hero or a poor youth seeing himself becoming rich and powerful.

Perhaps the greatest benefits derived from fantasy are temporary escape from painful environmental situations and achievement of solutions to problems that might not otherwise be solved. However, fantasy can be overdone to the point that people begin to "live in their heads" and thus lose touch with reality. People who begin to respond to fantasies as if they were real are in psychological trouble. It is probably not too harmful for a young man to imagine himself as quite rich and important but something else when he starts writing checks on his imaginary bank account.

Introjection

Introjection is a defense mechanism whereby people incorporate into their own personality structure the attributes of persons or institutions in their environment. A good example of introjection occurs when a person is taken as a political prisoner and a year or two later is released and appears to have been "brainwashed" by the captors; that is, the former prisoner appears to have accepted their ideals and ideas. "If you can't beat them, join them" is a popular concept that expresses the use of this defense mechanism. A young man who is beaten by a bully may subsequently become friends with him. The idea of peer pressure is also an expression of this defense mechanism.

The basic idea in introjection is to protect oneself from threatening circumstances by becoming attuned to the ideas and characteristics of the environment so as to lessen the threat. The advantage in using this mechanism is that it allows survival in situations that might otherwise be destructive. Perhaps the greatest disadvantage occurs when one is suddenly thrown into another culture or a different environment and those traits and behaviors that have been introjected may no longer be appropriate and instead create adjustment problems.

Reaction Formation

Reaction formation is a defense mechanism whereby people deny unacceptable feelings and impulses by adopting conscious behaviors that, at least on the surface, appear to be contradictory to the thoughts, feelings, and impulses being defended against. A reformed alcoholic may become a teetotaler and spend a great deal of time and effort preaching against the evils of alcohol. The sexually promiscuous parent may spend hours lecturing a teenager against the evils of sex. The "good Christian person" may be a malicious gossip, and the businessman who always complains about the poor morals of other businesspeople may be found to shortchange customers in one way or another. Some evidence indicates that public censors who protect us from the evils of sex and violence in movies, magazines, and television have a hard time not enjoying their jobs. The Shakespearean quote from *Hamlet* aptly summarizes this defense mechanism: "The lady doth protest too much, methinks." It is one thing to be genuinely concerned about a particular issue and another to be obsessed with it.

Undoubtedly, people with reaction formations control some of their less acceptable impulses. However, they would probably be much more comfortable with themselves and much more tolerant of other people if they could resolve the internal conflicts that make the use of reaction formation necessary.

Regression

Regression is a defense against anxiety or threatening situations that permits people to go backward in development to a time when they felt more at ease and more capable of handling the environment. It permits escape from the painful situations in the present and allows enjoyment of the relative peace and quiet of the stage of regression. Perhaps the most obvious case of regression is an adult who begins to behave in a childlike manner.

A common example occurs when a 3- or 4-year-old who has been toilet trained begins to wet the bed and use baby talk when a newborn is brought into the home. Another example at a more advanced age occurs when people become highly dependent and demanding when they are threatened. Regression frequently occurs when patients are hospitalized.

Another form of regression is seen when individuals have grown up and gotten into the business world. They subsequently decide to get out of the rat race and go back to a simpler form of living. Frequently, they go to rural areas to become farmers or, in some cases, choose to live in communes. The idea of "getting back to nature" expresses their desire to get back to a simpler time and to escape the complexities of a high-tech world.

Sublimation

Sublimation is a defense mechanism that allows an individual to divert unacceptable impulses and motives into socially acceptable channels. Rather than becoming a Peeping Tom or a simple voyeur, an individual may become an artist and draw nudes, a physician, or a photographer for *Playboy* magazine. In fact, *Playboy* magazine, at least in some circles, is a socially acceptable form of voyeurism. The popularity of X-rated videocassettes (which are said to account for a high percentage of all videocassette sales) suggests that satisfaction of voyeuristic impulses is substantial.

Other examples of sublimation are individuals with very strong, aggressive impulses who play football or hockey or participate in other physically violent activities that are sanctioned by society.

The advantages of sublimation are obvious in that sublimation allows expression of questionable desires and impulses in socially acceptable ways. The disadvantage might come with drives that are so strong that even sublimation is not sufficient to control the impulses and a person nevertheless engages in other extreme behaviors.

Restitution

The defense mechanism of restitution permits people to atone for behaviors they feel are unacceptable. For example, people who get their wealth by highly questionable means may become benefactors of an orphanage or otherwise contribute great sums of money to charity. This defense mechanism is sometimes referred to as *undoing,* and its aim is to reduce the guilt and anxiety people experience for having engaged in behaviors they now view as unacceptable.

Displacement

Displacement is a defense mechanism in which people transfer hostile and aggressive feelings from one object to another object or person. The classic example of this mechanism is the man who comes home from work after being chewed out by his boss and spies Fido lying in front of the door. Poor Fido gets a swift kick and slinks away wondering what in the world he did to deserve such treatment. Spouses and children, as well as pets, of course, are common targets of displacement.

The advantage of displacement is staying on good terms with the offending person and thus avoiding the possibility of being fired or otherwise facing the wrath of the offending person. If displacement becomes a way of life, however, alienation of friends or family members is probable.

The great efforts made today at improving communication between people in businesses and elsewhere attest to the importance of learning to convey feelings to people in on-the-job interactions. At home or at work, it is discomforting to be yelled at and not know why.

NEUROSIS AND PSYCHOSIS

The next step is to determine how these defense mechanisms are related to psychopathology. For all psychological disorders that are functional in nature (that is, not related to physical or organic causes), stressful situations are assumed responsible for the maladaptive behavior. Most authorities suggest that threat, anxiety, and malfunctioning defense systems are related to the development of abnormal behavior. Therefore, when an individual tries to use defense mechanisms to ward off feelings of anxiety or threat but cannot do so, either because the defense mechanisms are not strong enough or because they are generally inadequate, anxiety increases, as does inappropriate use of defense mechanisms. The individual who is unable to deal with anxiety-provoking problems through defense systems is likely to develop more and more inappropriate and maladaptive behavior, which results in the collapse of biological, psychological, and sociological functioning. At this point, "symptom formation" begins.

Depending on how well an individual's defense system is able to handle the threat and anxiety-generating stress on the individual's psy-

Table 3–1. **Characteristics of Neurosis and Psychosis**

Factor	Neurosis	Psychosis
Description	A neurosis causes a loss of personal efficiency and a decrease in activity. Some personality disorganization may be present. Neurotics frequently have some insight into the fact that they have emotional problems.	A psychosis is characterized by serious personality disorganization. Impaired memory, perception, and judgment are often apparent. Patients may have difficulty recognizing that they are emotionally ill.
Symptoms	Various complaints about nervousness, emotional upset, physical illnesses (with little organic basis), poor self-esteem, and feelings of worthlessness. Hallucinations do not occur.	Reality testing is impaired. Hallucinations, delusions, and bizarre bodily sensations occur frequently. A lack of reality contact is apparent.
Social elements	Social relationships are likely to show some deterioration but are not likely to be completely disrupted. Patient's behavior is not likely to be injurious to self or others.	Social relationships are likely to be significantly impaired and in some cases totally disrupted. Patients may show behaviors injurious to self or others.
Orientation	Patients usually oriented to time, place, and person. Patient's behavior probably does not seem especially peculiar.	Patients frequently disoriented as to time, place, and person. Patient's behavior may appear quite odd or peculiar.
Therapeutic measures factor	Usually treated in outpatient facilities, and many neurotic people receive no treatment at all. Only the most severe cases require hospitalization.	Frequently requires hospitalization but may be maintained in outpatient facilities.

chological structure, the individual may experience a mildly disruptive interpersonal relationship problem or may experience severe personality decompensation to the point of losing contact with reality.

The difference between mild and severe personality decompensation is generally described by the terms *neurosis* and *psychosis*. With a neurosis, the individual experiences mild interference with social relationships, occupational pursuits, and sexual adjustment. Neurotics are rarely dangerous to themselves or to society.

Neurotic patients usually maintain contact with reality, although there is often some distortion in the concept of reality. They usually realize they have some emotional problems and may have some insight into the nature of the problems. Neurotics are usually well oriented in time, person, and place and do not have delusions or hallucinations. They do often show symptoms such as obsessions, compulsions, phobias, and hysterical paralyses. Except in severe cases, neurotic patients do not require hospitalization, and many neurotic patients go through life without obtaining any help for their problems.

In psychosis, by contrast, patients frequently experience severe personality decompensation that interferes with vocational pursuits and interpersonal relationships, and, of course, contact with reality is poor. In fact, in most psychoses, there is a definite split between the reality of the world and reality for the patient. The patient frequently loses track of time, place, and person. Psychotic patients usually require hospitalization, and their behavior is sometimes injurious to themselves and other people. Psychotic patients rarely have any insight whatsoever into the nature of their behavior and, in fact, frequently insist that nothing is wrong with them and that they should be released. Table 3–1 summarizes the different characteristics of neurotic and psychotic patients.

This chapter has presented the concepts necessary to form a framework for the different types of mental illness. The next chapter discusses specific diagnostic categories and some of the problems inherent in the diagnostic process.

▼ KEY POINTS ▼

1. *Psychopathology* is a term used to indicate that a person is emotionally unable to deal with the stress and strain of everyday life.

continued on page 52

Key Points continued

2. A person whose defenses work adequately and who seems to be able to get along reasonably well in everyday life is said to be "adjusted."

3. Looking at behaviors in terms of a mental health continuum demonstrates that any given behavior has a socially acceptable range of occurrence and that either the absolute absence of that behavior or its constant presence might be seen as abnormal.

4. The degree to which a particular behavior is acceptable to individuals in a society is determined by how much of that particular behavior the society is willing to accept.

5. Even though a person is considered well adjusted by most friends and peers, it is unlikely that anyone is totally adjusted.

6. There are two major classifications for maladjustments: neurotic and psychotic.

7. The defense mechanisms are sometimes popularly called *adjustment* or *coping mechanisms,* but Freud saw them as ego defenses.

8. Defense mechanisms are used by almost everyone. They are used to help individuals maintain cherished beliefs about themselves and the world.

9. Repression is considered by many mental health experts to be the most common defense mechanism. People use repression when they "forget" or exclude from conscious thought those things they find too painful or anxiety provoking to remember.

10. Rationalization is a favorite defense mechanism for many people. It involves thinking up reasons for behavior that are more acceptable than the actual reason.

11. Denial of reality occurs when someone simply refuses to see what is obvious to everyone else.

12. In conversion reactions, the individual's emotional stress is unconsciously converted into physical complaints. The individual develops limitations related to physical factors for which no organic basis can be demonstrated.

13. Compensation is a mechanism whereby people try to cover up an area of weakness by showing a great deal of strength or excellence in another area.

Key Points continued

14. Projection is a defense mechanism that enables people to justify their own behavior and feelings by accusing others of having these same feelings and by blaming shortcomings on other people or objects. One of the easiest ways to spot this mechanism is to recognize the "blaming" theme that is usually present.

15. Fantasy is a defense mechanism that practically everyone employs.

16. Perhaps the greatest benefit derived from fantasy is that it permits temporary escape from painful environmental situations or helps achieve solutions to problems that might not otherwise be solved. However, fantasy can be overdone to the point that one begins to "live in one's head" and thus loses touch with reality.

17. Introjection is a defense mechanism whereby people incorporate into their own personality structure the attributes of people or institutions in their environment.

18. The basic idea in introjection is to protect the self from threatening circumstances by attuning the self to the ideas and characteristics of the environment and thus lessening the threat.

19. Reaction formation is a defense mechanism whereby a person denies unacceptable feelings and impulses by adopting conscious behaviors that, at least on the surface, appear to be contradictory to the thoughts, feelings, and impulses being defended against.

20. Regression is a defense against anxiety or threatening situations that permits people to go backward in development to a time when they felt more at ease and more capable of handling the environment.

21. Sublimation is a defense mechanism that allows an individual to divert unacceptable impulses and motives into socially acceptable channels.

22. The defense mechanism of restitution permits people to atone for behaviors they feel are unacceptable.

23. Displacement is a defense mechanism in which the individual transfers hostile and aggressive feelings from one object to another object or person.

24. Most authorities suggest that the concepts of threat, anxiety, and malfunctioning defense systems are very much related to the development of abnormal behavior.

continued on page 54

Key Points continued

25. The difference between mild personality decompensation and severe personality decompensation is generally described by the terms *neurosis* and *psychosis.*

26. With a neurosis, the individual experiences mild interference with social relationships, occupational pursuits, and sexual adjustment. Neurotics are rarely dangerous to themselves or to society.

27. In psychosis, the patient frequently experiences a severe personality decompensation that interferes with vocational pursuits and interpersonal relationships, and, of course, contact with reality is poor. In most psychoses, there is a definite split between the reality of the world and reality for the patient.

Annotated Bibliography

Agostinelli, B., Demers, K., Garrigan, D., and Waszynski, C.: Targeted interventions: Use of the mini-mental state exam. *Journal of Gerontology Nursing,* 1994, 20(8):15–23.

Discusses using the MMSE to assess global cognitive abilities as well as abilities and disabilities in daily living skills.

Boisen, A. T.: Personality changes and upheavals arising out of the sense of personal failure. *American Journal of Psychiatry,* 1994, 151(6):125–133.

The author suggests that neurosis and psychosis may be an attempt to reorganize the personality that can have positive results.

O'Connell, K. A.: Why rational people do irrational things: The theory of psychological reversals. *Journal of Psychosocial Nursing and Mental Health Services,* 1991, 29(1):11–14.

The reversal theory is applied to inconsistent and irrational behavior.

Puntil, C.: Integrating three approaches to counter resistance in a noncompliant elderly client. *Journal of Psychosocial Nursing and Mental Health Services,* 1991, 29(2):26–30.

Discusses how resistance is used by the elderly patient and how nurses can work through the resistance.

Roberts, S. J.: Somatization in primary care: The common presentation of psychosocial problems through physical complaints. *Nurse Practitioner,* 1994, 19(5):47–56.

Discusses how nurses can avoid extensive diagnostic evaluations and treatments through assessment of psychosocial problems in neurotic or psychotic patients who are expressing somatic complaints.

Taibbi, R.: Neurosis & psychoses: Giving problems a name. *Current Health,* 1994, 2:18–20.

The author briefly explains the difference between neuroses and psychoses and briefly discusses a few disorders.

Wilt, D. L., Evans, G. W., Muenchen, R., and Guegold, G.: Teaching with entertainment films: An empathetic focus. *Journal of Psychosocial Nursing,* 1995, 33(6):5–14.

Examines the use of two motion pictures with mental health themes as tools to facilitate the development of empathy in nursing students.

Post-Test

Matching. Match the defense mechanism in column B with the appropriate statement in column A. There is only one mechanism for each descriptive statement.

Column A

1. Denies unacceptable feelings and impulses by adopting conscious behaviors that are contradictory to the thoughts, feelings, and impulses.

2. Blames others for personal inadequacies or guilt feelings.

3. Refuses to see what is obvious to everyone else.

4. "Forgets" or excludes from conscious thought things too painful or anxiety provoking to remember.

5. Diverts unacceptable impulses into socially acceptable channels.

6. Is "undoing."

7. Transfers hostile and aggressive feelings from one object to another object or person.

8. Goes backward in development.

Column B

A. Repression

B. Displacement

C. Projection

D. Restitution

E. Denial

F. Regression

G. Reaction formation

H. Introjection

I. Sublimation

J. Fantasy

K. Suppression

L. Identification

M. Conversion

True or False. Circle your choice.

T   F   1. Emotionally healthy people accept themselves.

T   F   2. The inability to accept authority or make decisions for oneself is a sign of good mental health.

T   F   3. People's self-images are basically the ideas they have about what kind of people they are.

Post-Test

(continued)

T   F   4. Defense mechanisms are always healthy.

T   F   5. To be effective, defense mechanisms must be consciously used.

T   F   6. Psychotic patients rarely have insight into the nature of their behavior.

Fill in the Blanks. From the group of terms listed on the right, select the letter of the most appropriate term to complete the following sentences.

1. _____ is a term used to indicate that a person is no longer emotionally able to deal with the stress and strain of everyday life.

2. The person whose defenses work adequately and who seems to get along reasonably well in everyday life is said to be _____.

3. There are two major classifications of maladjustments: _____ and _____ maladjustment.

4. Defense mechanisms are sometimes called _____ mechanisms.

5. _____ is sometimes called the granddaddy of all the defense mechanisms.

A. Adjusted

B. Neurotic

C. Psychopathology

D. Denial

E. Coping

F. Psychotic

G. Repression

H. Insane

Multiple Choice. Circle the number or letter you think represents the best answer.

1. Mentally healthy individuals have the capacity to:
   a. Accept their strengths and weaknesses.
   b. Love others.

Post-Test

(continued)

   c. Have an effective conscience.
   d. Tolerate stress and frustration.
     (1) a and b.
     (2) a and c.
     (3) a, b, and c.
     (4) All of the above.

2. When observing behavior, the nurse should remember that behavioral symptoms:
   a. Have meaning.
   b. Are purposeful.
   c. Are multidetermined.
   d. Can easily be understood.
     (1) b only.
     (2) a and c.
     (3) a, b, and c.
     (4) All of the above.

   Situation: Mrs. White is in the hospital for diagnostic tests. She says to you, "Yesterday, my doctor told me he was referring me to a psychiatrist. There's nothing wrong with me that any psychiatrist can cure. I'm here to find out why I've been getting these backaches and that's all."

3. Mrs. White may be using the defense mechanism(s) of:
   a. Denial.
   b. Conversion reaction.
   c. Regression.
   d. A and B.
   e. B and C.

4. Your most therapeutic response to Mrs. White would be:
   a. "I can see why this would be upsetting, but don't worry. Everything will turn out all right."
   b. "I'm sure he had a good reason for suggesting this, so try not to be upset about it."
   c. "I have some time now. Could you tell me some of your feelings about seeing a psychiatrist?"
   d. "The x-rays of your back show nothing is wrong there."

5. Referral to a psychiatrist may be perceived by Mrs. White as a threat to her:
   a. Self-esteem.
   b. Security.
   c. Identity.
   d. Independence.

6. Many people experience compulsions in everyday life. In the following examples, which actions would be fairly normal (not neurotic)?
   a. Habitually emptying ashtrays in the living room before retiring.
   b. Carrying soap and towel around and washing their hands to the extent that no other activity is possible.
   c. Picking up every piece of paper they see all day.
   d. Having a morning routine in order to get to work on time.
      (1) a only.
      (2) b and c.
      (3) a and d.
      (4) All of these.

7. Mental processes and behaviors that serve to protect people's self-esteem by defending them against excessive anxiety are:
   a. General adaptation syndrome.
   b. Psychological adaptation processes.
   c. Defense mechanisms.
   d. Stressor factors.
   e. Flight and fight response.

8. Which of the following are true of defense mechanisms?
   a. Resolve intrapsychic conflicts.
   b. Minimize or eliminate anxiety.
   c. May operate unconsciously.
   d. May operate consciously.
   e. Are the same as mental mechanisms.
      (1) a, c, d, and e.
      (2) a, b, c, and d.
      (3) b, c, d, and e.

Post-Test

(continued)

(4) a, b, c, and e.
(5) All of the above.

9. A patient has been told by her physician that she needs surgery.
   This thought is very upsetting to her. She leaves the doctor's
   office and says to herself, "I won't think about it now. I'll do some
   shopping instead." She is utilizing which defense mechanism?
   a. Repression.
   b. Identification.
   c. Sublimation.
   d. Regression.
   e. Suppression.

10. A man is reprimanded by his boss. He comes home and proceeds
    to kick the family dog. This is an example of:
    a. Identification.
    b. Repression.
    c. Introjection.
    d. Suppression.
    e. Displacement.

11. Jane has done poorly on an examination. When asked about it,
    she replied, "I couldn't help it. I had planned to study all day
    Sunday and then my relatives came and stayed all day so I
    couldn't study." She is using the defense mechanism of:
    a. Compensation.
    b. Fantasy.
    c. Rationalization.
    d. Reaction formation.

12. Johnny was the shortest boy in the class and could never do well
    in athletics. However, he worked very hard at his studies and
    achieved the honor roll. The defense mechanism here is:
    a. Substitution.
    b. Fixation.
    c. Displacement.
    d. Compensation.

13. Mrs. Green is a patient who is scheduled for shock treatment.
    Ms. Jaynes, a new staff member, becomes very anxious and is
    unable to help with the treatment. She is using:

Post-Test

(continued)

a. Identification.
b. Denial.
c. Regression.
d. Suppression.

14. A patient is angry because he was hit by a car and incapacitated for several weeks. His wife is working and taking care of their three small children at home. He directs his angry energy into pounding designs into leather wallets. He then sends the small amount of money he earns from the wallets home, thus making him feel better. This is an example of:
    a. Displacement.
    b. Identification.
    c. Sublimation.
    d. Regression.
    e. Suppression.

15. A person who consciously acts ill to avoid an unpleasant experience is referred to as a:
    a. Neurotic.
    b. Hypochondriac.
    c. Malingerer.
    d. Procrastinator.

16. Which of the following is true of neurosis?
    a. Profound withdrawal from people.
    b. Impaired but not prevented occupational efficiency.
    c. Fragmentation of thought processes.
    d. Severe distortion in memory.
    e. May cause short-term memory problems.
       (1) a, b, c, and e.
       (2) b and e.
       (3) b, c, and d.
       (4) c, d, and e.

Post-Test

(continued)

17. Which of the following are true of psychosis?
    a. Possible delusions and hallucinations.
    b. No impairment in judgment.
    c. Awareness of personality disorder.
    d. Withdrawal from reality.
    e. Distorted affect.
       (1) All of the above.
       (2) b, d, and e.
       (3) a, c, and e.
       (4) a, d, and e.
       (5) None of the above.

18. Psychotic patterns of response are:
    a. Not as severe as neurotic disturbance.
    b. Involve minor defects in reality testing.
    c. Characterized only by hallucinating.
    d. Disturbances in total personality functioning.

CHAPTER

4

Legal and Ethical Considerations

OBJECTIVES: Student will be able to:

1. Define and give an example of *voluntary admission.*
2. Define and give an example of *involuntary admission.*
3. List the rights of voluntarily and involuntarily admitted patients.
4. State three specific things to be done in caring for the mentally ill that will reduce the likelihood of becoming involved in litigation.

Some experts call the present period in American history the "age of the consumer." Consumers have been insisting that they receive high-quality products and services for the money they pay. That fact has not been lost on the U.S. automobile industry, which had lost much of the American market to Japanese and German automobile manufacturers. The same is true of the electronics industry. In the 1990s, much of American industry has been scrambling to catch up.

So what do consumers' rights and preferences have to do with the mentally ill? Consider for a moment that patient care provided by a hospital or clinic is a service, and a costly one at that. Hospital room rates alone may run over $800 to $1000 per day. These prices often do not include special treatments, medications, psychotherapy, or other "ancillaries." Because mentally ill patients frequently are hospitalized for weeks at a time, it is not difficult to understand why people are demanding the best care. In addition, healthcare institutions are operating in a highly competitive market in which hospitals are closing because of insufficient demand. The lack of demand is not so much that the services are not needed as that many third-party payers are refusing to pay for mental health care or are very closely monitoring that care. Finally, many patients, or their families, readily seek legal advice if the care they receive is not satisfactory.

Fear of a lawsuit, however, should not be the motivating factor for providing high-quality care to patients. Rather, the obligation to honor the trust of patients is the professional and ethical commitment. Honoring this trust, and communicating effectively with patients, would practically eliminate lawsuits.

A major responsibility of individual members of the mental health team is to help other team members create the type of environment that provides both physical and emotional safety and comfort for patients. One step toward this type of environment is to treat all patients as unique individuals by taking measures to preserve their dignity and to respect the rights and privileges guaranteed them by law.

Most lawsuits against members of the mental health team center around a negligent act (negligence being seen as willful neglect, abuse, harassment, or failure to attend adequately to a patient). For example, if a patient who is experiencing confusion after electroconvulsive therapy (ECT) is allowed to take a shower unattended and subsequently falls and breaks a hip, the patient would very likely win a negligence suit. The reasoning is that the staff knew or should have known the patient was at risk because of treatment effects and should have attended the patient. If they neglected to do so, there may be an issue of liability.

The objective of this chapter is to provide basic guidelines to follow for working with mentally ill patients. These guidelines should help the mental health worker to avoid legal entanglements that might otherwise arise. Mental health workers must make themselves aware of the laws pertaining to the care of the mentally ill for the state where they practice because such laws vary considerably from state to state.

KNOW THE JOB RESPONSIBILITIES

Make sure you are familiar with the job description for your position. Know what you can legally do, and then learn to perform those procedures in a correct and skillful manner. Ask questions and tactfully refuse to do any task for which you have not been prepared. Be sure to read carefully the rules and regulations of the hospital or clinic, and thoroughly commit to memory those that are specific to the unit where you see patients. You should also familiarize yourself with the information in the procedure manual. Discuss with your supervisor any part of the procedure manual you do not understand completely. In many states you can be held legally responsible for any rules, regulations, and procedures that apply to patient care on your unit or the hospital in general, even if you do not "know" about a particular rule, regulation, or procedure. Make it your business to know. Be informed!

VOLUNTARY AND INVOLUNTARY ADMISSIONS

Familiarize yourself with the laws of your state regarding treatment of the mentally ill. In most states there are two main ways in which mentally ill patients are admitted for psychiatric care. When a person agrees that medical assistance is needed and agrees to be admitted to the hospital, it is said to be a voluntary admission. If an unwilling patient must be forced to enter the hospital, it is an involuntary admission (*involuntary admission* and *involuntary commitment* are considered to be interchangeable terms). Involuntary admissions require legal action. A judge, clinical psychologist, or physician (which one varies according to state law) who determines that a person is in danger of harming self or others has the responsibility of deciding whether to commit the person to a psychiatric hospital or mental health unit for evaluation or treatment.

The major reason for being aware of the difference between these two procedures is best illustrated when one is faced with a patient who has decided to leave the hospital. In the case of a voluntary admission, the patient who has decided not to continue treatment should be allowed to leave. Most hospitals ask patients to put their intentions in writing and then wait 24 hours before leaving. Patients who refuse to do so are usually asked to sign a legal form that states that they know they are leaving against medical advice and that the hospital is not responsible for their actions. In most states, however, patients cannot be required to sign such a form. If the person in charge of the unit believes such patients are likely to harm themselves or others if they leave, the charge person may detain them against their will for a period of 24 hours. During this time, legal procedures must be started in order to change the patient's admission status from voluntary to involuntary. A patient who has been involuntarily admitted should not be permitted to leave the hospital unless officially discharged by the attending physician (or psychologist in those states where psychologists have admitting and discharge privileges). Commitment is legally terminated upon discharge.

CONFIDENTIALITY

The issue of confidentiality is one of the more perplexing problems in mental health. It is widely accepted that therapeutic effectiveness depends on patients' willingness to discuss those private thoughts and feelings that frequently underlie their emotional maladaptation. In the process of treatment, patients sometimes reveal information about themselves or others that is incriminating and that, if made public, could result in disagreeable consequences to that patient. Generally speaking, mental health professionals are required to keep all information disclosed to them in confidence. Most patients realize that information given to one member of the mental health team is shared with the entire team, but staff should take great care not to imply to patients that what they say to one team member will be kept in complete confidence. That lesson was learned the hard way by one of the authors in what might be called an "early career growth experience."

A young patient, about 30 years old, had been doing quite well in therapy and was about ready to leave the hospital. The author was charting the patient's wonderful progress when the patient asked if she could say something that would be kept totally confidential. Perhaps distracted by the charting activity and lulled into a false sense of security by the patient's apparent progress (note the rationalizations), the author cheerfully said, "Sure." Big mistake! No sooner had the words left the author's mouth than the young woman said, "I've decided to kill myself. That's why I've been feeling so much better." That is what is called a therapeutic bomb! To make matters worse, when asked to be released from the commitment not to reveal the information about her suicidal intentions, the patient replied, "If you tell anyone, I will kill myself for certain." It is not difficult to see the bind. To break her confidence would risk the trust on which the therapeutic relationship was founded. Not protecting the patient against self-harm was unthinkable. The situation was resolved when the author was able to help the patient see the need to have the mental health team become aware of her decision so that appropriate therapeutic intervention could occur. The author has never made that error again.

DUTY TO WARN

Two other situations involving confidentiality require special attention. In addition to a responsibility to protect patients from themselves, caregivers have a "duty to warn." This responsibility was essentially established by a famous court case you might like to read if you have the opportunity. The case was *Tarasoff v. Regents of University of California* (1976). The essential elements of the case were that a patient told his therapist of his intent to kill his girlfriend. The therapist told the campus police of the patient's threat, but the patient was not arrested. He later killed Ms. Tarasoff. Her family filed suit and won, establishing thoroughly the responsibility of therapists to warn potential victims of threats made against them.

A new crisis currently abounds in this area of duty to warn. Do caregivers have the duty to warn partners of patients with AIDS, especially when the caregiver knows the patient is still sexually active and is not informing partners? This issue is hotly debated, but Gray and Harding (1988) say: "We believe that it is at the expense of the uninformed sexual partner's safety to keep confidential the information that the client has the AIDS virus. In our opinion, a sexually active, seropositive individual places an uninformed sexual partner (or partners) at peril, and the situation therefore falls under the legal spirit of the Tarasoff case and the ethical tenets of 'clear and imminent danger.'"

DUTY TO REPORT CHILD ABUSE

The other situation requiring violation of confidentiality is that of child abuse. Most states require professionals to report information about abuse of children, and there are legal penalties for not doing so. A patient's information about child abuse should be immediately discussed with the supervisor.

There is a difference between a patient's right to confidentiality and "privileged communication." The right to confidentiality is a general understanding that information will not be disclosed without the patient's permission. However, this right falls more under the rubric of ethics than under that of legality, and in many situations a court will order confidential information to be disclosed. Privileged communication, by contrast, is a legislated and specific right, honored by the courts, granting an individual the right to discuss matters with certain identified persons who cannot, by law, disclose that information without specific consent. Privileged communication is the right clients have to discuss information with their attorney. That right has been extended to physicians who are psychiatrists, psychologists, social workers, and nurses in some states. The right of privileged communication varies greatly from state to state, and learning whether it applies is important.

Court decisions generally seem to hold the position that the protective right of privileged communication and of confidentiality ends where the public peril begins. It is almost always in everyone's interest to gain the patient's permission to reveal a confidence. Indeed, some patients appear to disclose information with the intent of having the caregiver intervene. Most mental health facilities have written policies informing patients of the circumstances under which their right to confidentiality or privileged communication may be abridged. Patients who threaten to hurt themselves or others should be reported to the supervisor immediately. Failing voluntary disclosure by the patient, the supervisor will act upon the information in accordance with the procedures outlined by the agency, institution, and state in which the patient resides.

THE PATIENT'S CIVIL RIGHTS

American society values the rights of individuals and almost universally endorses the right of self-determination. All members of the psychiatric team must remember that patients admitted to the hospital on an involuntary basis do not necessarily lose any or all of their civil and legal rights. These patients do lose the right to leave the hospital without permission but in most states retain the right to vote, make contracts, drive a car, marry, divorce, write letters, and seek legal advice. As out-of-date laws are repealed in most states, the only way a patient can lose civil and legal rights is to be declared incompetent. This special legal procedure is not a routine matter for patients hospitalized on an involuntary basis. Once a patient is declared incompetent, it takes another legal procedure to declare them restored to competency. Discharge from the hospital is not sufficient.

Since the early 1970s, more and more of the court suits filed by mental health patients have dealt with what they considered to be infringements upon their basic human rights and freedoms as guaranteed to them by the Bill of Rights and the Civil Rights Amendments. Because hospitalized patients tend to be more vulnerable, they are more likely to have their rights violated.

Because of court rulings in the late 1960s and 1970s, thousands of patients have been released from state institutions and returned to a society ill prepared to meet their needs. This has led to conflict between society and the medical and legal professions. For example, many authorities attribute the substantial increase in the homeless population to the release of mental health patients and the refusal to hospitalize the ambulatory mentally ill. The laws governing mental health practices are in a state of flux, and many laws currently on the books are being challenged on the grounds that they are unconstitutional because they do not provide for due process.

ADEQUATE SUPERVISION OF PATIENTS

When patients are in your charge, be careful not to let your attention wander, not to be distracted, and not to allow yourself to be manipulated away from your duties. Be especially careful while taking a patient or a group of patients off the unit when a suicidal patient is under your supervision. A good rule to follow is that if you have more than one patient going off the unit, you should have more than one mental health worker with the group. Then, if something happens to a patient one staff member can stay with the group while the other staff member goes for help. It is generally not a safe practice to try to manage patient groups larger than 10.

INFORMED CONSENT AND A PATIENT'S RIGHT TO REFUSE TREATMENT

Generally speaking, patients have a right to refuse treatment or to withdraw from treatment once it is started. The constitutional basis is the patient's fundamental right to privacy and personal autonomy. Today's mental health professional walks a fine line between providing for patients' well-being and protecting their rights.

Except in extreme psychiatric emergencies, the mental health professional must explain all procedures and medications to the patient in such a manner that the patient can make an intelligent, informed choice as to whether to allow the procedure or take the medication. The patient's agreement must be written. The patient should be given information regarding expected outcomes, potential risks, and alternative treatment modalities.

Informed consent is not valid if a patient is coerced, under the influence of drugs or alcohol, or in such a state of agitation that it prevents free choice. If the staff feels a patient cannot make rational decisions regarding care, the proper authorities should be notified and incompetency proceedings initiated.

Patients so out of control that they must be restrained or secluded cannot give informed consent. Seclusion is not a punishment but a protective device that is used only when other methods (e.g., medication, talking) fail. If a restraint order is given, make sure the patient is checked at least every 15 minutes and that such checks are charted, including specifically that restraint contact points (such as wrists and legs) were examined. Stay with the patient if at all possible, or try to find a staff member or a family member who can stay.

DUE CAUTION

Caregivers have a responsibility to exercise due caution and protect patients from hazards. They should be constantly alert for potentially dangerous items on the unit. Remove these items when possible, and report any hazards to the supervisor. For example, a caregiver should pick up a nail file left by a visitor and report a torn screen to the head nurse. When repair workers or other technical personnel are on the unit, always check behind them to be certain they have not left anything patients can use to harm themselves, staff members, or other patients.

ETHICS

Ethical responsibilities differ from legal responsibilities in that they do not carry the force of legislative statute. They do, nevertheless, carry the force of professional expectation and professional honor. Ethical responsibilities are guidelines that sometimes address legal issues, but from the position of expectation rather than law. Very often ethical positions become law as they become widely accepted. For example, sex between patients and caregivers progressed from being frowned upon, to a violation of ethics, and to now being illegal in many states.

The Colorado Society of Clinical Specialists in Psychiatric Nursing adopted a set of guidelines in 1987, and a summary of the guidelines relating to respect for the rights of patients was presented in the *Journal of Psychosocial Nursing* (1990). The eight ethical guidelines related to patient rights are as follows:

1. The right to informed self-determination, when the client is rational;
2. The right to protection of self from his/her own limitations of reasoning and judgment, when the client is psychotic;
3. The right to an opportunity for treatment, including equity in the quality of treatment relative to all other clients;
4. The right to attain and maintain a sense of human worth;
5. The right to privacy in terms of the body and in regard to the emotional, intellectual, and spiritual dimensions of self;
6. The right to protection from physical and verbal abuse or misuse, including abusive behavior that carries sexual and/or emotional implications.
7. The right to expect a high quality of psychiatric nursing care, even when the client is incompetent to assess the nursing care; and
8. The right to expect that nursing care will be focused on each particular client's welfare to the greatest extent possible, even when such an individualized focus is in conflict with the welfare of the client's family, a group of clients, or society.

SUMMARY

This chapter has reviewed some of the legal and ethical issues involved in treating the mentally ill. The important things to keep in mind include paying attention to patients, addressing their concerns and needs, being aware of state laws, not guessing at responsibilities but *knowing* what they are, honoring confidentiality, and appreciating the need to communicate with patients about their concerns. Ethical issues are also important and require that those working with the mentally ill be aware of ethical considerations as well as legal ones. Chapter 8 discusses some communication techniques that may help caregivers manage their legal and ethical responsibilities.

▼ KEY POINTS ▼

1. In this "age of the consumer," patients expect and require that caregivers honor the trust they place in them to help them deal with their difficulties.

2. A major responsibility of individual members of the mental health team is to help other members of the team create the type of environment that provides physical and emotional safety and comfort for patients.

3. Specific legal and ethical responsibilities include:
   a. Know your job responsibilities. Be familiar with your job description and learn to perform procedures in a correct and skillful manner.
   b. Know the difference between voluntary and involuntary admissions. Voluntary admissions occur when a person agrees to be admitted to the hospital. Involuntary admissions occur when the admission is against the patient's will. Check your state law for specific criteria for involuntary admissions.
   c. Understand the importance of confidentiality. If certain information is not held in confidence, it could result in disagreeable consequences to the patient. Confidentiality is a general understanding that information will not be disclosed without written permission.
   d. Know your duty to warn. In addition to protecting patients from themselves, caregivers also have the responsibility to warn others of "clear and imminent danger."

---

continued on page 72

Key Points continued

e. Know how to report child abuse. Most states require that child abuse be reported.
f. Know that the patient has civil rights. Patients may lose their rights only upon being declared incompetent.
g. Understand the importance of adequate supervision of patients.
h. Know the patient's right of informed consent and the patient's right to refuse treatment.
i. Understand the difference between confidentiality and privileged communication. Privileged communication is a *legislated and specific right belonging to the patient* that specifies that certain persons (attorneys, psychologists, psychiatrists—differs according to state) may not disclose information given to them by the patient without the patient's permission.
j. Be aware of the responsibility to exercise due caution. Caregivers should be constantly alert for dangerous items on the unit and remove such items whenever possible.
k. Know your ethical responsibilities and that they differ from your legal responsibilities, which carry the force of legislative statute. Ethics carry only the force of professional expectations and honor but can result in serious professional consequences if violated.

Annotated Bibliography

Aroskar, M. A.: Ethics in nursing and health care reform: Back to the future. *Hastings Center Report,* May–June 1994, 11–12.

Discusses nurses' ethical tensions and nursing's participation in healthcare reform.

Colorado Society of Clinical Specialists in Psychiatric Nursing: Ethical guidelines for the Colorado Society of Clinical Specialists in Psychiatric Nursing. *Journal of Psychosocial Nursing and Mental Health Services,* 1990, 28(2):38–40.

Features guidelines on confidentiality, accountability, and competence.

Curtin, L. L.: Ethical concerns of nutritional life support. *Nursing Management,* 1995, 25(1):14–16.

Suggests institutional development of clear, explicit, and publicly available policies in regard to how and by whom decisions are made on a patient's behalf.

Gray, L. A., and Harding, A. K.: Confidentiality limits with clients who have the AIDS virus. *Journal of Counseling and Development,* 1988, 66:219–233.

Discusses the limits of confidentiality with AIDS patients who continue to be sexually active.

Kain, C. D.: To breach or not to breach: Is that the question? A response to Gray and Harding. *Journal of Counseling and Development,* 1988, 66:224–225.

Further examines the issues presented by Gray and Harding regarding patients who are HIV positive and the duty to warn high-risk partners.

Klop, R., Van Wijmen, F., and Philipsen, H.: Patients' rights and the admission and discharge process. *Journal of Advanced Nursing,* 1991, 16:408–412.

Discusses the information standard for patient's rights, which includes informed consent, informed referral, and informed discharge.

Leong, G. B., Eth, S., and Silva, J. A.: The Tarasoff dilemma in criminal court. *Journal of Forensic Sciences,* 1991, 36(3):728–735.

Legal, clinical, and ethical issues associated with the Tarasoff duty to warn.

Melia, K. M.: The task of nursing ethics. *Journal of Medical Ethics,* 1994, 20:7–11.

Discusses various and debatable ways toward which nursing ethics should be directed. The author favors ethics with a more patient/client-led perspective.

Oldaker, S.: Legal and ethical issues: Ethics in academia. *Journal of Professional Nursing,* 1995, 11(5):261.

Discusses nurses' responsibility in maintaining educational ethics and standards.

Olsen, D. P.: Ethical cautions in the use of outcomes for resource allocation in the managed care environment of mental health. *Archives of Psychiatric Nursing,* 1995, 9(4):173–178.

Explores the potential ethical pitfalls from an outcome-based system.

Sofaer, B.: Enhancing humanistic skills: An experiential approach to learning about ethical issues in health care. *Journal of Medical Ethics,* 1995, 21:31–34.

Examines various ways to teach ethics. The author favors an experiential technique to teaching ethics as opposed to role play or other offered techniques.

Stolte, K., Myers, S., and Owens, W.: Career scope: South Central. *Nursing Management,* 1995, 25:87–92.

Discusses healthcare reform as an ethical dilemma.

Sullivan, E. J.: Ensuring clinical experiences: Is managed care a threat? *Journal of Professional Nursing,* 1995, 11(5):262.

Expresses a negative opinion about HMOs by assuming there will be a decrease in available clinical experience because of the financial demands of managed care.

Post-Test

The following situations provide an opportunity to apply the information in this chapter to situations typical on a psychiatric unit. The five statements below describe actions taken by a mental health staff member. Some are appropriate, and some are inappropriate. Mark an *A* by those you believe to be appropriate and an *I* by those you believe to be inappropriate.

_____ 1. A patient approaches the staff member saying that he is tired of being cooped up and that he is going to leave the hospital. The staff member immediately notifies his supervisor, checks the patient's chart, and finds that the patient is a voluntary patient. The staff member then notifies the patient's physician, who asks the patient to sign a statement saying that he is leaving the hospital against medical advice. The patient signs the form and is permitted to leave.

_____ 2. Mr. Colbert is allowed to continue to carry his small pocketknife, even though he had threatened to use it on a fellow patient. The team member assigned to care for Mr. Colbert decided that the patient had just been angry and had not really meant what he said.

_____ 3. A patient, being very angry, screamed and yelled and called one of the staff several bad names. An hour later the patient became totally unmanageable and had to be restrained. In helping to apply the restraint, the staff member who had been verbally abused used more force than necessary to get the patient to settle down. Later, when the patient's arm began to swell, the staff member decided on his own to apply hot compresses to the area to reduce the swelling.

_____ 4. The staff member assigned to Mr. Goldstead, a patient who was confused as a result of a series of ECT treatments, was helping him bathe. Another staff member opened the door and asked the attendant to help him move another patient, stating it would take only a minute or two. Mr. Goldstead's attendant asked the other staff member to find someone else to help.

Post-Test

(continued)

_____ 5. A staff member who happened to be a very good bowler was demonstrating his bowling techniques to the 10 patients that he had taken to the bowling alley. When a patient asked to return to the unit, he was permitted to do so in the company of another patient.

After responding to the above statements on your own, discuss with your classmates what makes each of these appropriate or inappropriate.

True or False. Circle your choice. (Some answers may vary according to the laws of your state. Have you read the laws of your state?)

T   F   1. A patient cannot be legally detained in the hospital if he admitted himself voluntarily, even though he is still very ill.

T   F   2. Involuntary admission and commitment are considered the same thing.

T   F   3. A patient under a voluntary admission can be held against her will for 72 hours.

T   F   4. When a patient is admitted involuntarily, he automatically loses his civil and legal rights.

T   F   5. It is not necessary for a patient admitted involuntarily to give her consent to special treatment or procedures.

T   F   6. A temporary commitment permits a patient to be hospitalized from 90 to 180 days.

T   F   7. Patients have the right to be present at the court hearing for their commitment.

T   F   8. A patient who is committed by court action retains all of his civil rights except the right to leave.

T   F   9. A legally committed patient has the right to conduct business.

T   F   10. A guardian is always assigned to a person who is declared legally incompetent.

T   F   11. Malpractice is a kind of negligence.

T   F   12. Communication between husband and wife is not considered privileged.

Post-Test

(continued)

T   F   13. A patient who enters a psychiatric hospital
                retains all legal and civil rights except the right
                to leave.

T   F   14. The patient's nearest relatives may institute a
                commitment proceeding.

Matching. Select the appropriate term from column B for each
statement in column A.

Column A	*Column B*
_____ 1. Violation of civil rights.	A. ECT
	B. Restraining patients
_____ 2. Does not have right to leave hospital without permission.	C. Involuntary patient
	D. Reading patient's mail
_____ 3. Must have special signed consent form for voluntary patient.	E. Incompetency hearing
_____ 4. May leave hospital without physician's permission.	F. Voluntary patient
_____ 5. Special court procedure.	

Short Answer. Answer the following questions as briefly as
possible.

1. *Negligence* is defined as _____ .

2. Define the difference between voluntary and involuntary
   admission.

   _____

   _____ .

3. If you are unable to answer a patient's question correctly, the best
   thing to do is

   _____ .

Post-Test

(continued)

4. What would be the main reason for placing a patient in seclusion?

   _____ .

5. Most lawsuits involving members of the mental health team are usually centered around

   _____ .

Understanding the Patient's Diagnosis

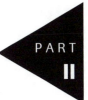

PART

II

Introduction to Diagnostic Considerations

OBJECTIVES: Student will be able to:

1. Define and describe the role, functions, and limitations of diagnoses.
2. Define and describe the *DSM-IV,* the fourth edition of the *Diagnostic and Statistical Manual of Mental Disorders.*
3. Recognize symptoms associated with various nonpsychotic mental disorders.

A diagnosis is used primarily by members of the treatment team as a shorthand method of describing a group of behaviors which might be expected from a particular person. In general social conversation, people often speak in shorthand and say they are upset, angry, sad, awful, hurt, stubborn, or some other such term that indicates a particular pattern of behavior. That is, one word or a few words differentiate one behavioral or feeling state from another. People expect a certain set of behaviors from those who say they feel hurt and a different set of behaviors from those who say they are happy. That same idea applies in the professional setting. A diagnosis that describes a patient as depressed simply passes along the information that the patient is having trouble sleeping, has lost interest in life, has a poor appetite, may cry a great deal, is generally unhappy, chooses to be alone much of the time, finds little or no pleasure in life, and perhaps has undergone a recent loss.

In mental health settings, diagnoses are necessary so that the health insurance company can classify the particular disorder the patient has and determine if reimbursement can be made to treatment personnel and to the hospital or clinic. The advent of diagnosis-related groups (DRGs) as a basis for third-party reimbursement has also affected the need for accurate diagnosis and assessment. All categories of mental illness fall within one of nine DRGs, and a fixed amount of money is paid for each illness depending on its DRG classification. In the "new" healthcare climate—that is, with the great emphasis on cost containment, treatment effectiveness, and alternative healthcare delivery systems—the newest trend is toward selecting specific providers who can demonstrate clear effectiveness with certain diagnostic groups through outcome data.

As of this writing, there are few solid data on outcomes of specific treatments in the mental health field, but there will be more in the near future. The authors believe that within the next 10 years there will be prescribed, fairly universal treatment protocols for specific mental disorders. This prospect raises a hue and cry about "cookbook" medicine, but, as the authors have gone around the country speaking and attending national conferences, there is evidence that protocols for treatment are being given a great deal of attention.

By contrast, interestingly, there is considerable sentiment in the mental health field to do away with assigning diagnoses to patients. They are criticized as inaccurate, misleading, and potentially damaging. In many cases, these criticisms are valid. Patients treated over a period of years have sometimes had as many as five or six diagnoses. Of course, the diagnostic changes may have been warranted because patients do change how they respond to life circumstances, but the reason for different diagnoses is frequently that different professionals tend to have favorite diagnostic categories for certain classes of behavior. In some cases the professional doing the diagnosing simply pays special attention to a different set of factors or behavioral characteristics than did other persons who diagnosed the same patient. Except for some rather specific diagnoses, the reliability of diagnostic categories from one professional to another may be low, largely due to the inexact nature of the diagnostic process.

A notable attempt has been made by the American Psychiatric Association to reduce the inexactness of the diagnostic process. That attempt has been ongoing since the first *Diagnostic and Statistical Manual* was published in 1952. The fourth edition *Diagnostic and Statistical Manual (DSM-IV)* of the American Psychiatric Association is the latest in the attempt to further reduce subjectivity in assigning diagnoses. Specific patient behaviors are given significant weight, and psychodynamic formulations are given very little consideration. The *DSM-IV* is intended to be based more on research data than on the consensus of expert committees, as was the case for previous editions of the *DSM* (Widiger, Frances, Pincus, Davis, and First, 1991). Although this work has had a significant impact on and has substantially improved the diagnostic process, there are still problems with reliability in assigning diagnoses.

DIAGNOSTIC CATEGORIES

The differences between the nonpsychotic disorders (usually called *neurotic* disorders) and the psychotic disorders are presented in Table 3–1, on p. 50. Briefly, the difference between neurosis and psychosis is the degree of disorganization in the patient's thought processes, the degree of social disruption caused by the symptoms, the degree of reality testing or the ability to distinguish between what is and is not real, and the kinds of treatment procedures needed to manage the symptoms.

Nonpsychotic (Neurotic) Patterns of Abnormality

The differences listed in Table 3–1 are pertinent to the discussion of the specific diagnostic categories, in this and the next two chapters, within the broad categories of the neurotic and psychotic disorders. Of course, the origins of neurotic and psychotic behaviors vary according to one's theoretical persuasion.

To stick with the concept of the mental health continuum, with its emphasis on behavior, neurotic conditions have their basis in past events, the interpretation of those events, and past learning situations. Symptom formation provides neurotic persons with primary gain in that the symptoms provide a means of escaping the anxiety they feel. In many cases symptom formation provides secondary gain, such as sympathy, sick leave, or financial benefits in the form of disability income or workers' compensation.

Frequently, in order to help patients conceptualize their emotional symptoms, the authors encourage them to look at their "neurotic behavior patterns" rather than their "neurosis" when they ask, "Am I neurotic?" "Neurotic behavior patterns" are behavior patterns that are self-defeating in some way; they cause isolation, loss of friends, loss of energy, loss of self-efficacy, or the like. Then patients can see their symptoms as more discrete and isolated and thus more manageable. Patients who see their symptoms as some huge, global, unmovable, unmanageable mass of psychological ineptness are less likely to risk working on the symptoms because the task appears hopeless. Once they see their "neurosis" as a maladaptive behavior pattern that can be isolated and defined, the task becomes more manageable, and they become hopeful of ridding themselves of their discomfort. As the saying goes, "Nothing succeeds like success," and small successes at controlling maladaptive behavior patterns encourage patients to try even harder. They are almost always, in our experience, able to achieve a much more satisfactory lifestyle.

All neurotic symptoms exhibited by a patient are unlikely to fall into any one diagnostic category, and it is not particularly unusual for symptoms to change over time from one category to another. Also, different symptoms may be dominant at different times. However, there are recognizable symptom patterns or complexes that are identifiable. *Identifiable* means that the behavioral elements of that symptom complex are often found together and represent a response or reaction to stressful conditions. Next are several of these identifiable symptom complexes that have been placed in diagnostic categories and labeled— individually, simply "the diagnosis." The number preceding the diagnostic label is the diagnostic code in the *DSM-IV*.

Anxiety Disorders

The *DSM-IV* lists 11 different diagnostic categories for anxiety. The two that reflect general anxiety symptoms are:

> (1) 300.02 Generalized Anxiety Disorder
> (2) 300.00 Anxiety Disorder, Not Otherwise Specified

People suffering from the anxiety disorders are usually tense, anxious, and worried but unable to say exactly why they feel that way. There is a sense of general apprehension or, as the *DSM-IV* says, an "apprehensive expectation." Again, depending on one's theoretical orientation, the causes of anxiety disorders are varied, but they are almost always associated with either an internal (psychological, biological, or chemical) or external (environmental) stressor.

Anxiety patients frequently have a history of having been faced with childhood situations and other life situations that did not provide firm, supportive approval or disapproval of behavior. In addition, they have frequently found themselves in situations in which they were uncertain of what was expected of them. In other cases, they were given instructions and directives accompanied by such extreme inflexibility and drastic or fear-inducing consequences that they are unable to achieve any flexibility in how they respond. To respond any way other than the way they were taught creates so much stress that anxiety symptoms appear and force compliance. Compliance reduces the stress, and the symptoms (anxiety) go away.

Psychodynamically oriented therapists often cast anxiety in terms of interpersonal conflicts that occur among a person's basic psychological drives and impulses and the threat of losing control of those impulses. Anxiety is also seen as stemming from a state of perpetual uncertainty. When a person is uncertain of what is going to happen, a general fear of the environment often develops, accompanied by a low frustration level and a tendency to view the world as a hostile, cruel place. These feelings frequently cause anxious neurotic patients to be uncertain of themselves, even in minor stress situations, and to have difficulty concentrating. Humans seem to need a fair degree of certainty in their lives, probably because knowing what is going to happen gives people the ability to predict their circumstances, and the ability to predict circumstances gives people a comfortable degree of control. Perhaps that is why anxiety is often described as a disease of control, or, more to the point, a lack of control. When presented with an anxious patient, the authors always look for the patient's perceived lack of control, and treatment is aimed at helping that patient gain or regain a sense of control through a combination of therapeutic techniques selected on the basis of the particulars of the patient's situation.

Let's look at a brief example. A young woman is engaged to be married. She is quite happy as she goes about planning her wedding some 5 months away. One evening she notices her fiancé is rather quiet and withdrawn. When she asks, he denies anything is wrong and says he's just tired. A few days later he doesn't call and is not at home when she calls him—all night. The next day she calls him at work and wants to know where he had been. He doesn't answer and demands to know if she is checking up on him. Finally, he apologizes, says he was out with the "boys," and agrees to pick her up that night, which he does 3 hours late. At first she is angry, but, when she sees he is not responding to her anger, she suddenly feels hot all over, her hands get cold, and her heart begins to beat faster. Her breathing becomes difficult, and she feels nauseated. Finally, she asks the big question, "Do you still love me?" He says, "Yes, I guess I'm just not feeling too good myself." In various forms, this behavior pattern repeats itself for 3 more weeks. Now she is distraught, not sleeping well, and distrusts what her fiancé tells her. She cannot predict when he is going to show up for a date, cannot predict what kind of mood he will be in if he does show, cannot predict how he will behave, has questions about whether he still loves her, and cannot predict whether the wedding will occur.

Within a month she is having daily headaches and intermittent nausea and cannot go to sleep at night, concentrate or attend to her job, or seem to get anything done. She worries constantly and is losing weight. She also feels depressed, is extremely irritable, and is critical toward others. She is short with her mother and father as well as her friends, and nothing pleases her. Her life feels out of control. Treatment requires helping her re-establish control by making some decisions about how she is going to deal with her fiancé's behavior. Is she going to tolerate his behavior and hope he will change before the wedding date, or is she going to confront him and risk losing whatever is left of the relationship? Everyone knows what she "should" do, but who hasn't tolerated such situations much longer than they "should" have, hoping things would straighten out?

As in this woman's situation, anxiety may affect practically all aspects of life. Frequently, in order to avoid anxiety-producing situations, neurotically anxious individuals restrict their daily activities so severely that they have very limited lives. They are usually unaware of their reasons for restricting their activities; they know only they feel more comfortable in highly structured and familiar surroundings. In the process of reducing anxiety, however, they give up many of the satisfactions life has to offer through relationships with other people and with the environment in general.

As people try to restrict their lives, they may experience strong anxiety reactions or anxiety attacks that include sweating, difficulty breathing, and increased heart rate. Many anxious individuals become dizzy, experience dry mouth, and feel that they are dying. Frequently such patients come to the emergency room complaining of heart attacks. In such cases, hospital admission and treatment often ensue.

The *DSM-IV* lists six symptoms related to a diagnosis of generalized anxiety disorder, at least three of which must be present (for more days than not) for a period of 6 months to make the diagnosis. The six symptoms are as follows:

(1) restlessness or feeling keyed up or on edge
(2) being easily fatigued
(3) difficulty concentrating or mind going blank
(4) irritability
(5) muscle tension
(6) sleep disturbance (difficult falling or staying asleep, or restless unsatisfying sleep)

(Warning: It is not unusual for nursing or other mental health students to have three or more of these symptoms on test day!)

Phobic Disorders (Phobic Neuroses)

Anxiety in phobic disorders is usually experienced when the individual with the phobia comes in contact with the feared situation, object, or condition. Phobias are usually described as a persistent and irrational fear of some object, place, or condition. Some of the more common phobias are related to high places, thunderstorms, closed places, being alone, crowds, darkness, and, recently, sexually contracted diseases. Interestingly, fear of public speaking is the most frequently reported phobia.

In the psychodynamic view, the particular object of an individual's phobia is usually not actually related to that object but represents a displacement of anxiety from the original cause to the phobic object. The phobia helps by allowing the individual to avoid the anxiety-provoking situation. For this reason, the phobia is thought to have symbolic significance to the individual. For example, a psychodynamic view might hold that a young man who is fearful of his hostile impulses, which involve fantasies about shooting his father, may develop a phobia of guns. He is not actually afraid of guns but displaces his fear of killing his father to guns. By avoiding all guns, he tries to avoid the anxiety associated with thoughts of killing his father. If untreated, a phobic person's fears may generalize to other related areas and may lead to increased isolation from relationships. Currently, the cognitive-behavioral approaches substantially ignore such formulations and deal primarily with the symptoms. The cognitive-behavioral approaches are quite effective for a large number of patients.

In all phobias, the basic elements are a persistent, strong, and irrational fear of some object or situation. Because of the tendency for a phobia to generalize or to become associated with objects other than the original phobic object, it sometimes is difficult to discover the symbolic significance of a particular phobic reaction. From a therapeutic standpoint, phobias often generate feelings of dependency and helplessness in people, who are likely to need support and encouragement from the treatment team. Also, phobias protect the individual from anxiety, and the individual does not understand the phobia any better than anybody else, and probably not as well as members of the treatment team. Except under controlled treatment procedures, utilizing well-established cognitive-behavioral techniques, exposure to the phobia is not helpful to the patient. Reassurance, support, and acceptance of the patient, as well as application of the aforementioned treatment procedures, are necessary for the patient's return to adequate functioning.

The *DSM-IV* lists five categories of phobic neurosis, including panic disorder:

(1) 300.21 Panic Disorder with Agoraphobia
(2) 300.01 Panic Disorder without Agoraphobia
(3) 300.22 Agoraphobia without History of Panic Disorder
(4) 300.23 Social Phobia
(5) 300.29 Specific Phobia

Briefly, panic disorder is a condition wherein the patient experiences sudden onset of extreme anxiety during which many of the symptoms of anxiety already discussed appear in an exaggerated form. Although the symptoms may last from a few minutes to, in rare cases, hours, there is often a period of a minute or two in which the patient has extreme fear of dying or "going crazy." Often there is intense fear of having another attack, which increases the discomfort and worry of the patient.

Agoraphobia, which can occur with or without panic symptoms, is a fear of being in a place, situation, or condition from which the patient feels escape will be difficult, impossible, or embarrassing. One of the most frequent of the symptoms reflecting agoraphobia is some patients' refusal to leave their homes or go into a crowded store or mall. Many patients restrict their lifestyle significantly or cannot go places unless someone accompanies them.

Obsessive-Compulsive Disorders

300.3 Obsessive-Compulsive Disorder

Another group of diagnostic symptoms within the category of anxiety-related disorders is that of the obsessive-compulsive disorder. Patients experiencing an obsessive-compulsive disorder are unable to prevent thoughts or ideas they do not wish to think about or are unable to keep from engaging in some repetitive behavioral act. The patients usually recognize the fact that the thoughts or behaviors are irrational but are unable to prevent them. Importantly, these patients recognize the obsessions or compulsions are a result of their own thought processes and thus do not ascribe them to something or someone outside themselves.

As with most other disorders, specific behavioral characteristics are associated with obsessive-compulsive patients. They tend to be neat, perfectionistic, usually rather rigid, and sometimes obstinate.

They very often have difficulty making up their minds and thus are unable to make decisions effectively. These patients may tend to blurt out particular statements or words and seem unable to control themselves. They may also show a strong need for structure or for doing things in a specific way, at a certain time, or in a certain position. Although obsessive thoughts include a wide range of subjects, the most common concerns are about bodily functions, right and wrong, religion, and suicidal thoughts. A key feature of the obsessive thoughts is that they are unwanted but persistent, even though the patient is frustrated by their presence.

Patients who are experiencing compulsive disorder have a strong desire to repeat some particular behavior or action or to repeat a series of behaviors. Frequently the patients believe something drastic will happen to them if they do not carry out their rituals, and the rituals are designed to prevent that occurrence. However, an objective observer would have difficulty understanding how the ritual could prevent the occurrence of the dreaded event because it does not appear to be realistically related to the event.

One patient had a particular series of behaviors he felt he had to complete before going to bed each night. If he did not complete his routine, he believed something terrible would happen to him, and his anxiety level would become so high he could not sleep. His ritual included crossing his left leg over his right leg twice, lacing his left shoelace inside his shoe, and placing the left shoestring across the laces of the shoe. He would also face the door and bow three times, as well as recite a short poem he had learned. Eventually, with therapy, he was able to relinquish most of his ritual, but he maintained some of the behaviors and added others from time to time.

Of course, many people engage in minor obsessive-compulsive behavior patterns when they are under stress or wish to accomplish a certain goal. As long as the obsessive-compulsive behavior patterns are relatively temporary and help them obtain their goals, there is probably no cause for great concern. However, when the behaviors begin to unduly restrict a person's behavior, treatment is indicated.

In dealing with obsessive-compulsive patients in a treatment center, nurses must recognize that they are highly sensitive to stressful or threatening situations. These patients try to rearrange their environment in an attempt to impose structure and rigidity so that they can control what happens. If they believe they can control their environment, they feel safer. The rituals and the behaviors of obsessive-compulsive individuals are designed to help them adjust to the dangers and threats that they perceive as being all about them. Kindness, reassurance, and tolerance are necessary staff behaviors for treating these patients.

Post-Traumatic Stress Disorder

> **309.81 Posttraumatic Stress Disorder**

Post-traumatic stress disorder is a complex of symptoms that occur in association with a psychologically painful or distressing event. To meet *DSM-IV* criteria, the event must have included the person's having witnessed or been confronted with an event that involved actual or threatened serious injury or death or a threat to the physical integrity of the person, *and* the person must have responded to the event with intense fear, helplessness, or horror. The event associated with the development of the disorder is thus, by definition, traumatic. Usual symptoms include the general anxiety symptoms discussed earlier, and, in addition, the patient tends to re-experience the event repetitively through "flashbacks" (dissociative symptoms), nightmares or distressing dreams, or feelings of "reliving" the event or events. In extreme cases, patients may have illusions or hallucinations during which the experience is re-created, and they feel they are actually back in the situation.

To qualify as a post-traumatic stress disorder, patients must experience the symptoms for more than a month. The disorder is not uncommon, to varying degrees, in persons who have been raped, nearly killed in some way, or involved in terroristic actions or war-related activities. Symptoms may occur almost immediately or be delayed for years. Symptoms may come and go and may be rekindled by seeing similar events or symbols of the distressing event. The "anniversary" reactions refer to the exacerbation of symptoms around the time of the occurrence of the distressing event. The *DSM-IV* uses a new classification for symptoms of less than 4 weeks' duration. The new category is 308.3 Acute Stress Disorder. This disorder is diagnosed when the symptoms occur within 4 weeks of the disorder and last from 2 days to 4 weeks.

Somatoform Disorders

The somatoform disorders are a group of five disorders with the central feature of mimicking physical disorders, for which no physiological basis can be found. Two additional groups cover somatoform type disorders that do not fit into one of the five established categories. These disorders include the following:

(1) 300.7 Body Dysmorphic Disorder
(2) 300.11 Conversion Disorder
(3) 300.7 Hypochondriasis
(4) 300.81 Somatization Disorder
(5) 307.xx Pain Disorder
(6) 300.81 Undifferentiated Somatoform Disorder
(7) 300.81 Somatoform Disorder Not Otherwise Specified

Conversion Disorder (Hysterical Neurosis, Conversion Type).
At one time many people believed that being struck blind, speechless, or with a paralysis of some sort was due to the wrath of God or to demonic possession. However, such explanations for the sudden onset of blindness, paralysis, or mutism have given way to more sophisticated explanations. Most people no longer believe that babies are "marked" at birth because the mother was frightened by a bear or scared by a devil or because she had evil thoughts during her pregnancy. Perhaps, because of increased educational levels, such explanations for behavioral characteristics in people have changed, although we still see many patients who suffer conversion disorders.

A conversion disorder is an attempt by people to defend themselves from some anxiety-provoking situation by unconsciously developing symptoms of a physical disorder that has no underlying organic, or physical, basis. Although the symptoms are psychogenic in origin, they are quite real to the patient. The basic characteristics of this disorder are that patients lose the ability to perform some physical function that they could perform before the onset of the disorder. The lost function is usually symbolically related to some situation that produces stress or anxiety for the individual. The patient may lose sensitivity to some area of the body, be unable to hear or talk, have unusual sensations such as tingling or burning, or lose the ability to perform some motor function such as walking or moving an arm or a hand. *Primary gain* is achieved by keeping the anxiety-provoking need or conflict out of awareness, and *secondary gain* is sometimes achieved through sympathy from the family or friends of the individual, and the symptoms are thus reinforced. Such persons are usually first seen by a physician who can find no physical basis for the symptoms. They are often referred to a neurologist, whose tests are also negative. As a last resort, the patient is then referred to a psychologist or a psychiatrist.

To illustrate, one of the authors treated a young woman who had suddenly become paralyzed from the waist down and was unable to walk. The patient was 18 years old and had already been seen by her family physician and by a neurologist, neither of whom could discover any physical basis for the paralysis. In reviewing the patient's history, the psychological factors leading to the paralysis were fairly clear-cut. The patient had a younger sister who contracted polio at age 2 and was disabled by the disease. She died at age 15. Because of the sister's disability, most of the family's efforts and attentions were focused on this child, and the older girl received little attention. Consequently, she developed some rather strong hostile feelings toward her sister. Of course, her hostility could not be expressed directly, and the patient suffered severe guilt feelings for the hostility she felt.

A few months after her sister died, the patient was involved in an accident in which she was hit by a falling tree limb. The patient did not suffer any significant injury as a result of the accident, and no medical follow-up was required. However, several months later, the patient developed the paralysis. The patient's family, afraid that another tragedy was about to befall one of their children, became quite concerned and showed the patient a great deal of sympathy and attention. Several weeks of treatment were required for both the patient and her family before she was able to walk again.

Conversion disorders are not common. They constitute less than 5 percent of all neurotic reactions. Only those who work in a hospital or clinic setting may ever see a patient in this diagnostic category. Of course, a great many people have headaches, stomach aches, and minor aches and pains that may be related to emotionally stressful situations. Only when they become severely debilitating do they significantly affect a person's life.

Perhaps the most important aspect of conversion disorders is that they are caused by situations an individual perceives as highly stressful and by the person's need to escape from the anxiety and stress created by that situation. The pain or the paralysis that may develop is real to the individual, and the fact that it is psychogenic in origin does not diminish the effect of the condition.

Because there is no apparent organic dysfunction, people frequently assume that the patient is faking or that the paralysis or the pain is not real. However, the particular conversion reaction has meaning to the patient, and, whether or not members of the treatment team understand it, patients are not helped by derogatory comments about their illness or by being told that the illness is "all in your head."

Body Dysmorphic Disorder. This disorder is one in which people become preoccupied with the idea that something is wrong with their appearance, but the imagined defect is not apparent to an objective observer. The complaints often are related to the face, skin, or other exposed body areas. Frequent trips to plastic surgeons are not uncommon. If the preoccupation with the imagined defect reaches delusional status, the diagnosis is delusional disorder, somatic subtype, because delusions are psychotic rather than neurotic in nature.

Hypochondriasis. The hallmark of the hypochondriac is a preoccupation with the idea that they have some horrible or debilitating disease and nobody will help them. Despite complete medical clearance and reassurance from their physician, hypochondriacal patients are never quite comfortable that they have been adequately evaluated. If they had been properly evaluated, they reason, the physician would have found the disease process causing their concern. Such patients, under pressure, can usually admit some possibility that they are wrong and are misinterpreting the symptoms. Yet the appearance of any small symptom or sensation sets them off again, certain that this time their fears are justified. These patients often have medicine cabinets full of medicine and often see multiple physicians in their search for the disease process they are so certain is present. Patients sometimes have their anxiety focused in this particular way due to having had some true illness or by having been associated with a family member or friend who has such an illness. These patients are often angered by any suggestion that they should seek mental health treatment.

Somatization Disorder. The major difference between hypochondriasis and somatization disorder is that hypochondriacs tend to be preoccupied with having some *particular* disease process, whereas the somatization disorder patient focuses on a variety of symptoms without ascribing them to any particular disease process. Somatization disorder patients have a long history of multiple problems for which no suitable organic cause can be established. Symptoms usually begin before age 30. To qualify for this diagnosis, the patient must have complaints of at least eight different physical symptoms spread across four categories (at least four pain symptoms, two gastrointestinal symptoms, one sexual symptom, and one pseudoneurological symptom). Their symptoms list is often presented with drama and flair, and there is a long, involved medical history that can be overwhelming. The nurse has the feeling of not knowing where to start because so many things are wrong.

Pain Disorder. Somatoform pain disorder is characterized by the patient's preoccupation for 6 months or more with pain for which no physical cause can be demonstrated. The concentration of attention to the pain is evident in that patients want to talk about little else and are often irritated that no one appreciates the intensity of their pain. Pain becomes the central focus of their existence and tends to govern or control much of their activity. The pain may not be consistent with any known pattern of physical pathology or may mimic known pain such as angina or sciatica. There may be direct evidence of the role of psychological factors when development of the pain follows or is connected with some environmental event that serves an emotional conflict or need. If the pain intensifies each time the patient's wife tells him he needs to get out of the wheelchair and begin to use crutches, the pain may be serving the patient's dependency needs. Sometimes pain allows patients to avoid activities and situations to which they are averse, and sometimes other evidence for secondary gain is clear. In some cases there is no apparent psychogenic role. Care must be taken with somatoform pain patients to avoid unnecessary medication and medical procedures. The *DSM-IV* divides this diagnosis into two categories: pain disorder associated with psychological factors and pain disorder associated with both psychological factors and a general medical condition.

Dissociative Disorders

Dissociative Disorders (Hysterical Neurosis, Dissociative Type). Dissociative disorders form an interesting diagnostic group even though they, too, account for less than 5 percent of all neurotic reactions. The dissociative disorders are like the conversion disorders in that they frequently occur in the same personality type, and both disorders serve to protect the individual from an especially stressful situation. Amnesia, fugue, depersonalization, and identity disorder (previously multiple personality disorder) are the major categories of dissociative reactions and reflect the major feature of this disorder, which is a disturbance in the proper integration of memory, consciousness, and identity. The five *DSM-IV* categories are as follows:

> (1) 300.14 Dissociative Identity Disorder
> (2) 300.13 Dissociative Fugue
> (3) 300.12 Dissociative Amnesia
> (4) 300.6 Depersonalization Disorder
> (5) 300.15 Dissociative Disorder Not Otherwise Specified

Multiple personality, now called *dissociative identity disorder,* is perhaps the most famous of all dissociative disorders, given the number of television shows, movies, and novels about people who suffer from this disorder. In clinical practice there are few actual cases of true multiple personalities, although in the last few years many clinicians have come to believe that it is not nearly so rare as once was thought. The disorders appear almost always to originate in childhood and in association with a trauma of some kind, particularly physical and sexual abuse, and they are rarely discovered until adulthood. The number of personalities can range from 2 to more than 100.

In dissociative identity disorders, an individual usually shows evidence of having two or more identifiably different patterns or characteristic ways of responding to the environment. Each of these identifiable ways of responding is operationally defined as a different personality. Usually each individual "personality" within the patient is a complete personality system of its own, and the patient responds to the particular personality that is conscious at any given time by allowing that personality system to dominate the patient's behavior or reactions to the environment. In many cases, but not all, some or all of the various personalities are aware of the others, and they may communicate internally. Some personalities are assigned roles such as "the worker," "the socializer," or "the protector," and different personalities may be in control at various times in the patient's life. The personalities are often very different from each other; astoundingly, research indicates that different personalities may have different psychological profiles as well as different physiological characteristics (such as eyeglass prescriptions and asthma).

One of the most frequent ways dissociative identity disorders are discovered is that a patient comes to therapy for some reason other than multiple personalities, and in the course of therapy the existence of alternative personalities is uncovered. Frequently, the tipoff comes when the therapist discovers time gaps or time periods for which the patient has no memory. Another tipoff occurs when the therapist recalls something said to him or her by the patient, but the patient has no recollection of it. This is a complex disorder to diagnose and to treat and should not be undertaken by persons without specific training in treating dissociative identity disorder.

Dissociative Fugue. In dissociative fugue, patients not only have amnesia but also combine the amnesia with flight, leaving the area where they live or work. Fugue is usually precipitated by some socially or environmentally stressful situation from which patients attempt to remove themselves both mentally and physically. The removal, however, is unconscious rather than conscious in that patients are usually unaware of where they came from and are unable to recall any former identity. When the episode is over, the patient usually is unable to recall events occurring during the episode. A key feature in the diagnosis of fugue is that the travels of the person appear to be purposeful rather than aimless.

Dissociative Amnesia. *Amnesia* is the sudden and temporary forgetting of information about one's life or environment. There are four basic types of amnesia: (1) localized, (2) selective, (3) generalized, and (4) continuous. In localized amnesia, the patient usually forgets specific information for a specified but undetermined length of time. For example, a patient may forget his or her name or a particular period of time in life, such as a traumatic event, a stressful operation, or an unhappy family situation. In selective amnesia, the patient cannot remember certain things that occurred during a specific time period. In generalized amnesia, patients do not recall anything about their lives. It is also referred to as *global amnesia.* In continuous amnesia, the patient is unable to recall information from some particular time or event to the present.

Amnesia is typically precipitated by a psychologically stressful event or situation, is usually fairly brief in duration, and often ends suddenly. The patient is usually able to regain all the lost information, and repeat experiences of amnesia are rare.

Mood Disorders

The *DSM-IV* handles mood disorders differently than the other classifications of disorders in order to avoid duplication of diagnostic categories. Mood disorders include mood disturbances falling in a range from very depressed mood to elation and disorders in which both extremes occur within the same individual. Mood disorders are divided into two categories of bipolar disorder (bipolar I disorders and bipolar II disorders) and one category of depressive disorder.

Bipolar Disorders. The *DSM-IV* categories of bipolar disorders are as follows:

(1) 296.6x Bipolar I Disorder, Most Recent Episode Mixed
(2) 296.4x Bipolar I Disorder, Most Recent Episode Manic
(3) 296.40 Bipolar I Disorder, Most Recent Episode Hypomanic
(4) 296.0x Bipolar I Disorder, Single Manic Episode
(5) 296.5x Bipolar I Disorder, Most Recent Episode Depressed
(6) 296.7 Bipolar I Disorder, Most Recent Episode Unspecified
(7) 296.89 Bipolar II Disorder
(8) 301.13 Cyclothymic Disorder
(9) 296.80 Bipolar Disorder Not Otherwise Specified

(The *x* is a placeholder for indicating severity characteristics of the disorder, such as mild, moderate, with or without psychosis, and the like.)

In the bipolar disorders, diagnoses are based on the nature of the moods experienced by the individual. In the "mixed" category, the patient has had one or more manic episodes and one or more major depressive episodes. Manic episodes are characterized by strongly elevated mood, expansive mood, or irritability, accompanied variously by inflated self-esteem or grandiosity, decreased need for sleep, pressured speech or being hyperverbal, racing thoughts, distractibility, increased psychomotor agitation, or engaging in behaviors carrying a high risk for harm or painful consequences. A common behavior in mania is the spending spree. Patients buy things they do not need and cannot use. They may give money away, believing they have an unlimited supply. They may sing and dance and preach and engage in promiscuous sexual behavior, and they may believe they are managing everything just fine. However, there is marked impairment in social and occupational functioning, and manic patients are often hospitalized. Psychotic features also occur, usually in the form of delusions or hallucinations of inflated worth, power, identity, or special relationship with some famous person or deity. A lesser debilitating form of mania is called *hypomania* and is usually distinguished from mania by the fact that the symptoms are the same but not as severe and do not result in substantial impairment in social and occupational functioning.

In depressive episodes, patients show depressed mood characterized by feelings of sadness, sometimes irritability, and what are commonly called the *vegetative* signs of depression, including a loss of appetite or overeating, inability to sleep or sleeping too much, decreased energy, anhedonia (inability to experience pleasure), loss of interest in activities, and weight loss or weight gain. In addition, depressed patients experience excessive guilt, feel worthless, helpless, and hopeless, and have trouble maintaining attention and concentration. There is frequently withdrawal from friends and acquaintances, and patients sometimes lock themselves away from the world and refuse to answer the telephone or the door if someone knocks. Psychomotor retardation or agitation is also seen, along with indecisiveness. Suicidal ideation is common and represents the most immediate and serious threat in depressed persons.

In cyclothymia, the symptoms described for mania and major depressive episodes occur but are of lesser intensity and meet the definition for hypomanic disorder rather than full mania. The symptoms involve both depressive episodes and hypomanic episodes. Some researchers maintain that cyclothymia is simply a mild form of bipolar disorder.

Depressive Disorders. The *DSM-IV* adds two other categories of mood disorder: one related to a medical condition that is supposed to account for the mood disturbance, and a category that supposes that the disturbed mood is due to the ingestion of some chemical substance.

(1)	296.2x	Major Depressive Disorder, Single Episode
(2)	296.3x	Major Depressive Disorder, Recurrent
(3)	300.4	Dysthymic Disorder
(4)	311	Depressive Disorder Not Otherwise Specified

These diagnostic categories describe those mood disorders that have only elements of depressed mood and do not include a history of manic or hypomanic episodes. In the "single episode" category are included patients who have never had either a manic, hypomanic, or previous depressive episode. If the patient has previously had a depressive episode, the "recurrent" category is used. Dysthymia bears much the same relationship to major depression that hypomania bears to mania; that is, the symptoms are of the same nature but are not as severe. This, of course, makes for some difficulty in deciding in some cases if the person has a dysthymia or a major depression. To make this diagnosis, the mood disturbance must have been present for 2 years (1 for children and adolescents) with no more than 2 months of that time being symptom free. The not otherwise specified category is for those patients with depressive symptoms that do not qualify for one of the other mood disorders.

The next chapter discusses the psychotic disorders. Self-test questions for Chapters 5, 6, and 7 can be found at the end of Chapter 7.

▼ KEY POINTS ▼

1. A diagnosis is used primarily by members of the treatment team as a shorthand method of describing a group of behaviors that might be expected from a particular person.

2. In mental health settings, diagnoses are necessary so that the health insurance company can classify the patient's particular disorder and determine if reimbursement can be made to treatment personnel and to the hospital or clinic.

3. The advent of diagnosis-related groups (DRGs) as a basis for third-party reimbursement has also affected the need for accurate diagnosis and assessment.

Key Points continued

4. All categories of mental illness fall within one of nine DRGs, and a fixed amount of money is paid for each illness depending upon its DRG classification.

5. The difference between neurosis and psychosis is the degree of disorganization in the patient's thought processes, the degree of reality testing (the ability to distinguish between what is and is not real), and the kinds of treatment procedures needed to manage the symptoms.

6. The *DSM-IV* lists nine different diagnostic categories for anxiety. The two that reflect general anxiety symptoms are generalized anxiety disorder and anxiety disorder not otherwise specified.

7. Anxiety patients frequently have a history during childhood and other life situations that did not provide firm, supportive approval or disapproval of behavior.

8. Anxiety in phobic disorders is usually experienced when the individual with the phobia comes in contact with the feared situation, object, or condition. Phobias are usually described as a persistent and irrational fear of some object, place, or condition.

9. Cognitive behavior approaches deal primarily with the symptoms.

10. The *DSM-IV* lists five categories of phobic neurosis including panic disorder: (1) panic disorder with agoraphobia, (2) panic disorder without agoraphobia, (3) agoraphobia without history of panic disorder, (4) social phobia, and (5) specific phobia.

11. Panic disorder is a condition wherein the patient experiences sudden onset of extreme anxiety, during which many symptoms of anxiety appear in an exaggerated form.

12. Agoraphobia, which can occur with or without panic symptoms, is fear of being in a place, situation, or condition from which the patient feels escape is to be difficult, impossible, or embarrassing.

13. Obsessive-compulsive disorders fall within the category of anxiety-related disorders. Patients experiencing an obsessive-compulsive disorder are unable to prevent repetitive thinking about unwanted thoughts or ideas, or are unable to keep from engaging in repetitive behavior.

14. Post-traumatic stress disorder is a complex of symptoms that occur in association with a psychologically painful, distressing, or threatening event.

continued on page 100

Key Points continued

15. The somatoform disorders have the central feature of mimicking physical disorders, but no physiological basis can be found. They include (1) body dysmorphic disorder, (2) conversion disorder, (3) hypochondriasis, (4) somatization disorder, and (5) pain disorder.

16. Two additional groups cover somatoform-type disorders that do not fit into one of the five established categories: undifferentiated somatoform disorder and somatoform disorder not otherwise specified.

17. A conversion disorder is an attempt to defend the self from some anxiety-provoking situation by unconsciously developing symptoms of a physical disorder that has no underlying organic or physical basis. Conversion disorders are not common.

18. In body dysmorphic disorder, people become preoccupied with the idea that something is wrong with their appearance, but the imagined defect is not apparent to an objective observer.

19. The hallmark of hypochondriacal disorder is preoccupation with the idea that one has some horrible or debilitating disease and that nobody will help.

20. The major difference between hypochondriasis and somatization disorder is that hypochondriacs tend to be preoccupied with having some particular disease process, whereas the somatization disordered patient focuses on a variety of symptoms without ascribing them to any particular disease process.

21. Somatoform pain disorder is characterized by the patient's preoccupation for 6 months or more with pain for which no physical cause can be demonstrated.

22. There are five dissociative disorders listed in the *DSM-IV:* (1) dissociative identity disorder, (2) dissociative fugue, (3) dissociative amnesia, (4) depersonalization disorder, and (5) dissociative disorder not otherwise specified.

23. Dissociative identity disorder, previously called *multiple personality disorder,* appears almost always to originate in childhood and in association with a severe trauma of some kind, particularly physical and sexual abuse, and is rarely discovered until adulthood.

24. In dissociative fugue, patients not only have amnesia but also combine the amnesia with flight by leaving the area where they live or work. Fugue is usually precipitated by some socially or

Key Points continued

environmentally stressful situation from which patients attempt to remove themselves both mentally and physically.

25. Dissociative amnesia is the sudden and temporary forgetting of information about one's life or environment. There are four basic types: (1) localized, (2) selective, (3) generalized, and (4) continuous.

26. Mood disorders are divided into two categories of bipolar disorder (bipolar I disorders and bipolar II disorders) and one category of depressive disorder: (1) bipolar I disorder, most recent episode mixed; (2) bipolar I disorder, most recent episode manic; (3) bipolar I disorder, most recent episode hypomanic; (4) bipolar I disorder, single manic episode; (5) bipolar I disorder, most recent episode depressed, (6) bipolar I disorder, most recent episode unspecified, (7) bipolar II disorder, (8) cyclothymia, and (9) bipolar disorder not otherwise specified.

27. In bipolar disorders, diagnoses are made depending upon the nature of the moods experienced by the individual. In the "mixed" category, the patient has had one or more manic episodes and one or more major depressive episodes.

28. In depressive episodes, patients show depressed mood characterized by feelings of sadness, sometimes by irritability, and by what are commonly called the *vegetative* signs of depression.

29. In cyclothymia, the symptoms described for mania and major depressive episodes occur but are of lesser intensity and meet the definition for hypomanic disorder rather than full mania.

30. The *DSM-IV* also adds two *categories* of mood disorder; one category supposes some medical condition that is believed to be responsible for the mood disturbance and a second category that supposes that the disturbed mood is due to the ingestion of some chemical substance. Diagnostic classifications include: (1) major depression, single episode; (2) major depression, recurrent; (3) dysthymia, and (4) depressive disorder not otherwise specified.

Annotated Bibliography

Agostinelli, B., Demers, K., Garrigan, D., and Waszynski, C.: Targeted interventions: Use of the mini-mental state exam. *Journal of Gerontology Nursing,* 1994, 20(8):15–23.

The authors have found the MMSE to be a stable measure for global assessment of cognitive abilities; it also gives clues to specific functional abilities and disabilities of daily living skills.

American Psychiatric Association: *Diagnostic and Statistical Manual of Mental Disorders, ed. 4.* Washington, D.C.: APA, 1994.

Barth, F. D.: Obsessional thinking as "paradoxical action." *Bulletin of the Menninger Clinic,* 1990, 54:449–511.

Utilizes Schafer's theory of obsessional thinking as paradoxical action and a case example to illustrate the treatment and resistance to treatment of persons suffering from obsessive-compulsive disorder.

O'Connell, K. L.: Schizoaffective disorder: A case study. *Journal of Psychosocial Nursing,* 1995, 33(10):35–40.

Provides diagnostic criteria for the diagnosis of schizoaffective disorder and discusses using lithium as a means of affective treatment for schizoaffective disorder.

Pollack, L. E.: Improving relationships: Groups for inpatients with bipolar disorder. *Journal of Psychosocial Nursing and Mental Health Services,* 1990, 28(5):17–22.

Discusses the use of group therapy to improve social skills of patients with bipolar disorder.

Roberts, S. J.: Somatization in primary care: The common presentation of psychosocial problems through physical complaints. *Nurse Practitioner,* 1994, 19(5):47–56.

Discusses using a careful and holistic assessment of somatic complaints and psychosocial aspects to avoid extensive diagnostic evaluations and treatment.

Rogers, B.: Socio-economic status, employment and neurosis. *Social Psychiatry and Psychiatric Epidemiology,* 1991, 26:104–114.

Explores the social, occupational, and educational status of persons suffering from neurosis.

Shealy, A. H.: Attention-deficit hyperactivity disorder—etiology, diagnosis, and management. *Journal of Child and Psychiatric Nursing,* 1994, 7(2):24–34.

Discusses the developmental disorder and how it affects patients at home, at school, and with peer relationships and how it persists through adolescence and continues into young adulthood. Provides diagnostic criteria for assessment.

Simoni, P. S.: Obsessive-compulsive disorder: The effect of research on nursing care. *Journal of Psychosocial Nursing and Mental Health Services,* 1991, 29(4):19–23.

Defines obsessive-compulsive disorder and presents concepts for nursing care and intervention.

Turner, D. M.: Panic disorder: A personal and nursing perspective. *Journal of Psychosocial Nursing,* 1995, 33(4):5–8.

Discusses biologic etiology, health and social consequences, diagnosis, and treatment, as well as nursing implications.

Whitley, G. G.: Ritualistic behavior: Breaking the cycle. *Journal of Psychosocial Nursing and Mental Health Services,* 1991, 29(10):31–35.

Presents treatment strategies for working with patients with obsessive-compulsive disorders.

Widiger, T., Frances, A., Pincus, H., Davis, W., and First, M.: Toward an empirical classification for the DSM IV. *Journal of Abnormal Psychology,* 1991, 100(3):280–288.

The empirical basis for the *DSM-IV* is discussed, and a historical perspective of past editions of the *DSM* is presented.

The Psychotic Diagnostic Categories

OBJECTIVES: Student will be able to:

1. Discuss three different categories of psychosis.
2. Identify several characteristics of persons suffering from psychoses.
3. Identify the largest single group of psychotic patients.
4. Name and list characteristics of several different types of schizophrenia.
5. Discuss the five major types of delusions associated with delusional (paranoid) disorders.
6. Relate the reasons paranoid patients are sometimes considered the most difficult to manage.

The psychoses are generally divided into two categories, the organic psychoses and the functional psychoses. Organic psychoses are caused by some disorder of the brain for which physical pathology can be demonstrated. The functional psychoses are psychotic disorders caused by psychological stress; that is, they occur in response to psychological stresses and in the absence of demonstrated neurological pathology. In both categories, patients exhibit bizarre behavior and are obviously ill. People are more likely to notice a psychotic patient than to notice a patient with a neurosis because of the bizarre quality of a psychotic person's behavior. This is largely due to the fact that the psychotic patient's behavior differs greatly from the so-called "normal" behavior of human beings.

A third category of psychotic reactions is sometimes used when mental health teams wish to differentiate psychotic reactions caused by toxic substances. They are called *toxic psychoses* and are generally caused by the ingestion of drugs or poisons of some type.

In psychotic reactions, as opposed to neurotic reactions, the patient is not dealing with objective reality. The reality the individual experiences is unique to him or her and is not the same reality that a mentally healthy person experiences. To psychotic patients, the spiders they see on their arms are real and the person to whom they talk, who is unseen by others, is also real. The voices that psychotic patients hear are real to them, and they are sincerely convinced that they are Jesus Christ or Napoleon or a prophet or an FBI agent or that their food or water is being poisoned. Arguing with patients or trying to logically demonstrate that their perception of reality is in error is of very little benefit. Staff members' "logical" arguments appeal to a reality that does not exist for the patients. They just do not see the world in the same way that staff members do.

Contrary to what many people in the general population believe, a very large percentage of patients admitted to hospitals with a psychotic disorder recover and are able to once again function effectively. After a sufficient period of recovery, many patients suffering from psychotic disorders are able to resume their lives and make good adjustments subsequent to hospitalization. However, far too many, for reasons not yet understood, become chronically ill and live with a reality that is incompatible with adequate social and occupational productivity.

Because the differences between neuroses and psychoses have been discussed previously, what follows is a description of the different functionally (nonorganically) based psychotic categories of the *DSM-IV*.

SCHIZOPHRENIC DISORDERS

(1) 295.20 Schizophrenia, Catatonic Type
(2) 295.10 Schizophrenia, Disorganized Type
(3) 295.30 Schizophrenia, Paranoid Type
(4) 295.90 Schizophrenia, Undifferentiated Type
(5) 295.60 Schizophrenia, Residual Type

In general, most authorities are uncertain about why people develop schizophrenia. Hereditary factors have been linked to schizophrenia, and research suggests that individuals may be predisposed to develop schizophrenia under stressful environmental conditions. Factors such as family behavioral patterns and other sociological and cultural differences have been designated as contributing factors in schizophrenia. It seems more likely, however, that schizophrenia is the result of a complex relationship between biologic, psychological, and sociological factors.

Schizophrenic reactions may occur suddenly, in which case they are referred to as *acute schizophrenic reactions*. They may also be of long duration and develop slowly over a rather lengthy period. In this latter case, they are called *chronic schizophrenic reactions*.

Schizophrenia is the largest single diagnostic group of psychotic patients. Approximately 1 percent of the people in the United States suffer from schizophrenia as it is now defined by the *DSM-IV*. As is obvious from the preceding list, there are many different classifications of schizophrenia. However, the overriding characteristic in the schizophrenias is the bizarre nature of the thought content and process. The thought content of schizophrenics tends to include both delusions and hallucinations that are so patently strange or bizarre as to defy all logic. Schizophrenic patients may believe the television is giving them messages from God or the president or the CIA. A patient of one of the authors believed he was receiving messages from aliens in outer space through the fillings in his teeth, and another patient believed himself to be dead. Patients sometimes believe thoughts are being inserted into their heads against their will, that others can read their thoughts or are stealing their thoughts, and that they are being controlled by or are controlling forces outside themselves. They may think that some force such as "x-rays" or radio waves have somehow disturbed their bodies and are causing their tissues to rot or to have some other equally illogical outcome.

Disturbances in the process of schizophrenics' thinking are revealed in how verbalizations are processed and organized. This disturbance in cognitive processing is called a *formal thought disorder*. Patients who demonstrate it may be extremely tangential and unable to answer questions in a relevant way. *Tangential* means that their associations may be quite loose; that is, their thoughts are not logically related or expressed, and they jump from one subject to another. In addition, they may show flight of ideas, may be incoherent and use neologisms (words that are just made up and have no real meaning in the language), may talk all around an issue and give so many nonessential details that they have trouble getting to the point they wish to make (circumstantiality), and may demonstrate echolalia (echoing what is said to them), mutism, thought blocking, posturing, poor abstraction abilities, and a supreme lack of awareness that they are communicating poorly. Their perceptions are often bizarre and include delusions and hallucinations. Affect (emotional tone) is often flat or inappropriate, with giggling or unpredictable laughing or crying. There is often a loss of a sense of personal individuality, with patients unsure of their relationship to the world and their place in it. Some patients become preoccupied with questions about the meaning of life and other esoteric concerns. Schizophrenic patients often have difficulty with impulse control, especially while acutely ill, and they may lack the ability to appreciate the social consequences of their behavior. Most schizophrenic patients show very limited insight and may show very poor judgment. They have impairment in social relationships and impairment in their ability to get organized to perform tasks and accomplish goals. Suicide is also a serious risk in schizophrenic patients.

Catatonic Schizophrenia

The catatonic schizophrenic is quite striking because of the extreme nature of the person's withdrawal. Catatonic patients may refuse to eat, will not speak, and may remain motionless for hours or days. The two phases of catatonia are the stuporous phase, in which the patient is motionless, and catatonic excitement, in which the patient over-reacts, shouts, talks, paces, and appears quite manic. Patients may alternate between these phases, sometimes quite rapidly, but most seem to show a preference for one or the other. One particularly interesting and clear diagnostic indicator of catatonia is that of posturing or catatonic rigidity. In this condition, a patient refuses to allow his or her body position to be altered. In "waxy flexibility," when the patient's hand or some other body part is placed in some particular position, even an uncomfortable one, she or he tends to maintain that position. It is as if the patient were made of soft, warm wax and can be molded into almost any position. Catatonia is fairly rare but dramatic in its presentation and easy to recognize.

Paranoid Schizophrenia

The paranoid schizophrenic often shows much hostility and suspicion and may show a great deal of overt aggression. The "glaring" intensity of many paranoid schizophrenic patients has sometimes led people to refer to the "paranoid stare" as a characteristic. These patients sometimes relate in an intense, overbearing way, and the anger and hostility are often apparent as the patient talks and interrelates with others. Paranoid schizophrenic patients tend to be rather well organized in their delusions and hallucinations, and those phenomena are usually organized around a single idea or theme. They do not seem as strange or bizarre as the other types of schizophrenic patients, and therapists often speak of these patients' ability to "reconstitute" quickly; that is, they can sometimes pull themselves together quickly, and, with only brief exposure to the patient, a nurse who did not know about the illness might wonder why the patient was in treatment. Sometimes these patients appear so well organized, and their delusional material so logical, that nurses must talk to family or others who know the patient to verify what is and is not fact. However, after being around the patient for a while, the nurse can recognize the preoccupation with whatever is the central theme to the illness.

Disorganized Schizophrenia

In disorganized schizophrenia, patients may appear manic and have bizarre mannerisms. They often laugh and giggle inappropriately and are preoccupied with trivial things. They represent one of the most severely disorganized personality structures in the schizophrenic group. Delusions and hallucinatory phenomena, when they occur, tend to be random and very poorly presented. In talking with this group of patients, the nurse recognizes right away that something is tremendously wrong, and it is usually difficult to make any emotional contact with the disorganized schizophrenic. The withdrawal is extreme, and others can never be comfortable that any emotional contact has been made with the patient. These patients suffer the most social isolation over time because they tend not to have significant remissions, and their course is often chronic. To be assigned this diagnosis, a patient must demonstrate disorganized speech, disorganized behavior, and a flat or inappropriate affect.

Undifferentiated Schizophrenia

In undifferentiated schizophrenia, there are prominent delusions or hallucinations, incoherence, or other evidence of grossly disorganized behavior that does not meet the criteria for other types of schizophrenia or meets the criteria for more than one.

Schizophrenia, Residual Type

In residual type schizophrenia, there is an absence of prominent symptoms such as hallucinations or delusions, but there remains evidence of attenuated or reduced symptoms characteristic of schizophrenia. For example, the individual may continue to demonstrate eccentric or odd beliefs or may reflect unusual or peculiar perceptual processes.

295.70 Schizoaffective Disorder

In a previous edition of this book, we stated that this diagnostic entity was included more out of obstinacy than anything else. In the *DSM-III-R,* the previous edition of *DSM,* it was classified under "Psychotic Disorders Not Elsewhere Classified." This category had been deleted from the schizophrenic disorders because mood disorders had been thought to be distinguishable from thought disorders. We are happy to report that the *DSM-IV* has reinstated the category.

In schizoaffective schizophrenia, a significant thought disorder is apparent, along with significant mood variation. These patients may at first appear to be merely depressed or manic, but further inquiry reveals a basic personality disorganization. The framers of the *DSM-IV* require that this disorder be diagnosed only when the symptoms of the mood disorder are present for a substantial portion of the total duration of the active and residual periods of the illness *and* when there have been delusions or hallucinations for at least 2 weeks in the absence of prominent mood symptoms. The authors have found this diagnosis very useful with a select group of patients who clearly seem to have disorders that cannot be classified purely as a mood disorder or as a schizophrenic disorder but have elements of both.

297.1 Delusional Disorder

The *DSM-IV* uses the term *delusional disorder* for this diagnostic category in order to escape the multiple implications inherent in the term *paranoid.* This disorder is separate from that of paranoid schizophrenia and is differentiated largely on the basis of the lack of bizarreness and mental disorganization seen in the paranoid schizophrenic. Auditory or visual hallucinations are not usually a part of the clinical picture for the delusional disordered patient, and they are not often seen as eccentric or strange. For the most part, the delusions involve situations that occur in real life, such as poisoning, having a disease, sexual infidelities, deception, or being stalked.

Five general themes make up the bulk of the delusional material in this disorder.

1. *Erotomanic.* This is the category of delusion so often played out on the nightly news. Sometimes referred to as "fan obsessions," movie and television stars often find themselves the target of delusional people who are convinced the star needs them for one reason or another or that the star loves them but just does not realize it. Any person of public prominence may be a target of persons with erotomanic delusions simply because of his or her public stature, but star status is not a requirement to become a target. Targets may be a boss, a neighbor, or even a stranger. The person suffering the delusion may try to contact the target in a number of ways, including calling, writing, or stalking. Such experiences often frighten the target and have sometimes resulted in the target's death, as in the case of actress Rebecca Schaffer from the television program *My Sister Sam,* but the motivation is not usually sexual gratification. For whatever reason, perhaps because of social conditioning, men more often pursue their delusions to the point of contact with police than do women.

2. *Grandiose type.* Persons suffering from grandiose type delusions usually act on a strong belief that they are somehow special or have been assigned a special project by some very important figure. They sometimes believe they have been entrusted with a secret that will save the world or humanity, have invented some marvelous new device with fantastic potential, or have developed special knowledge or abilities of great value. If they believe themselves to be some living person of great importance, they believe that the actual person is a fraud or imposter and may go to some lengths to try to prove it. One area that seems particularly attractive for delusional persons is religion, and a person who is adept enough at managing such a delusion can attract a lot of followers. Some years ago Jim Jones not only convinced many of his followers to go with him to Guyana but also convinced them to participate in a mass suicidal destruction of his entire following. The adults gave poisoned Kool-Aid to their children and then drank it themselves. Hundreds of people died at the religious commune.

3. *Jealous type.* In this delusion the patient comes to believe that a spouse or lover is engaging in a relationship with another person. To make this diagnosis, there cannot be objective cause for the concerns. The authors have seen instances in which the patient's spouse is rarely out of sight, but the patient persists in believing the spouse is unfaithful. The patient finds small clues and "evidence" that are taken as proof of the imagined relationship. This "evidence" often throws the patient into an angry outrage,

and the patient may become physically abusive and violent toward the spouse or lover. The patient often plays detective and follows the object of concern in an effort to prove the validity of the suspicion—and looking that hard often uncovers some tiny bit of information that can be construed as consistent with the delusional belief.

4. *Persecutory type.* These patients are often disliked by staff members, other patients, family members, and everyone else in general because they are so very difficult to get along with and frequently quite hostile. They are often resentful and usually mistrust the motives of almost everyone. Frequently they are overly concerned with issues of right and wrong and rigid in their beliefs and expectations. They go to ridiculous extremes to right an imagined wrong or to avenge an imagined slight, and thus they frequently threaten to take legal action. Their delusions often include being poisoned, plotted against, or ignored, having their ideas stolen, or in some way having been deprived of something that is rightfully theirs. Persons with persecutory type delusions can be frightening and do sometimes act out violently against those they believe responsible for their torment.

5. *Somatic type.* The *DSM-IV* recounts that the most frequent manifestation of paranoid somatic delusions is that patients believe that some part of the body is emitting a foul odor, that they have some type of parasite living within them, or that some type of infection or perhaps some type of insect is inhabiting their bodies. There may also be a perception, with no objective evidence, that some part of the body is malformed or misfunctioning. Such patients usually are diagnosed when they visit a family doctor or other specialist for attention to their somatic complaint.

A major difference between delusional (paranoid) patients and paranoid schizophrenics is that the delusional patient usually has better intellectual control and is able to make more appropriate intellectual and social responses. Compared with paranoid schizophrenics, delusional patients are usually more reality oriented. Except in the area of their delusions, their intellectual capacities are much better organized, and they are able to present their feelings in a much more effective manner.

One of the most important things for a mental health worker to recognize is that paranoid delusional patients have significant difficulty recognizing their own hostilities and anger and that they tend to project their anger onto others. Such patients use the defense mechanism of projection to prevent themselves from having to recognize their own anger and hostility. Frequently the paranoid patient deliberately does something to anger a staff member or a fellow patient in order to confirm the delusion that other people do not like or are angry at the patient. If the staff member or fellow patient responds in an angry fashion, the paranoid patient feels that the original belief was correct and justified.

In general, paranoid patients are often difficult to manage. However, they represent a very small percentage of psychiatric patients, probably less than 1 percent of all psychiatric admissions.

The next chapter discusses the personality disorders and sexual disorders. Questions for Chapters 5, 6, and 7 are at the end of Chapter 7.

▼ KEY POINTS ▼

1. The psychoses are generally divided into two or three categories, the organic psychoses and the functional psychoses.
   - Organic psychoses are caused by some disorder of the brain for which physical pathology can be demonstrated.
   - Functional psychoses are psychotic disorders that occur in response to psychological stresses and in the absence of demonstrated neurological pathology.
   - Psychotic reactions in a third category are caused by toxic substances. In all categories, the psychotic patient's behavior differs a great deal from the so-called "normal" behavior of human beings.

2. The following are descriptions of the different functionally (nonorganically) based psychotic categories of the *DSM-IV*.

Schizophrenic Disorders

(1) 295.20 Schizophrenia, Catatonic Type
(2) 295.30 Schizophrenia, Paranoid Type
(3) 295.10 Schizophrenia, Disorganized Type
(4) 295.90 Schizophrenia, Undifferentiated Type
(5) 295.60 Schizophrenia, Residual Type

3. The overriding characteristic in the schizophrenias is the bizarre nature of the thought content and process.

continued on page 114

Key Points continued

4. Most authorities are uncertain about why people develop schizophrenia. It is likely that schizophrenia is the result of a complex relationship between biologic (genetic), psychological, and sociological factors.

5. Schizophrenia is the largest single diagnostic group of psychotic patients. Approximately 1 percent of the people in the United States suffer from schizophrenia as it is now defined by the *DSM-IV.*

6. Disturbances in the process of schizophrenic thinking show up in how verbalizations are processed and organized. Problems in content, speed of thinking, and ease of flow are characteristic. Associations may not be logically related (looseness of associations), and patients may show flight of ideas.

7. There are two phases of catatonic schizophrenia:
   • The stuporous phase in which the patient is motionless.
   • Catatonic excitement, during which the patient is overreactive, shouts, talks, paces, and appears quite manic. One clear diagnostic indicator of catatonia is that of posturing or catatonic rigidity, which is sometimes called *waxy flexibility.*

8. Paranoid schizophrenic patients often show much hostility and suspicion and sometimes a great deal of overt aggression.
   • Paranoid schizophrenic patients tend to be rather well organized in their delusions and hallucinations, and those phenomena are usually organized around a single idea or theme.
   • They may not seem as strange or bizarre as the other types of schizophrenic patients until one hits upon their particular delusional system.

9. In disorganized schizophrenia, patients may appear manic and have bizarre mannerisms. They often laugh and giggle inappropriately and are preoccupied with trivial things. Their behaviors appear random and disorganized. They also may be withdrawn and difficult to contact emotionally. These patients tend not to have significant remissions, and their course is often quite chronic.

10. In undifferentiated schizophrenia, there are prominent delusions or hallucinations, incoherence, or other evidence of grossly disorganized behavior that does not meet the criteria for other types of schizophrenia or meets the criteria for more than one.

Key Points continued

11. In schizoaffective schizophrenia, a significant thought disorder is apparent, along with a significant mood variation.

Delusional (Paranoid) Disorder

12. This disorder is differentiated from paranoid schizophrenia largely on the basis of the lack of bizarreness and lack of mental disorganization seen in the paranoid schizophrenic. Delusional patients are not often seen as eccentric or strange beyond their unique or unconventional belief system.

13. There are five general categories of delusions:
    - Erotomanic type
    - Grandiose type
    - Jealous type
    - Persecutory type
    - Somatic type

14. The erotomanic type is sometimes referred to as "fan obsessions." Movie and television stars often find themselves the target of delusional people who are convinced the star needs them for one reason or another or that the star loves them but just doesn't realize it. Men more often than women pursue their delusions to the point of contact with police.

15. In the grandiose type, persons usually act on a strong belief that they are somehow special, like Jesus Christ or God or the president, or have been assigned a special project by some very important figure.

16. In the jealous type delusion, the patient comes to believe that a spouse or lover is engaging in a relationship with another person. To make this diagnosis, there cannot be objective cause for the concerns.

17. Persons suffering from persecutory delusions often experience delusions about being poisoned, plotted against, or ignored, having their ideas stolen, or in some way being deprived of something that is rightfully theirs. They are often difficult to get along with, frequently hostile and resentful, and usually mistrust the motives of almost everyone.

18. Persons suffering from somatic delusions believe that some part of the body is emitting a foul odor or that they have some type of

continued on page 115

Key Points continued

parasite, infection, or insect inhabiting their bodies. There may also be a perception, with no objective evidence, that some part of the body is malformed or misfunctioning.

19. A major difference between delusional (paranoid) patients and paranoid schizophrenics is that the paranoid patient usually has better intellectual control and is able to make more appropriate intellectual and social responses. Paranoid patients have significant difficulty recognizing their own hostilities and anger; they tend to project their anger onto others and are often difficult to manage. However, they represent a very small percentage of psychiatric patients and probably account for less than 1 percent of all psychiatric admissions.

Annotated Bibliography

Buchanan, J.: Social support and schizophrenia: A review of the literature. *Archives of Psychiatric Nursing,* 1995, 9(2):68–76.

Examines social support as a protective factor that facilitates coping and competence in schizophrenic patients.

Chapman, T.: The nurse's role in neuroleptic medications. *Journal of Psychosocial Nursing and Mental Health Services,* 1991, 29(6):6–8.

Neuroleptic medications for the treatment of schizophrenia often have adverse side effects. Patients were allowed to express their attitudes concerning the need for these medications.

Dauner, A., and Blair, D.: Akathisia: When treatment creates a problem. *Journal of Psychosocial Nursing and Mental Health Services,* 1990, 23(10):13–17.

Explains the symptoms and dangers of akathisia (a side effect of antipsychotic medications) and gives several case examples of patients suffering from these symptoms.

Dzurec, L. C.: How do they see themselves? Self-perceptions and functioning for people with chronic schizophrenia. *Journal of Psychosocial Nursing and Mental Health Services,* 1990, 28(8):10–14.

Research study describing the relationship between the self-perceptions of schizophrenic patients and their level of daily functioning.

Ehmann, T. S., Higgs, E., Smith, G. N., Altman, T. S., Lloyd, D., and Honer, W. G.: Routine assessment of patient progress: A multiformat, change-sensitive nurses' instrument for assessing psychotic inpatients. *Comprehensive Psychiatry,* 1995, 36(4):289–295.

Discusses using the Routine Assessment of Patient Progress scale to incorporate both interview and observational data into the assessment process.

O'Connell, K. L.: Schizoaffective disorder: A case study. *Journal of Psychosocial Nursing*, 1995, 33(10):35–40.

Presents a case scenario with schizoaffective symptoms and treatment. Provides a table illustration of the *DSM-IV* criteria for the diagnoses of schizoaffective disorder.

Roberts, S. J.: Somatization in primary care: The common presentation of psychosocial problems through physical complaints. *Nurse Practitioner*, 1994, 19(5):47–56.

Discusses using a careful holistic assessment to avoid extensive evaluations and treatment for those with psychosocial problems and poor coping skills that result in somatic delusions.

Siever, L. J., and Others: Eye movement impairment and schizotypal psychopathology. *American Journal of Psychiatry*, 1994, 151(8):1209–1215.

Discusses the close and parallel relationship between schizophrenia and schizotypal personality.

CHAPTER

7

Personality Disorders and the Sexual Disorders

OBJECTIVES: Student will be able to:

1. Discuss the significance of personality disorders to the lives of people who have them.
2. Identify four characteristics of persons with personality disorders.
3. Understand and express the reasons personality disordered persons are often shunned by treatment personnel.
4. Name several different types of personality disorders.
5. Name two major categories of sexual disorders.
6. Identify several characteristics of persons who experience sexual disorders.

This category includes patterns of behavior that are neither psychotic nor neurotic but are nonetheless substantially maladaptive. There is little information about the cause of personality disorders, but, as usual, such factors as genetics, environment, culture, and maturation may play roles. Personality disorders are used to describe behavior patterns that are usually long-standing and frequently are apparent from early adolescence. Because personality disorders are often not seen as being as "serious" as neurotic or psychotic conditions, and perhaps because they are so prevalent in our society, the significance of such disorders is often overlooked.

Perry and Vaillant (1989) make the point that a number of "saints, artists, revolutionary heros and true innovators" had personality disorders. They also point out that a large percentage of prison inmates, welfare recipients, and persons "known in lay terms as bad, deviant, sinning, cranky, or n'er-do-well [sic]" are among the personality disor-

119

dered. They enumerate four characteristics shared by persons with personality disorders:

1. An inflexible and maladaptive response to stress.
2. A disability in working and loving that is generally more serious and always more pervasive than that found in neurosis.
3. Elicitation of problematic responses by interpersonal conflict.
4. A particular capacity to "get under the skin" of and distress others.

Personality disorders are differentiated from personality "traits" primarily on the basis of the degree of maladaptation and personal discomfort created by the personality characteristics. Patients with personality disorders have difficulty managing emotionally intense situations, have trouble managing anger, and want others to adapt to their demands rather than adapt themselves to the demands of others. They tend to view people as difficult to live with, have trouble seeing their own faults and problems, and tend to blame others when things go wrong. People with personality disorders tend to ask what is wrong with the world rather than what is wrong with them.

Because of these characteristics, persons with personality disorders tend to be shunned by treatment personnel. They are difficult to treat, reject efforts to help, do not see their need for change, and are irreverent and sometimes openly contemptuous toward the caregiver. These characteristics are not endearing, and their resistance to change, regardless of what mode of therapy is used, often makes them less than favorites as patients. There is often a perception that personality disorders are untreatable, but it would be unreasonable to assume that an enduring personality adaptation would remit as readily as, say, a phobia, which creates a lot of discomfort for the affected person. Personality-disordered patients often see their personality characteristics as consistent with getting their needs met and as necessary to deal with an uncaring world. Given that mind-set, it is not surprising they are reluctant to change.

Personality disorders are divided into three "clusters" in the *DSM-IV*.

Cluster A: The Odd and the Eccentric
  (1) 301.0 Paranoid Personality Disorder
  (2) 301.20 Schizoid Personality Disorder
  (3) 301.22 Schizotypal Personality Disorder

Cluster B: The Dramatic, Emotional, or Erratic
(1) 301.7 Antisocial Personality Disorder
(2) 301.83 Borderline Personality Disorder
(3) 301.50 Histrionic Personality Disorder
(4) 301.81 Narcissistic Personality Disorder

Cluster C: The Anxious, Fearful, or Introverted
(1) 301.82 Avoidant Personality Disorder
(2) 301.6 Dependent Personality Disorder
(3) 301.4 Obsessive-Compulsive Personality Disorder

PARANOID PERSONALITY DISORDER

Paranoid personalities are decidedly unlikable for the most part. They are angry, prone to misinterpret the actions and intentions of almost everyone, hold grudges (seemingly forever), are quick to blame others for everything, and seldom accept responsibility for the circumstances they have created. They tend to react with rage and vindictiveness when they feel they have been wronged and are quick to resort to threats of legal action. They are quite vigilant and seem afraid of anything "foreign" or poorly understood. Paranoid personalities have difficulty finding humor in the world, especially if it is at their expense. These patients have great difficulty with love and intimacy but curiously perceive that they are desired by those they fear will hurt them. Nurses must always be sensitive to the paranoid personalities' lack of trust, insistence on being treated with dignity and honor, and propensity for misinterpreting friendly overtures that infringe too much on their need for emotional distance. Paranoid personalities are quite aware of the roles people are supposed to play and may react strongly when someone begins to play "one up" or to assume more responsibility than her or his assigned role would dictate. Finally, these patients are always looking for evidence that they have been slighted, ignored, taken advantage of, or otherwise exploited—and they usually find such evidence. Patients with paranoid personality traits are likely to take very personally any event that seems to them to be demeaning, and almost anything can be interpreted in that fashion by these patients.

SCHIZOID PERSONALITY DISORDER

The hallmark of the schizoid personality is a rather marked withdrawal from social contact. Such withdrawal encompasses most aspects of these patients' lives and severely limits their social interactions, which tend to be meager or nonexistent. These patients are usually seen as quiet, strange, lonely, and alienated. They seem to reject social contact and shun social gatherings and prefer, instead, the fantasy and self-involvement that seem more controllable and safer. These patients have a difficult time handling anger and rarely show that emotion in other than passive ways. They often prefer jobs that take them away from society and may be seen as "the strong, silent type," although they are seldom romantic figures because they are too nerdish to carry off the role. They sometimes revel in "deep and meaningful" issues, which translates into obscure and unusual interests. They have difficulty forming close, warm, and intimate relationships and usually function poorly sexually. On the positive side, these patients are well organized intellectually and emotionally and often succeed in occupational endeavors, even though their occupational efforts usually involve solitary jobs.

SCHIZOTYPAL PERSONALITY DISORDER

Schizotypal personality-disordered people differ from schizophrenics in that, although clearly odd and eccentric, they do not show the florid bizarreness and have not experienced an episode of outright psychosis. Instead, schizotypal patients show subtler forms of perceptual distortion such as magical thinking, depersonalization, and believing they have special abilities such as clairvoyance or a sixth sense or are capable of mental telepathy. Schizotypal patients may have myriad social fears and preoccupations and many strikingly odd beliefs and experiences. They often have shown ritualistic or repetitive mannerisms and may hold many unconventional attitudes and beliefs. Their speech often contains unusual use of language, and others must be careful to understand the context in which the schizotypal patient uses the language. These patients are usually more comfortable with their own thoughts and feelings than in interactions with others. Some authorities consider such people as palm readers, astrologers, and religious cult leaders to be among those suffering from schizotypal personality disorder.

ANTISOCIAL (SOCIOPATHIC) PERSONALITY DISORDER

Although many factors are important in determining a person's personality structure, the antisocial personality-disordered person often has a history of a chaotic family life and of not being required to live within defined limits, including not having to face the consequences of his or her behavior. There is usually a history of a distant parent-child relationship that lacked warmth, intimacy, and genuine emotion or a history of parental deprivation that resulted in inadequate exposure to social controls. Severe conflicts between parents may also lead to the development of antisocial behavior because such conflicts leave the growing child with no choice but to learn to manipulate in order to avoid being rejected by one or both parents.

This personality type is thought to make up as much as 3 percent of the male population and 1 percent of the female population. It is characterized primarily by a lack of responsiveness to social norms and rules. Such individuals fail to develop a concern for the welfare of others and use relationships to get their own needs met. There is little or no concern for what effect their behavior might have on others, and they seldom feel remorse or guilt.

Persons with antisocial personality disorders are frequently friendly, outgoing, likable, intelligent people who can be quite charming. Their relationships with others, however, tend to be quite superficial because they lack the capacity for deep emotional responsiveness. Sexual activity is usually for the sake of sex and not a means of expressing affection or intimacy. Sexual activity is carried out with many different people and usually with little regard for the partner's satisfaction.

Other characteristics worthy of mention include their use of physical intimidation and aggression, physical fighting, lying, stealing, arson, inability to maintain employment, extreme conflict with any kind of authority, blatant exploitation of relationships including spouse and child abuse, lack of forethought, engagement in high-risk behaviors, lack of regard for the rights of others, and continual justifying or rationalizing of their actions. They refuse to accept responsibility for their actions and always make undesirable outcomes someone else's fault. Antisocial personality-disordered people have great difficulty learning or profiting from experience. They are unreliable, untruthful, undependable, and insincere. Because they do not feel "responsible," they are often impulsive and seek immediate gratification of wants and perceived needs. Little thought is given to delaying gratification of immediate needs, wants, or wishes, even though doing so might be beneficial in the long run.

A large number of people have antisocial traits that, as with most other personality characteristics, vary in number and severity. Antisocial personality disorders are found in all professions, although most manage to contain their acting out behaviors because they are intelligent enough to be aware of the external controls placed on them by society. They avoid acting out not because of internal values or controls but because they do not wish to be punished. It is also true that the more intelligent an individual with antisocial personality disorder, the better he or she is able to find socially acceptable ways to meet needs and wants.

Antisocial personalities generally have a very low frustration tolerance and find it difficult to work at any task for a prolonged period. They are easily bored and continually seek excitement. When they are unable to manipulate their environment to meet their wishes, they may threaten suicide. Many antisocial personality-disordered persons die by accident as a result of a manipulative suicidal gesture. Such a case occurred when a girl broke up with her boyfriend. He tried to get her to come back to him, and, when she refused, he impulsively told her he was going to kill himself. He jumped in his car and, in full view of the girl, headed straight for a high bank at the edge of a large lake. Although he tried to swerve away before he got to the edge, the car turned over and rolled over the bank into the water. He was trapped inside the car and drowned before he could be rescued.

The antisocial personalities usually come to treatment as a result of having been "caught" in some fashion. They may have committed either a minor or a major crime, in which case they are sent for evaluation by the court. They may have attempted suicide or been required to seek treatment by an employer or family member. They can be expected to continue their manipulative ways with the clinic or hospital staff and to show very little positive change. Antisocial behavior patterns are difficult to alter and show poor response to one-on-one therapeutic intervention. External controls are necessary to control their acting out behavior and often represent the only means of effectively controlling their behavior. Their lack of adequate socialization often prevents guilt and desire for approval from being effective controlling mechanisms.

In summary, antisocial personality-disordered patients are often well liked by staff members but very difficult to treat. They are often helpful and friendly and provide the staff with a lot of verbal reinforcement. They learn to speak the language of psychology and can often report personality dynamics as thoroughly as the therapist. They can make great promises and build great dreams, but, when the time comes to face reality, they can usually be found going merrily on their charming way and never giving a thought to the lies told, the hearts broken, or the misery created in their wake. These individuals are said to burn out at about age 40, if they live that long, and may become depressed. They seldom present voluntarily for treatment before this age and then present themselves for treatment of their depressive symptoms, not their antisocial symptoms.

BORDERLINE PERSONALITY DISORDER

Borderline personality disorders are also difficult to treat. This group of patients have gotten a lot of attention in such movies as *Fatal Attraction* and *Basic Instinct.* This disorder occurs much more frequently in women than men; estimates range from 2:1 to 5:1. It seems to have its genesis in a temperamental inclination toward a poor ability to handle strong emotion. This deficit leads the person to have difficulty responding effectively and consistently to stressful environmental events and results in behavior that appears unstable to the casual observer.

This extreme affective instability—which includes an unstable identity and relationships, and difficulty maintaining a stable mood— defines this disorder. Probably the characteristic about borderline patients that is most easily recognized is their very poorly controlled anger, which they often vent indiscriminately and aggressively. The unrelenting anger is often directed at themselves in the form of repeated suicidal attempts, drug abuse, and self-mutilation. It is sometimes directed at others in the form of screaming, shouting, hitting, or even more physically damaging attacks with various weapons in extreme cases. Their anger outbursts and other affective displays are unpredictable and often outrageous.

The instability in identity is demonstrated in borderline patients' inability to make solid progress toward career goals, an inability to define what they wish to do with their lives, and difficulty in identifying their sexual orientation. In discussing such issues with borderline patients, a caregiver often feels overwhelmed and unsure of where to start in the face of such a broad range of emotional difficulties. Should therapy start with anger management or by addressing the deep loneliness and emptiness expressed by the patient or with the extreme fear of rejection and abandonment so painfully felt by the patient?

Borderline patients, much more than other diagnostic groups, use the defense mechanism of splitting. *Splitting* refers to the idea of splitting people into totally good or totally bad groups, according to how they are experienced by the observer. Because of the peculiarities of their perceptual processes, borderline patients tend to see people as all good or all bad and thus have difficulty appreciating the complexities of human relationships. Just because a person does one or two things one disagrees with does not mean that person is all bad. All people have good and not so good, or even bad, characteristics, and they learn to integrate those characteristics into healthy, well-functioning personalities. To the borderline patient, however, people are either all good or all bad, depending on how they experience others' ability to meet their dependency needs and how others fit into their fantasies about rejection, nurturance, and abandonment. They tend either to overidealize people and see them as impossible to reach or to devalue them and reject them as bad.

Treatment for borderline personality disorders is difficult because of the extreme demands these patients place on a therapist. Their anger, often directed at the therapist, is difficult to manage, as are their often repetitive attempts at self-mutilation, seduction, and self-destruction. They show brief periods of psychosis; deep depressions and dissociative episodes are not infrequent. Borderline patients often drop out of treatment because they are angered by confrontation and cannot tolerate the structure and expectations for change inherent in the therapeutic process. Long-term therapy seems to offer the only likelihood for substantial change.

HISTRIONIC PERSONALITY DISORDER

In many ways the histrionic personality-disordered person is captured by the drama, or perhaps the melodrama, of life. To the patient with a histrionic personality, emotions are much more important than thought processes. They live for and by their feelings, and their needs for attention and excitement are often exaggerated. Some of our best entertainers, writers, and artists have histrionic personality disorders, and some of the liveliest and most likable people have, to varying degrees, histrionic personalities. They pay great attention to physical attractiveness, like to be the center of attention, and do not do well when out of the limelight. Histrionic personalities manipulate others with emotional displays and often are unaware of their hidden agendas of getting dependency needs met or avoiding painful affect.

A characteristic of histrionic personality-disordered patients is the amount of attention they give to how they dress and how they present themselves to the public. Although not outright lying, they often embellish reality just enough to enhance their status with others. They are dramatic, often exhibitionist, and often overtly seductive in their approach to others. When confronted with these behaviors or asked to acknowledge them, however, they protest that they meant no such thing by their actions and state their resentment for such an interpretation of their intentions. Even so, these patients live for approval and acceptance and go to great lengths to attain them. As with all diagnostic categories, histrionic types vary from mildly to severely histrionic, and the degree of disturbance in social relationships depends on the degree of histrionic symptoms. At the more severe end of the spectrum, they express anger over the fact that their demands to be the center of attention are frustrated, demand constant reassurance of their worth, and constantly seek praise, even when it is unwarranted. Histrionic personalities do not like introspection. They would much rather bask in the light of someone else's flattering impression of them than deal with the reality of their needs when they are alone.

NARCISSISTIC PERSONALITY DISORDER

Although histrionic personality disorder is more prevalent in women, narcissistic personality disorder is more prevalent in men. Both of these personality disorder categories reflect a need for attention and approval from others as well as a need for admiration. People with narcissistic personalities are convinced that they are special and are upset when their "specialness" is questioned. They are not plagued by self-doubt; rather, they suffer from a sense of entitlement. *Entitlement* refers to the idea that whatever good things one wants should come to one just because one is there. No effort should be required because it is enough that one's wonderful presence is available to receive whatever one wishes to have.

Having such a wonderful view of themselves would understandably create problems for such people when they are criticized or demeaned in any fashion. Narcissistic personalities often react to criticism with extreme anger, frustration, and depression. They have a very unstable sense of self-worth and overreact to any suggestion that they may not be as wonderful as first thought. Everyone has a need to be wonderful, but narcissistic personality-disordered persons need to be wonderful all the time. The paradox is that narcissistic personalities have a difficult time allowing warranted praise they receive to become a part of how they see themselves and thus do not accept it as being true. That puts them on a treadmill of always having to do more and more to prove how wonderful they are. Underneath the superficial shell of self-confidence and invulnerability are people struggling with a deep sense of worthlessness and strongly held feelings of inferiority.

At its worst, narcissistic personality disorder can create strong problems for its hosts. They are accused of being willing to "sell their souls for that promotion" and of having little regard for the rights of those around them, taking credit for other people's ideas, believing their needs are special and deserve special consideration, being consumed with thoughts of success, status, image, and power, and of lacking empathy, as shown by difficulty understanding why other people do not like them. They often envy the accomplishments of others and have great difficulty tolerating others' success, especially when it exceeds their own.

Treatment usually focuses on helping narcissistic personalities to stabilize their self-esteem and learn to accept reasonable limitations in themselves and others. As with all other behaviors, certain aspects of the narcissistic personality disorder can be helpful, and those possessed of the less damaging of those behaviors do well because they believe in themselves and epitomize the phrase "them that say it can't be done should get out of the way of them who are doing it."

AVOIDANT PERSONALITY DISORDER

Persons afflicted with avoidant personality disorder rarely come to anyone's attention because they stay as far away from people and social events as their life demands allow. They are quite uncomfortable in new and unfamiliar situations and have little sense of adventure. They avoid social relationships out of a fear of rejection and lack of acceptance and feel comfortable only with family and friends they have known over a long time. These patients are often overly concerned about saying or doing something that would result in embarrassment for themselves and are similarly concerned with what others think of them. They are easily hurt by criticism and quick to anticipate disapproval. They tend to overestimate the probability of various happenings and use that overestimation to justify not doing what could otherwise be done. They often put themselves down and are eager to please others in an effort to fend off the anticipated rejection. Anxiety about rejection causes them to refuse to make their needs known, and thus their needs often go unmet because no one knows about them. Intimacy is made difficult by their fear of becoming vulnerable with exposure. Anticipation of rejection often leads to their perception of others' rejection when none was intended. Work achievement is made difficult by their shyness and introverted social relationship style. Treatment usually centers around establishing a good relationship with the therapist, gaining group support, and assertiveness training. A lot of role-playing may be desirable to reduce the likelihood of failure when the patient tries to exercise assertiveness skills.

DEPENDENT PERSONALITY DISORDER

Persons with dependent personality disorders are very much a mixed blessing for those around them. On the one hand, they are devoted and often sacrifice everything to satisfy the needs of their families, lovers, or friends. They always let others make decisions and rarely disagree with what others want to do. They tend to be thoughtful and considerate of others and try to change anything for which they are criticized.

On the other hand, they have great difficulty being alone, are often easily frightened, try to get others to make decisions for them, feel unable to manage even mundane tasks outside the home, and never take leadership positions. In fact, they try never to make a decision for which they could be criticized. They go along with a decision with which they privately disagree but cannot say so for fear of rejection. These patients may agree to do jobs or duties others shun because those tasks are dirty, demeaning, or otherwise seen as undesirable. They do so in an effort to win favor or acceptance and approval. Patients with dependent personalities have trouble with social relationships because they put so much into them and rely on them so much that they are crushed when a relationship ends and feel overwhelmed with the task of finding someone else on whom to depend. These patients tend to be pessimistic, filled with apprehension, misgivings, and self-doubt, and skeptical about their ability ever to function except in the shadow of some person they perceive to be competent. They become so invested in doing things for others that they may have great difficulty doing only for themselves. In seeking to be therapeutic with these patients, nurses might do well to remember that, no matter how clear it is to the caregiver that the patient's tolerance for abusive behavior is destructive, great care must be given to appreciate the patient's attachment issues. Dependent patients fear a loss of attachment more than anything else, and, in that context, "even a bad love is better than no love at all."

OBSESSIVE-COMPULSIVE PERSONALITY DISORDER

Most successful people have elements of the obsessive-compulsive personality style. In its less pathological manifestation, it is the heart of achievement. It allows its host to stick to the job until it is completed, and completed right. Attention to detail is assured, and order and organization always allow opportunity to finish a task on time. So what if rigid adherence to the rules and "doing it the right way" took all the fun out of it! Life was not meant to be fun anyway. Life is much too serious to be fun, and so is everything else. There is no room for pleasure, which is for the no-goods out in the world who will never accomplish anything. The rules are what is important, along with bathroom habits, lists of what needs to be done today, keeping everything clean, neat, and orderly, and being on time. And, of course, setting unreasonable goals is only proper. Without unreasonable goals, people will never achieve what they do achieve while reaching for unreachable goals. In addition, a person must always check and double-check every detail because to make a mistake, even a small one, would be an intolerable error. Great attention must be given to every detail, and, in discussions of situations or decisions, every aspect of the decision must be beaten to death. Even then a decision must be made with caution: Commitment to a decision prematurely might result in a wrong decision. New information may come along at any time and render the decision inadequate, along with the person responsible for the decision. Somewhere there is a "right" solution, and obsessive-compulsive people are determined to find it and relieve their anxiety. The preoccupation with being right and perfect is only proper in view of the fact that perfection is a fact and must be discovered.

The foregoing paragraph has actually been a test. For those reading it who think the authors have taken too great a license with the presentation of serious professional material, you are now official members of the OCD club!

For those charter members of the obsessive-compulsive disorder club, the authors offer the following: Obsessive-compulsive personality disorder patients are highly perfectionistic, are preoccupied with details, insist that everything be done the right way, forsake social and personal pleasure to ensure occupational success, are indecisive because of the fear of being wrong and thus being rejected, tend to be overly rigid in their thought processes and expectations of others, have a difficult time expressing affection, finding pleasure, laughing, playing, or otherwise having a good time, tend to be stingy, and are pack rats (that is, they never throw anything away).

Treatment usually centers around getting patients away from thinking processes because they are already overly introspective and "think" everything into oblivion. The problem is they are unable to get to their emotions and then do not manage them well when they do get to them. Obsessive-compulsive patients are prone to power struggles and are control addicts. Try to avoid these struggles by focusing on how the patient feels. The patient always wins the power struggle.

PASSIVE-AGGRESSIVE PERSONALITY DISORDER

Passive-aggressive personality disorder (now classified under personality disorder not otherwise specified) describes a set of behaviors that people generally find annoying in others but sometimes engage in themselves. These behaviors are usually associated with social or occupational roles and expectations but tend to be pervasive and resistant to change without direct intervention. Passive-aggressive patients have a lot of resentment and anger and find themselves in the bind of not being able to express that resentment and anger in a direct manner for fear of rejection, punishment, or disapproval. Instead, the anger and resentment are expressed through passive resistance to demands and expectations. The person is always late for deadlines but always has a good "reason" or is apologetic to the point of eliciting acceptance of the behavior.

At other times passive-aggressive patients sulk, pout, "drag their heels," or perform poorly when asked to do something they do not want to do. They frequently display chronic anger toward authority by ridiculing or speaking derogatorily of persons in authority. They are often chronic complainers who find something wrong with everything. They feel they are required to do more with less than anybody else in the world and are certain that they could do their bosses' jobs better than their bosses. They rarely offer solutions for problems but can find more problems than anybody can possibly solve. When efforts are made to solve problems, it soon becomes apparent that, no matter what is done, nothing can satisfy the complainer. Passive-aggressive people are tied to their resentments in such a way that they know no other way to respond. They sometimes become scapegoats because others recognize their resistance but become victims of the very behavior they dislike in the patient. Others reject passive-aggressive patients by ignoring them or by making jokes about their behavior. These patients sometimes feel a need for revenge but, in keeping with their style, exact that revenge by passive resistance rather than by acting out their frustrations. Treatment is difficult in that patients wish to become dependent on the caregiver and resent frustration of that need. They experience encouragement toward independence as rejection, but supporting that need also supports the very behaviors for which they are seeking treatment. These patients insist on their right to do as they please. Trying to change that attitude starts a battle that is difficult to finish.

PSYCHOSEXUAL DISORDERS

The diagnosis of a sexual deviation is reserved for those persons who fail to develop what society deems appropriate patterns of sexual behavior. What is appropriate is determined by the society in which a person lives, and there is usually some distinction between the relatively nonaggressive forms of sexual deviations, such as voyeurism, and the highly aggressive and dangerous sexual deviations such as masochism and sadism.

Many sexual behavior patterns that were considered deviant in the past are not considered deviant by most people in our present society. Masturbation—the manual or mechanical stimulation of one's genitals for the purpose of obtaining sexual pleasure—is a notable example of this change. Masturbation is not considered abnormal unless it totally replaces sexual activity with another person. Homosexuality—being sexually attracted to a person of the same sex—is another example of sexual behavior that was at one time considered deviant but is now generally understood to represent a nonpathological expression of sexual preference.

Many people have the misconception that violent, unrestrained behavior is characteristic of sexual deviates. Actually, much of the research indicates that most persons with sexual disorders are rather reserved and timid and have a great deal of difficulty interacting effectively with people of either sex. The more serious and persistent the sexual deviations, the more difficulty individuals are likely to experience in other areas of their lives. The major deviations are defined in the following paragraphs. If more in-depth information is desired, a good abnormal psychology text should be consulted.

The usual designation for what the general public considers to be sexual disorders is *paraphilia*. These disorders involve sexual activity and arousal patterns not common to the general population. The other main category of problems in the sexual arena is that of *sexual dysfunctions*. This second category involves problems with adequacy of desire or problems in carrying through the usual sexual response cycle from attraction through desire, arousal, and intercourse, to orgasm. The sexual dysfunctions category is reserved for disorders within the usual pattern of sexual arousal and functioning. The paraphilias, on the contrary, include those disorders that involve arousal patterns and activities outside those common to most adults in the society.

302.3 Transvestic Fetishism

In transvestic fetishism, sexual gratification is obtained by wearing clothing of the opposite sex (cross-dressing). This disorder is sometimes associated with transsexualism. Transsexualism is coded as a gender identity disorder in the *DSM-IV* and involves a more drastic form of changing one's sexual identity by actually changing the anatomic structure of the individual to that of the opposite sex.

302.4 Exhibitionism

Exhibitionism involves the attainment of sexual gratification by exposing one's genitals to another person. Male exhibitionism involves the display of the male genitals, primarily to women or children. There are few reported cases of female exhibitionism. However, females who are exhibitionists may find a socially appropriate outlet for exhibiting themselves, such as becoming strippers.

302.84 Sexual Sadism

Sexual sadism occurs when a person is able to obtain sexual gratification only through the mechanism of inflicting physical or mental pain on another individual. The most deviant example of this category is the person who can receive sexual pleasure only from drawing blood from the tortured individual or even causing someone's death. Sadism is often practiced with a masochistic partner, although in many cases the sadist gains satisfaction only when the partner fears the impending sadistic acts. Manifestations of this disorder can range from fairly mild behavior such as spanking or paddling, to low-level bondage, and to stabbing, strangulation, and other forms of mutilation to the point of death.

302.83 Sexual Masochism

Sexual masochism refers to the attainment of sexual satisfaction by being physically or mentally abused. Inflicted pain becomes a source of pleasure and sexual excitement and is sometimes self-inflicted. Masochism may range from something as simple as needing a "caveman" approach to sexual activity to the necessity for severe punishment or humiliation before sexual gratification is achieved. It is diagnosed only when such punishment is necessary for sexual fulfillment.

302.82 Voyeurism

Voyeurism is the term used when sexual gratification is obtained from observing the sexual organs of others or as a result of watching others in the act of sexual behavior or sexual intercourse. Many people enjoy viewing the nude bodies of members of the opposite sex, which is not pathological voyeurism unless the voyeuristic desires exceed the individual's desire for intercourse.

302.81 Fetishism

Fetishism occurs when a material object, usually some article of clothing such as a bra or shoes, belonging to members of the opposite sex (or in some cases the same sex) produces sexual gratification and fulfillment for an individual. Masturbation is commonly associated with the object, which is used as a primary means of sexual arousal.

302.2 Pedophilia

Pedophilia occurs when an adult, usually male, has some form of sexual relationship with a child. This sexual activity may be either heterosexual or homosexual and is said to occur frequently among persons who are unable to obtain sexual gratification with adults because of fears of inadequacy or impotence. There are two subtypes of pedophiles: the exclusive type and nonexclusive type. Exclusive types are attracted only to children, whereas nonexclusive types are attracted to both children and adults. The children may be victimized with a wide range of sexual activities, including behaviors that would be normal if both partners were adults, as well as behaviors related to sexual sadism to the point of death. In some cases the child molestation is limited to members of the perpetrator's family. In such cases, the diagnosis specifies that the pedophilia is limited to incest.

302.89 Frotteurism

Frotteurism is a disorder in which sexual arousal occurs in response to rubbing against or touching someone who does not consent to the touching. The individual usually chooses a crowded public place where the frottage can take place in a way that confuses the victim about who is doing the touching and from which the perpetrator can escape or claim the touching was an accident if he is caught. The frotteur usually engages in strong fantasy activity while pressing his penis against the victim and experiences an instantaneous erection. Frotteurs can often reach excitement to the point of ejaculation within 60 to 90 seconds. If ejaculation occurs, the frotteur quickly disengages. Otherwise he may try again.

▼ KEY POINTS ▼

Personality Disorders
1. The personality disorders include patterns of behavior that are neither psychotic nor neurotic but nonetheless substantially maladaptive. Personality disorders involve behavior patterns that

Key Points continued

are usually long-standing and frequently apparent from early adolescence.

2. Persons with personality disorders typically demonstrate the following characteristics:
   - An inflexible and maladaptive response to stress.
   - A disability in working and loving that is generally more serious and always more pervasive than that found in neurosis.
   - Elicitation of problematic responses by interpersonal conflict.
   - A particular capacity to "get under the skin" of and distress others.

3. Patients with personality disorders have difficulty managing emotionally intense situations, have trouble managing anger, and want others to adapt to their demands rather than adapting themselves to the demands of others. They tend to view people as difficult to live with, have trouble seeing their own faults and problems, and tend to blame others when things go wrong. Individuals with personality disorders tend to ask what is wrong with the world rather than what is wrong with them. Because of these characteristics, persons with personality disorders tend to be shunned by treatment personnel.

4. Personality disorders are divided into three clusters in DSM-IV:

Cluster A: The odd and the eccentric
(1) 301.0   Paranoid Personality Disorder
(2) 301.20 Schizoid Personality Disorder
(3) 301.22 Schizotypal Personality Disorder

Cluster B: The dramatic, emotional, and erratic
(1) 301.7   Antisocial Personality Disorder
(2) 301.83 Borderline Personality Disorder
(3) 301.50 Histrionic Personality Disorder
(4) 301.81 Narcissistic Personality Disorder

Cluster C: The anxious, fearful, and introverted
(1) 301.82 Avoidant Personality Disorder
(2) 301.6   Dependent Personality Disorder
(3) 301.4   Obsessive-Compulsive Personality Disorder

continued on page 136

Key Points continued

5. Paranoid personalities are angry, are prone to misinterpret the actions and intentions of almost everyone and hold grudges (seemingly forever), are quick to blame others for everything, and seldom accept responsibility for the circumstances they have created. These patients are always looking for evidence that they have been slighted, ignored, taken advantage of, or otherwise exploited, and they usually find such evidence.

6. The hallmark of the schizoid personality is a rather marked withdrawal from social contact. These patients are usually seen as quiet, strange, lonely, and alienated, and they seem not to desire social contact. They have difficulty forming close, warm, and intimate relationships and usually function poorly sexually. Nonetheless, these patients are well organized intellectually and emotionally.

7. Schizotypal patients show more subtle forms of perceptual distortion, such as magical thinking, depersonalization, or thinking that they have special abilities, such as clairvoyance or a sixth sense, or are capable of mental telepathy. Schizotypal patients may have myriad social fears and preoccupations, feature many strikingly odd beliefs and experiences, and often show ritualistic or repetitive mannerisms.

8. Antisocial personality disorder is characterized primarily by a lack of responsiveness to social norms and rules. Such individuals have little or no concern for what effect their behavior might have on others, and they seldom feel remorse or guilt. They have great difficulty learning or profiting from experience and are unreliable, untruthful, undependable, and insincere. There is usually a history of a distant parent-child relationship that lacked warmth, intimacy, and genuine emotion, or a history of parental deprivation resulting in inadequate exposure to social controls. Additionally, antisocial behavior patterns are difficult to alter and show poor response to one-on-one therapeutic intervention. External control (incarceration, probation, hospitalization) of these individuals' acting out behavior is necessary and often represents the only means of effectively altering their behavior.

9. Patients with borderline personality disorder have a poor ability to handle strong emotion. It is this extreme affective instability—which includes an unstable identity, unstable relationships, and difficulty in maintaining a stable mood—that defines borderline personality.

Key Points continued

Unpredictable angry outbursts and often outrageous affective displays are also characteristic of borderlines, who may feature brief periods of psychosis, deep depressions, and dissociative episodes, as well as self-defeating or dangerous acting out. Impulsiveness is also a problem.

10. For the histrionic personality, emotions are much more important than thought processes. They live for and by their feelings, and their needs for attention and excitement are often exaggerated. They pay great attention to physical attractiveness, like to be the center of attention, and do not do well when out of the limelight. These patients live for approval and acceptance and go to great lengths to attain them.

11. Like histrionic personality disorders, persons with narcissistic personality disorder reflect a need for attention and approval from others, as well as a need for admiration, but often do not want to truly earn their achievements. They are extremely sensitive to the evaluations of others. Narcissistic personalities are convinced that they are special, tend to be grandiose, and suffer from a sense of entitlement. They often exaggerate accomplishments and abilities. They tend to lack empathy. Underneath the superficial shell of self-confidence and invulnerability is a person struggling with a deep sense of worthlessness and strongly held feelings of inferiority.

12. Persons afflicted with avoidant personality disorder stay as far away from people and social events as their life demands allow. They avoid social relationships out of a fear of rejection and lack of acceptance, feeling comfortable only with family and friends they have known for a long time. Avoidant personalities often put themselves down and are eager to please others in an effort to fend off the anticipated rejection. Work achievement is made difficult by their shyness and introverted social style.

13. Persons with dependent personality disorder are devoted and often sacrifice everything in order to satisfy the needs of their families, lovers, or friends. They almost always let others make decisions and rarely disagree with what others want to do. They have great difficulty being alone, are often easily frightened, and never take leadership positions. These patients tend to be pessimistic, filled

continued on page 138

Key Points continued

with apprehension, misgivings, and self-doubt; they are skeptical about their ability ever to function except in the shadow of some person they perceive to be competent.

14. Patients with obsessive-compulsive personality disorder are highly perfectionistic, are preoccupied with details, and insist that everything be done the "right way." They forsake social and personal pleasure to ensure occupational success, are indecisive because of their fear of being wrong and thus of being rejected, tend to be overly rigid in their thought processes and expectations of others, have a difficult time expressing affection or finding pleasure, tend to be stingy, and are pack rats. These patients are also prone to power struggles and are control addicts.

15. Passive-aggressive patients have a lot of resentment and anger and find themselves in the bind of not being able to express that resentment and anger in a direct manner for fear of rejection, punishment, or disapproval. Instead, the anger and resentment are expressed through passive resistance to demands and expectations. They frequently display a chronic anger toward authority by ridiculing or speaking derogatorily of persons in authority. They are often chronic complainers who find something wrong with everything. This category is not included in *DSM-IV.*

Sexual Disorders

1. The diagnosis of a sexual deviation is reserved for those persons who fail to develop what society deems appropriate patterns of sexual behavior.

2. There are two categories of sexual disorders.
   - The *sexual dysfunctions* category is reserved for disorders that are within the usual pattern of sexual arousal and functioning.
   - The *paraphilias* include those disorders that involve arousal patterns and activities outside those common to most adults in the society.

Paraphilias

1. In transvestic fetishism, sexual gratification is obtained by wearing clothing of the opposite sex (cross-dressing).

2. Exhibitionism involves the attainment of sexual gratification by exposing one's genitals to another person.

3. Sexual sadism is obtaining sexual gratification only by inflicting physical or mental pain on another individual.

Key Points continued

4. Sexual masochism refers to the attainment of sexual satisfaction by being physically or mentally abused. It is diagnosed only when such punishment is necessary for sexual fulfillment.

5. Voyeurism occurs when sexual gratification is obtained from observing the sexual organs of others or as a result of watching others engage in sexual intercourse or other sexual behavior.

6. Fetishism occurs when a material object, usually some article of clothing, produces sexual gratification and fulfillment for an individual.

Annotated Bibliography

American Psychiatric Association: *Diagnostic and Statistical Manual of Mental Disorders, ed. 4.* Washington, D.C.: APA, 1994.

Barstow, D. G.: Self-injury and self-mutilation. *Journal of Psychosocial Nursing,* 1995, 33(2):19–22.

Provides a brief cultural history of self-injury and self-mutilation and the function these behaviors play in the disorder. Discusses staff responses and treatment approaches for intervention in the disorder.

Black, D. W., Baumgard, C. H., and Bell, S. E.: A 16 to 45 year follow-up of 71 men with antisocial personality disorder. *Comprehensive Psychiatry,* 1995, 36(2):130–140.

A study concluding that antisocial personality disorder is chronic and associated with ongoing psychiatric, medical, and social problems.

Daum, A. L.: The disruptive antisocial patient: Management strategies. *Nursing Management,* 1995, 25(8):46–51.

Explains strategies for intervention with the antisocial patient while managing typical staff responses to the patient's behavior.

Long, K., and Long, R.: Treating obsessive-compulsive disorder. *Nurse Practitioner Forum,* 1995, 6(3):136–137.

Discusses the neurobiologic treatment of obsessive-compulsive disorder with serotonin-reuptake inhibitors.

Meyer, J. K., and Levin, F. M.: Sadism and masochism in neurosis and symptom formation. *Scientific Proceedings,* 1988, 789–804.

Presents several theories on the development of sadism and masochism and provides case examples for further study.

Miller, C. R.: Creative coping: A cognitive-behavioral group for borderline personality disorder. *Archives of Psychiatric Nursing,* 1995, 8(4):280–285.

Describes a specific cognitive-behavioral group therapy in conjunction with other structural elements.

Perry, C., and Vaillant, G.: Personality Disorders. In: Kaplan, H., and Sadock, B. (eds): *Comprehensive Textbook of Psychiatry, ed. 5.* Baltimore: Williams & Wilkins, 1989, 2:1352.

Quality Assurance Project: Treatment outlines for paranoid schizotypal and schizoid personality disorders. *Australian and New Zealand Journal of Psychiatry,* 1990, 24:339–350.

Presents treatment outlines for paranoid, schizotypal, and schizoid personality disorders that utilize advice from expert committees, review of the literature, and the opinions of practicing psychiatrists.

Siever, J. L., and Others: Eye movement impairment and schizotypal psychopathology. *American Journal of Psychiatric Nursing,* 1994, 151(8):1209–1215.

The authors suggest there is qualitatively poor tracking associated with schizotypal personality disorder or schizotypal features.

Widiger, T. A., and Weissman, M. M.: Epidemiology of borderline personality disorder. *Hospital and Community Psychiatry,* 1991, 42(10):1015–1020.

Presents information on the prevalence, incidence, and sex ratio of patients diagnosed with borderline personality disorder. Also provides information on further testing designs that can be utilized.

Post-Test

Chapters 5, 6, and 7: Understanding the Patient's Diagnosis

Matching. Match the diagnoses listed in column B with the appropriate symptoms listed in column A.

Column A

1. Person feels tense, anxious, or worried but unable to pinpoint exactly why.

2. Engages in repetitive behavioral acts.

3. Adult engages in sexual relationship with a child.

4. Abnormal continuous grief over a lost one.

5. General symptoms exhibited are inappropriate affect, autism, and inability to deal with reality.

6. Able to obtain sexual gratification only by inflicting pain on others.

7. Show signs of grandiosity and persecution.

8. Loss of hearing with no physical basis

9. Sometimes called *split personality* by the general public.

Column B

A. Obsessive-compulsive disorder

B. Paranoid disorder

C. Conversion disorder

D. Anxiety disorder

E. Dysthymic disorder

F. Schizophrenia

G. Dissociative disorder

H. Pedophilia

I. Sexual sadism

Post-Test

(continued)

True or False. Circle your answer.

T   F   1. Diagnostic categories are helpful only for insurance purposes.

T   F   2. Diagnosis is necessary because from it the mental health worker is able to predict the exact behavior that will be exhibited by the patient.

T   F   3. Anxiety disorders constitute approximately 30 to 40 percent of all neurotic disorders.

T   F   4. Obsessive-compulsive people feel that if they are not allowed to carry out their rituals, something drastic will happen to them.

T   F   5. The patient with a diagnosis of organic psychosis usually exhibits more bizarre behavior than the patient with a functional psychosis.

T   F   6. Arguing with psychotic patients in order to make them realize their thinking is not logical is a major role of the mental health worker in caring for psychotic patients.

T   F   7. *Schizophrenia* basically means "split personality."

T   F   8. Paranoid patients are usually disliked by everyone.

T   F   9. Paranoid patients are usually the easiest of all psychiatric patients to accept and manage.

T   F   10. Some authorities feel that the manic phase of a bipolar disorder is a defense against anxiety.

T   F   11. Sexual deviates tend to be violent and unable to control their behavior.

T   F   12. Sexual sadism is often performed with a masochistic partner.

T   F   13. Paraphilia refers to individuals who obtain sexual gratification only with children.

Short Answer. Answer the following questions as briefly and specifically as possible.

1. Phobias are usually described as _____

2. Give three of the basic behavioral characteristics associated with the obsessive-compulsive patient.

Post-Test

(continued)

a. _____

b. _____

c. _____

3. List three of the personal traits one would expect to see in a patient with a diagnosis of dysthymic disorder.

a. _____

b. _____

c. _____

4. One of the most important things a mental health worker can do in caring for the patient with a diagnosis of dysthymic disorder

is _____ .

5. What is the basic difference between an organic psychosis and a functional psychosis?

_____

_____

6. Briefly discuss the difference between sexual disorders and sexual dysfunctions.

_____

_____

_____

Multiple Choice. Circle the letter or number you think represents the best answer.

1. The person diagnosed as paranoid schizophrenic presents all the following symptoms except:
   a. Waxy flexibility.
   b. Extreme suspiciousness.
   c. Delusions of persecutions.
   d. Hallucinations.

2. The most common characteristics of schizophrenia are:
   a. Apathy and autistic thinking.

Post-Test

(continued)

   b. Flat affect, autistic thinking, ambivalence, and associative looseness.
   c. Ambivalence, ideas of reference, autistic thinking, and associative looseness.
   d. Confabulation and intuition.

3. All of the following statements are generally true of schizotypical personality except:
   a. The patient is often eccentric.
   b. Delusions and hallucinations are rare.
   c. They often become vagrants, wandering from place to place picking up menial jobs.
   d. The onset is sudden.

4. All of the following are considered possible causes of schizophrenia except:
   a. Disturbed mother-infant relationship.
   b. A poorly adjusted family situation.
   c. The precipitating factor may be a situation calling for close interaction with another human being.
   d. Abnormalities in the way the brain is formed.

5. Fifty percent of the resident population of long-term mental hospitals is composed of patients with a diagnosis of:
   a. Senile brain disease and cerebral arteriosclerosis.
   b. Schizophrenia.
   c. Alcohol intoxication or addiction.
   d. Personality disorders.
   e. Psychosis.

6. Antisocial individuals usually:
   a. Profit from their mistakes.
   b. Assume responsibility for their own conduct.
   c. Do not feel shame for their conduct.
   d. Are responding to hallucinations.

7. In relating to an antisocial patient, the mental health worker should anticipate that rapport will be established:
   a. Without difficulty within a few days.
   b. With difficulty over a long period of time.

Post-Test

(continued)

   c. With difficulty but within a few days.
   d. Without difficulty within a few hours.

8. Mr. Green is a 24-year-old patient who has been diagnosed as an antisocial personality. Your primary responsibility for him will most likely be to:
   a. Set firm and consistent limits on his behavior.
   b. Help him to develop insight.
   c. Encourage him to get involved in ward activities.
   d. Arrange opportunities for him to develop stronger superego controls.

9. Situation: Mrs. M is a 23-year-old newlywed admitted to a psychiatric hospital after a month of unusual behavior that included eating and sleeping very little, talking or singing constantly, charging hundreds of dollars worth of furniture to her father-in-law, and picking up dates on the street. In the hospital, she monopolized conversation, insisted on unusual privileges, and frequently became demanding, bossy, and sarcastic. She had periods of great overactivity and sometimes became destructive. She frequently used vulgar and profane language. Mrs. M had formerly been witty, light hearted, and the "life of the party." Her many friends say she was ladylike in spite of her fun-loving ways and a kind, sympathetic person. The symptoms Mrs. M exhibited are suggestive of which of the following diagnostic entities?
   a. Manic bipolar disorder
   b. Schizophrenic disorder
   c. Paranoid disorder
   d. Major depression

10. Exaggerated mood swings from deep depression to wild excitement are seen in:
   a. Anxiety disorders.
   b. Schizophrenic disorders.
   c. Mixed bipolar disorders.
   d. Paranoid disorders.

Post-Test

(continued)

11. Which of the following are characteristic of the obsessive-compulsive disorder?
    a. Flexibility.
    b. Enjoyment of people.
    c. Excessive conformity to standards.
    d. Easily relaxed.
    e. Expresses self with difficulty.
       (1) a, c, and e.
       (2) c, d, and e.
       (3) b and d.
       (4) c and e.
       (5) None of the above.

12. One of the major personality characteristics of an obsessive-compulsive patient is:
    a. Dependency.
    b. Self-depreciativeness.
    c. Impulsiveness.
    d. Orderliness.

13. The symptom that characterizes paranoia in its true form is:
    a. Bizarre hallucinations.
    b. Inappropriate affect.
    c. Severe depression.
    d. Systemized delusions.

14. The major defense mechanism utilized in paranoid thinking is:
    a. Reaction formation.
    b. Rationalization.
    c. Compensation.
    d. Sublimation.
    e. Projection.

15. Malingering differs most significantly from a conversion disorder in that the malingerer:
    a. Unconsciously simulates illness to avoid an unpleasant situation.
    b. Converts anxiety arising from some conflictual situation into somatic symptoms.

Post-Test

(continued)

   c. Seems unconcerned and shows no anxiety about the disabling symptoms.
   d. Simulates illness on a conscious level to avoid intolerable alternatives.

16. The term that best describes the reaction of an individual who makes an emotional response through an organic illness is:
   a. Neurotic reaction.
   b. Organic reaction.
   c. Psychosomatic reaction.
   d. Psychotic reaction.

17. Another problem neurotic patients suffer is:
   a. Memory loss.
   b. Indecision.
   c. Disorientation.
   d. Hallucinations.

18. People suffering from neuroses usually complain of:
   a. Hallucinations, delusions, and fatigue.
   b. Fatigue, fears, and physical complaints.
   c. Fatigue, rejections, and dissociation.
   d. Flight of ideas, illusions, and disorientation.

19. Which of the following are characteristic of pedophiles?
   a. Only attracted to children of the opposite sex.
   b. Never engage in sexual activity with children in their own family.
   c. Never engage in sexual activity with adults.
   d. Often are unable to engage in sexual activity with adults due to fear of inadequacy or impotence.
   e. Are also sadistic
     (1) a, b, and c.
     (2) a and d.
     (3) d only.
     (4) c only.

20. When an individual obtains sexual gratification by rubbing or touching someone who does not consent and who is often unaware of the person touching them, the act is known as:

Post-Test

(continued)

    a. Voyeurism.
    b. Fetishism.
    c. Paraphilia.
    d. Frotteurism.

21. When severe punishment or humiliation is needed for sexual fulfillment, the condition is known as:
    a. Sexual sadism.
    b. Sexual masochism.
    c. Frotteurism.
    d. Fetishism.

22. When an individual obtains sexual gratification by dressing up in clothing of the opposite sex, the condition is known as:
    a. Transvestic fetishism.
    b. Homosexuality.
    c. Frotteurism.
    d. Exhibitionism.

Therapeutic Treatment Activities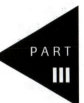

Dear Mom and Dad,

Since I left for nursing school I have been remiss in not writing and I am sorry for my thoughtlessness in not having written before. I will bring you up to date now, but before you read on, please sit down. You are not to read any further unless you are sitting down. Okay?

Well, then, I am getting along pretty well now. The skull fracture and the concussion I got when I jumped out of the window of my dormitory when it caught on fire shortly after my arrival here are pretty well healed now. I only spent two weeks in the hospital and now I can see almost normally. I only get those sick headaches once a day. Fortunately, the fire in the dormitory and my jump were witnessed by an attendant at the gas station near the dorm and he was the one who called the fire department and the ambulance. He also visited me in the hospital and since I had nowhere to live because of the burned-out dormitory, he was kind enough to invite me to share his apartment with him. It's really a basement room but it's kind of cute. He is a very fine boy and we have fallen deeply in love and are planning to get married. We haven't got the exact date yet, but it will be before my pregnancy begins to show.

Yes, Mom and Dad, I am pregnant. I know how much you are looking forward to being grandparents, and I know you will welcome the baby and give it the same love and devotion and tender care you gave me when I was a child. The reason for the delay in our marriage is that my boyfriend has a minor infection that prevents us from passing our premarital blood tests and I carelessly caught it from him.

I know that you will welcome him into our family with open arms. He is kind and, although not well educated, he is ambitious. Although he is of a different race and religion than ours, I know your often-expressed tolerance will not permit you to be bothered by that.

Now that I have brought you up to date, I want to tell you that there was no dormitory fire, I did not have a concussion or skull fracture, I was not in the hospital, I am not pregnant, I am not engaged, I am not infected, and there is no boyfriend in my life. However, I am getting a D in Psychology and an F in Anatomy and Physiology, and I want you to see those marks in their proper perspective.

Your loving daughter,
Susie

CHAPTER 8

Communication

OBJECTIVES: Student will be able to:

1. Define *communication.*
2. Differentiate between verbal and nonverbal communication.
3. List major objectives in developing a therapeutic relationship.
4. List 10 techniques useful in communicating more effectively with patients.
5. List at least eight major factors that should be used to maintain accurate and complete charting.

Communication, a key factor in the development of any therapeutic relationship, occurs on both a verbal basis and a nonverbal basis. Verbal communications are transmitted through the spoken or written word, and nonverbal communications are transmitted through behavior. Regardless of the mode of transmission, the aims of all forms of communication are to provide information, receive information, or exchange information.

WRITTEN COMMUNICATION

When using written communication, the writer provides information without the benefit of feedback; therefore, if the one to whom the message is written does not understand the message, successful communication has not been achieved. For example, if a staff member charts that a patient is "hostile" and Dr. Jones reads the chart after that staff member has gone off duty, he really does not know what happened and probably will not have a clear understanding of what the staff member meant by "hostile." This is especially true if Dr. Jones sees the patient sitting calmly in the day room visiting and chatting with other patients. In order to discuss the behavior with the patient, Dr. Jones must understand what the staff member meant by "hostile."

One means of clarifying and making written communication more explicit is to use description. Instead of saying that the patient is "hostile," it would be better to write exactly what the patient said or did, for example, "The patient is walking up and down the hall cursing" or "When other patients walk by, Mr. Brown screams at them and tries to hit them." This note tells the doctor exactly what the patient has been doing. Because unclear written communications are likely to result in either no information or misinformation, descriptive writing is extremely important.

VERBAL COMMUNICATION

Most people know how to communicate verbally because nearly everybody converses daily. Unfortunately, people frequently do not think before they talk and are unaware of what they are communicating to other people. Verbal communication, therefore, is largely effective because it is easy to talk, and feedback can alert the speaker to the possibility that the desired message is not being communicated. For example, a person listening to someone speak may question what has been said, challenge a statement, ask for clarification of a point, or add to a statement, thus facilitating effective communications.

A frequent error people make when communicating verbally occurs when they say things they do not mean. A mother says to her son who has misbehaved, "I'm not going to love you any more." Obviously the message being sent is not true. A mother is not going to stop loving her child because he misbehaved. The message she wanted to communicate was "I do not like the way you are behaving. I love you, but I want you to change your behavior." When people say things they do not mean, the messages they send may be misunderstood and cause interpersonal relationship problems. Communications such as these, if consistent over a long enough period, may contribute to mental illness by further isolating people from each other.

NONVERBAL COMMUNICATION

Some authorities believe that nonverbal communication is the most accurate form of communication. People communicate nonverbally via their behavior and their body posture. People who are depressed may slump, walk with their heads down, and look gloomy. These behaviors send a message to all those who come in contact with this person: "I don't feel well; I'm depressed." Remember the song that says, "If you're happy and you know it, then your face will surely show it"? When people are happy, their faces generally show it. They also express their feeling of well-being when they walk at a brisk pace with their head up and shoulders thrown back. Behavior thus often indicates state of mind, and mentally ill patients are no exception. Their behavior expresses a great deal about their feelings. When a nurse walks into Mr. Brown's room and says, "How are you feeling this morning?" the patient may respond by saying that he feels fine. If, however, while stating this, he is lying in a fetal position with the covers drawn up to his shoulders and refuses to have his room light turned on, his nonverbal behaviors indicate that he is not feeling well.

Why would Mr. Brown respond, "I'm feeling fine," when he is obviously not? There are several possibilities. Perhaps Mr. Brown is afraid that, if he says he is not feeling well, the physician will not let him go home on Friday as planned. Mr. Brown may have heard a nurse standing outside his door complaining to another staff member about the floor being overloaded with patients, thus causing the staff to be overworked. Therefore, Mr. Brown is afraid to say he feels bad because that might put another burden on the nurses.

All people have said things they did not mean, and patients are no exception. Because nonverbal communications convey attitudes, feelings, and reactions much more clearly than verbal communications, they are generally more accurate. Nurses must, therefore, always be alert to nonverbal clues that may actually be a better indication of the patient's true feelings than the words said.

STAFF-PATIENT RELATIONSHIPS

In establishing a therapeutic relationship, the first step is to make initial contact with the patient. Obviously, in talking to a patient for the first time, the nurse cannot expect that patient to relate his or her life history. People are generally cautious about meeting someone new. They are not sure what the new person's attitude will be toward them and are uncomfortable if the new person is too pushy, overly friendly, or too inquisitive. Mentally ill people are often very sensitive individuals who have been hurt in their interpersonal relationships many, many times. The people they have trusted may have often let them down. They may have shared their personal problems with individuals who seemed to care but ultimately responded in a way that caused the patient to feel laughed at, ridiculed, degraded, or otherwise treated unkindly. They may not trust people because their experiences have taught them that people cannot be trusted.

It follows, then, that a primary objective of early staff-patient contacts is to establish a relationship that promotes mutual trust. A step is made in that direction when a staff member is honest and straightforward with patients. For example, if staff members do not know the answer to a patient's question, they should tell the patient they do not know the answer but that they will try to find the answer for him or her. When a staff member makes such a promise, care should be taken that adequate follow-up is done. Staff members should consider carefully what they tell patients they will do for them. Casual remarks and half-hearted offers are often taken seriously. Because a person can never be sure what the events of the day will bring, a thoughtful response to make to a patient who asks to go for a walk might be "It looks as though my schedule is free this afternoon and unless something unusual interferes, I'll go for a walk with you around four o'clock." If something does interfere, one might then say to the patient, for example, "I'm really sorry, but Dr. Jones is making rounds and I can't leave the unit now" or "I've been called to a staff meeting so we can't go for a walk this afternoon. I'll be back around five o'clock" or "Is there something special you wanted to talk about with me? If not, we'll try to take that walk tomorrow."

When a staff member is beginning to develop a trusting and therapeutic relationship with a patient, frequent contacts of short duration are often best. At the first meeting, staff members should introduce themselves, tell the patient their title (nurse, nursing assistant, social worker, and so forth), and then explain their purpose for approaching the patient. A mental health worker on a hospital unit might say, "I'm Jane Doe, a mental health technician. I work the three to eleven shift, and I'm assigned to take care of you this evening. If you need anything, or want to talk, or have any questions, I'll be happy to help." Then engage the patient in a discussion of some neutral topic. If the patient was watching television or reading the newspaper, some very neutral comment about the program, a sporting event, or the weather forecast reported in the paper is appropriate. Try to have a short, pleasant conversation, and then leave the patient for a while. Later, try to interest the patient in some social activity such as playing cards, checkers, or having a cup of coffee with another person.

Staff members should work toward helping all patients realize that the staff is sincerely interested in them and their problems. Patients need to feel important, and there are two key approaches to helping make them feel that way: First, the very fact that a staff member would want to spend time with them helps patients to feel important. Patients often see mental health workers as authority figures and as special persons. Thus, many patients are surprised when a staff member says, "I would like to sit and talk with you for a while." Patients' self-esteem is frequently so poor that they may have a difficult time accepting that someone as important as a staff member would want to talk with them or could actually be concerned about their problems.

Another way for a staff member to honor patients' importance is to make sure time with them is not spent in talking about one's own personal life. Talking about oneself or unloading one's own personal problems on a patient says to that patient that the staff member is self-centered and not interested in anyone else.

There are other reasons, of course, why staff members should not talk about their own personal lives. Mentally ill patients sometimes use the personal information given to them to justify ill feelings toward the very staff member who shared the information with them. They may also use the information to gossip with other patients. Telling depressed patients about one's own burdens in an attempt to help them understand that they are not the only people with problems may make them even more depressed. They may even feel that they should not add to the staff member's load by discussing their own problems.

Telling a patient one's address or telephone number is not a good idea, even if the patient insists. When a patient makes such personal inquiries, a staff member might respond by saying, "What makes you ask?" and then attempt to involve the patient in a discussion directed toward the patient's problems. The staff member might also say, "This time is for you to talk about your problems" or "It would be more helpful if you would talk about yourself." This approach is especially important in the first few patient-staff contacts, when the patient may be unclear about the relationship and the purpose of the discussions. If all else fails, staff members may simply say that they are not permitted to discuss personal information. Learning about boundaries is important for both patients and staff.

Dating patients is also an unwise practice for staff members, even after patients have been discharged from the hospital. One never knows when a patient might need to return to the hospital, and it is extremely difficult and often unethical to mix personal and professional relationships. If a patient's efforts to establish a social relationship persist, a staff member might need to respond in the following manner: "I'm sorry, but it's hospital policy that staff members not see patients socially." A hospital is an impersonal object toward which a patient can ventilate anger without causing any great harm.

Because spending time with patients is one of the most therapeutic activities in which a staff member can engage, it is important to make the most of each opportunity. A 5-minute visit may seem much longer to the patient if the staff member seems relaxed and unhurried and discusses topics that are important to the patient.

When talking with patients, the staff member should pull a chair close or sit beside them on the sofa. Pay attention to what the patient is saying. Do not fidget in the chair, tap your feet, or wring your hands. Adopt a pleasant, sincere, interested attitude that says to the patient, "I'm here to talk to you, and I'm interested in what you have to say." Try never to stand over a patient. To do so makes one appear rushed, and the patient may become anxious and uncomfortable. If you are in a hurry, let the patient know when there will be time to talk.

Because time with patients is limited, a staff member's verbal communication must be as effective as possible. Using goals can help. Such goals are determined by the purpose for contact with a patient and may be further influenced by the amount of time available, the nature of the information to be communicated, and one's attitude toward the patient. For example, if a staff member is to tell Mr. Jones about a test he is going to have the next day, then the goal of the conversation is to familiarize Mr. Jones with that test. He has to be told when the test is scheduled and whether he has to make any special preparations for the test. He should then be encouraged to ask questions for clarification and to express any feelings or concerns he might have about the procedure.

The goals for this conversation are quite different from the goals of a conversation with a patient who is depressed and just wants someone to sit and listen. In this situation, the staff member's goals would probably be aimed toward supporting the patient while allowing the patient an opportunity to talk.

COMMUNICATION TECHNIQUES

Often when patients try to tell their physician, nurse, social worker, or mental health worker about their problems, their illness or inexperience at effective communication causes them to leave out important details or to skip from one subject to another before completing their original thoughts. Listed here are some techniques that staff members may find useful in helping mentally ill patients communicate more effectively.

1. The high anxiety level many mentally ill patients experience, plus their preoccupation with the things that are upsetting them and making them anxious, greatly decreases and narrows their attention span. They may appear confused and hear very little of

what is said to them. Staff members may have to repeat their names several times or reintroduce themselves each time they approach the patient. Staff members, therefore, should watch for behavioral or verbal clues that would indicate that a patient has not understood the intended message and thus cannot respond appropriately. Then again, some patients are acutely aware of all that is happening in their environment and would feel greatly insulted if a staff member kept repeating things over and over again.

2. Staff members need to use simple, direct statements and questions. Long, involved sentences and explanations may just confuse patients. Use the simplest language possible to convey the message. Avoid abstract statements such as "It's raining cats and dogs outside." A psychotic patient might take this statement literally and respond inappropriately.

3. Do not use indefinite pronouns such as *she, he, they,* and so forth. Be specific about the person being discussed. Encourage patients to do the same. Ask for clarification about the identity of the person the patient is discussing. For example, a patient might say, "She always belittles me. I can never do anything right." The staff member might respond by saying, "Who is she?" or "Who is it that you feel belittles you?" Remember, contradicting the patient's perceptions is usually not a good idea; rather, ask questions that gently lead patients to explore the development of their perceptions.

4. Psychiatric patients sometimes have difficulty trying to describe or explain things that happen to them. Because their interpretation of their experiences may be very different from what actually occurred, it is helpful to such patients if a staff member can assist them to more objectively describe their experience and then consider alternatives that were previously overlooked. If Mr. Green is unfriendly one morning, Mr. Jones may become upset because he believes Mr. Green is angry with him. If a staff member helps Mr. Jones see that Mr. Green is upset about a personal problem, Mr. Jones may be able to relax and feel less anxious.

5. Staff members often have to help patients maintain an orientation to the "here and now." Patients sometimes try to escape a problem by denying its existence or by talking about getting out of the hospital, Aunt Bee's new hat, or the possibility that a rich uncle may die and leave them a fortune. It is usually more beneficial for patients to deal with their real problems in an open manner than to smooth over them with wishes, dreams, and

fantasies. To learn to guide patients skillfully requires time, patience, and practice. Try not to expect yourself to be an expert from day one, but do be aware of how you sound to the patient as you provide therapeutic interchange.

6. Open-ended questions should be used to engage a patient in conversation or obtain general information. If a patient is asked, "Are you married?" the probable response is "Yes." The question is answered, but the conversation is over. By contrast, the patient cannot answer an open-ended statement such as "Mr. Jones, tell me about your family" with a simple "yes" or "no." He has to elaborate in his response, which begins a conversation that may lead to further discussion of related topics. Sentences such as "Tell me about yourself," "What happened to bring you to the hospital?" and "What have you done today?" are all examples of open-ended questions. The open-ended question also allows the patient some freedom in choosing what to discuss. Mr. Brown may choose a neutral topic when asked, "What has happened since we talked last week?" He may say that he got a nice birthday card from his mother, that he had a date, or that it was a nice weekend, all very safe subjects. Then again he may choose to tell you that he had a terrible fight with his girlfriend. In either case, Mr. Brown chose the topic and is, therefore, less likely to feel the staff member is prying or pushing him to discuss something that he is not ready to discuss.

7. Mentally ill patients may use mental health staff members as role models and pattern much of their behavior after that of the staff. Likewise, they may pattern their communication style after the style of the person with whom they are working. Therefore, it is important to be a good role model when communicating with patients as well as with other staff members.

8. Because patients sometimes take cues about staff members' expectations of them from the way a statement is phrased, words such as *can, could,* and *would* may create problems. A sentence beginning with *can* or *would* may lead patients to believe that they have some choice in the matter when they really do not. The patient who is asked, "Can you get up?" or "Would you come with me?" may say "No." If a patient must go somewhere for a treatment, it is probably best to say, "It's time for your treatment. Please come with me." From that statement, it is obvious that the patient is expected to cooperate. Most authorities agree that it is better not to offer a patient a choice when there is none. Offering a nonexistent choice may only anger the patient and create animosity.

9. Whenever possible, the patient should be consulted when the staff is developing the patient's care plan. If Mr. Jones likes to take his bath in the evening and there are no valid staff objections, his preference should be honored. This consideration helps Mr. Jones feel that the staff sees him as an individual whose personal concerns are important. As a general rule, no one is more interested in his well-being than the patient himself. Most patients feel better when they have some say in their own lives and control over themselves, even when they are ill.

10. Mentally ill patients sometimes have difficulty focusing on one topic at a time or may skip from one subject to another without ever finishing a thought. High levels of anxiety may make it difficult for them to concentrate. Skipping from subject to subject may also allow patients to avoid talking about a particular topic that makes them feel anxious. Helping patients improve their ability to discuss one topic at a time, especially if the topic involves an area of conflict, is important. If the topic of conflict can be discussed fully, the patient may gain a better understanding of it and even uncover some of the reasons behind the conflict.

11. Patients often relate to mental health staff members as authority figures and, therefore, may want staff members to make many or all their decisions for them. Having someone else make decisions for them does not help patients learn to deal more effectively with their problems or help them learn to be more responsible for their lives. Also, if patients do not like the outcome of decisions made for them by a staff member, the staff member is likely to receive the blame.

12. Silences often provoke anxiety, and both patients and staff members are likely to feel uncomfortable when they occur. However, both patients and staff members sometimes need a brief period of silence in order to collect their thoughts. Patients who are anxious may need time to organize what they are going to say or to decide exactly how they feel about something. Mental health workers need to be good observers to determine whether patients are silent because they are out of contact with reality, are uncomfortable with the subject matter, or simply need to collect their thoughts.

13. A good technique for working with patients who are communicating on a nonverbal basis is to help them identify their feelings. A staff member might say to a patient something like "Are you feeling anxious?" If the patient responds, "No, why?" one might say, "Well, I noticed you were swinging your

foot, and you've smoked six cigarettes in the last twenty minutes." Helping the patient become aware of nonverbal cues of anxiety may enable the patient to discuss such feelings verbally. Also, just as staff members observe patients for their nonverbal communications, patients also notice the nonverbal communication of staff members. If, during a conversation, one swings one's leg or twiddles a piece of clothing, the patient may believe that the staff member is bored, in a hurry, or wishes that the patient would get on with the topic of discussion.

14. When discussing painful or embarrassing subjects, patients need support and encouragement. Looking at the patient in a helpful, interested, concerned manner encourages the patient to continue. In addition, the nurse might occasionally say, "I see" or "Go on" or "I can understand that." Such statements also encourage the patient to continue talking and let the patient know that the staff member is listening and attentive to what is being said.

15. If the nurse does not understand something a patient said, it may be that the patient is not clear about the subject either. Ask for clarification: "I'm sorry, but I didn't hear the last thing you said" or "I don't understand what you mean. Please explain it to me." Do not make statements such as "You talk so low I can't understand what you are saying" or "The last statement you made was mean." Statements such as these run the risk of causing patients to feel intimidated and inferior, thus lowering their self-esteem and, therefore, possibly blocking further attempts to communicate.

16. Mental health workers should avoid emotionally charged words and incriminating statements. Statements such as "You know smoking can cause lung cancer" may cause a patient to become unduly upset. Leading questions such as "It doesn't hurt when you bend over, does it?" imply that a particular answer is expected and predispose the patient to admit or deny symptoms.

Communication is something people practice all their lives. Some seem to learn at an early age to be better at it than others. Fortunately, this skill can be improved at any age if one takes the time to learn and practice a few basic techniques such as the ones discussed in this chapter.

REPORTING AND RECORDING

One of the most important uses for good communication skills is reporting and recording information concerning patients. Pertinent information is kept in a legal document usually referred to as the patient's record or the patient's chart. Each patient's record should contain everything of significance pertaining to that patient. Accurate and complete charting and verbal reporting of observations encourage continuity of patient care by providing usable information about the patient to other team members.

The suggestions about effective communication techniques in this chapter, along with the specific instructions regarding charting listed next, should be helpful when reporting or charting observations about patients. *Above all, the cardinal rule is: If it's not written down, it didn't happen.*

1. Write or print legibly in ink. Be sure that notations are made on the correct patient's chart and that all notations are dated and signed.
2. Do not erase. If a mistake is made, draw one line through it and print the word *error* above the line.
3. Be concise, yet make the meaning of each sentence clear.
4. Be objective by providing a description of what the patient has said or done. Try to avoid interpreting the patient's behavior. Remember that behaviors taken out of context may seem bizarre but, when described relative to the situations in which they actually happened, may be quite normal and appropriate.
5. Use only the abbreviations approved by the institution.
6. Chart medications and treatments after they are given, not before. If a patient refuses to participate in an activity, take a medication, or allow a treatment, be sure to chart the refusal. Whenever possible, the patient's reason for the refusal should also be noted.
7. Report and record any sudden change in the patient's behavior.
8. Always record the time of occurrence of the event being recorded. Record events as soon after they happen as possible because important details may be forgotten if one waits several hours to write the report.
9. Accidents should be reported and recorded according to the policy of the institution. Thoroughness in writing such reports is extremely important because legal action may later require detailed information about the accident.

The following charts are provided as a guide to some of the factors that need to be observed and recorded in working with mentally ill patients. Many hospitals and clinics routinely use similar charts.

BEHAVIORS TO BE OBSERVED

Appearance

Personal Hygiene: clean _____ dirty _____
body odor _____
bathes self _____
requires help with bath _____
Dress: appropriate _____ inappropriate _____
neat _____ unkempt _____
dresses self _____ requires help dressing _____

General Behavior

cooperative _____ helpful _____ dependable _____
quiet _____ loud _____ excitable _____
overactive _____ depressed _____ listless _____
irritable _____ verbally aggressive _____
anxious (specify:_____)
complaints (specify:_____)
physically aggressive _____ temper tantrums _____
bites nails _____ uses obscene language _____
shows fear of others _____ pacing _____
seems overtly nervous _____ masturbates _____
sexually interested in staff _____
in other patients _____ expresses suicidal impulses _____
homicidal impulses _____

Body Behavior

staring into space _____ rigid, stiff movements _____
obviously tense _____ jerking spastic movements (tics) _____
frequent startled responses _____
holds one position for prolonged periods _____
seems to be in a trance _____
coordinated motor behavior _____ staggers _____
falls _____ slumps when sitting _____
good general posture _____ poor general posture _____

Verbal Behavior

Speech: slow _____ rapid _____ slurred _____
otherwise impaired _____
unintelligible _____ rambling _____
dramatic _____ talks to self _____
repeats words or phrases over and over _____
talks compulsively or constantly _____
talks very little _____ not at all _____

Thought Processes

Answers to questions: relevant _____
irrelevant _____
rambling _____
incoherent _____
Hears voices: threatening _____ ordering _____
accusing _____
Has visual hallucinations (specify:_____
_____)
Has visions (specify:_____
_____)
Has peculiar bodily sensations (specify:_____
_____)

BEHAVIORS TO BE OBSERVED *continued*

Has delusions (specify:_____
_____)

Ideas of: reference _____ persecution _____
conspiracy _____ people controlling _____
outside forces controlling _____
body destruction _____ famous people _____
having unusual powers _____
having a divine mission _____

Orientation

Oriented to: time _____ place _____ person _____
date _____ month _____ year _____
Able to recognize: staff _____ other patients _____
own room _____
Short-term memory: good _____ poor _____ bad _____
Long-term memory: good _____ poor _____ bad _____
frequently forgets who
he (she) is_____

PHYSICAL SYMPTOMS

Vital Signs

Temperature _____ Pulse _____ Respiration _____
B/P _____ Weight _____

Neck, Face, and Skin

Appearance: pale _____ rosy _____ clammy _____
hot _____ cold _____ sweaty _____
acne _____ scars _____ red spots _____
bruises or lacerations _____
smooth texture _____ rough texture _____

Mouth

Teeth: natural _____ dentures _____ clean _____
good hygiene _____ poor hygiene _____
Gums: good color _____ smooth _____
irritated or inflamed _____ wet _____
dry _____ chewed or bitten _____
Breath: clean _____ sour _____ fruity _____

Urine

Color: pale yellow _____ bloody _____ pus _____
dark _____
Odor: essentially odorless _____ foul odor _____

Urinary Habits

Voiding: voids easily _____ trouble voiding _____
voids too often _____
incontinent for urine _____

Stool

Consistency: liquefied _____ soft _____ hard _____
normal _____
Color: (brown, etc.)_____
Unusual odor _____ blood _____ mucus _____

continued

PHYSICAL SYMPTOMS *continued*

Pain	Area (leg, etc.)_____
	sharp _____ dull _____ stabbing _____ throbbing _____
	intense _____ mild _____ occasional _____ frequent _____
	continuous _____ first noticed (time) _____
	How long has patient had the pain
	(days, hours, etc.)?_____
Vomiting	Time (1 A.M., etc.)_____
	Color (yellow, etc.)_____
	Amount: little _____ moderate _____ much _____
	Consistency: watery _____ average _____ thick _____
	bloody _____
	Material vomited (breakfast, etc.) _____
Cough	When: continuously _____ moderately _____
	occasionally _____ mostly A.M. _____ P.M. _____
	day _____ night _____
	Type: dry _____ sputum produced _____ blood _____
	loud _____ soft _____ hacking _____
	whooping _____ hoarse _____
Sleep	Amount (7 hrs, etc.)_____
	day _____ night _____ sound _____
	moderate _____ light _____ fitful _____ disturbed _____
	restless _____ up a lot _____ sleeps easily _____
	sleeps with difficulty _____ needs sleep medication _____
Eating Habits	Appetite: very good _____ good _____ fair _____
	poor _____
	eats without assistance _____ needs assistance _____
	throws food _____
	Table manners: good _____ fair _____ poor _____
Medications	Takes meds without complaints _____
	"cheeks" meds _____ hoards meds _____ refuses meds __
	no side effects noted _____ side effects (specify:_____)

BEHAVIORS AND PROBLEMS FREQUENTLY SEEN

Anxiety Disorders

1. Increased heart rate, palpitations, increased blood pressure
2. Muscular tension, parasympathetic responses
3. Increased respirations to the point of hyperventilation
4. Weakness
5. Dilated pupils
6. Constipation

7. Dry mouth
8. Anorexia
9. Urinary frequency, diarrhea
10. Headaches
11. Nausea and vomiting
12. Decreased sexual functioning
13. Restlessness
14. Tremors
15. Accident proneness

Dysthymic Disorders or Major Depression

1. Poor personal hygiene
2. Decreased motor activity
3. Fatigue
4. Anxiety, restlessness
5. Low self-esteem
6. Decreased mental processes
7. Constipation
8. Increased or decreased appetite
9. Sleeping disturbances: increased or decreased sleep, early morning awakening
10. Suicidal verbalization or gestures

Manic Disorders

1. Increased agitation
2. Hyperactivity
3. Loose associations
4. Insomnia
5. Hostility
6. Acting out
7. Hallucinations
8. Delusions
9. Sexual acting out
10. Rapid speech

Psychotic Disorders

1. Hallucinations
2. Delusions
3. Inappropriate affect
4. Regressive behaviors
5. Withdrawn behaviors
6. Sleep disturbances
7. Disorganized, illogical thinking
8. Acting out
9. Aggressive or destructive behaviors
10. Suicidal verbalization or gestures
11. Poor personal hygiene

Neurological Disorders

1. Short attention span
2. Disorientation
3. Confusion
4. Confabulation
5. Poor immediate recall
6. Inappropriate or dramatic changes in social behavior
7. Poor judgment
8. Anger, hostility, or combativeness
9. Withdrawal
10. Inability to complete a task
11. Impaired ability to take care of activities of daily living

---

▼ KEY POINTS ▼

1. The aim of all forms of communication is to provide information, receive information, or exchange information.
2. One means of clarifying and making written communication more explicit is to use description.

Key Points continued

3. Verbal communication is largely effective because it is easy to speak and immediate feedback can alert one to the possibility that the desired message is not being communicated.

4. Some authorities believe that nonverbal communication is the most accurate form of communication. People communicate nonverbally via their behavior and their body posture.

5. A primary objective of early staff-patient or student-patient contacts is to establish a relationship that promotes mutual trust. A step is made in that direction when a staff member is honest and straightforward with patients.

6. When beginning to develop a trusting and therapeutic relationship with a patient, it is often advantageous to have frequent contacts of short to intermediate duration rather than trying to jump right into a heavy discussion of interpersonal issues.

7. Two key approaches to helping patients recognize their importance are (a) spending time with patients and (b) making sure time with the patient is spent *focusing on the patient.*

8. A 5-minute visit may seem much longer to the patient if the staff member seems relaxed and unhurried and discusses topics that are important to the patient.

9. When talking with patients, one should pull a chair close or sit beside them on the sofa but be careful not to invade their comfort zone. Pay attention to what the patient is saying. Do not fidget in the chair, tap your feet, or wring your hands. Adopt a pleasant, sincere, interested attitude.

10. Communication techniques useful in helping mentally ill patients communicate more effectively:
    a. Be aware of the patient's current attentional capacity.
    b. Keep verbalizations appropriate to the patient.
    c. Clarify specifics.
    d. Help patients develop an accurate understanding of environmental events.
    e. Help patients attend to reality.
    f. Use open-ended questions when appropriate.
    g. Model appropriate verbal responses.
    h. Do not appear to give patients a choice when you do not intend the patient to have one.

continued on page 168

Key Points continued

    i. Encourage patients to participate in developing their plans of care.

    j. Help patients focus on a single topic in order to explore it.

    k. Encourage independence and decision making on the part of patients.

    l. Be aware of the therapeutic implications of silence.

    m. Learn to interpret nonverbal behavior to patients.

    n. Support the patients' efforts at disclosure.

    o. Ask for clarification if something is unclear.

    p. Avoid leading questions and pronouncements.

11. One of the most important areas requiring good communication skills is reporting and recording information concerning patients.

12. When reporting or charting observations:

    a. Write or print legibly in ink.

    b. Do not erase.

    c. Be concise.

    d. Be objective.

    e. Use only the abbreviations approved by the institution.

    f. Chart medications and treatments after they are given, not before.

    g. Report and record any sudden change in the patient's behavior.

    h. Always include the time of occurrence of the event being recorded.

    i. Accidents should be reported and recorded according to the policies of the institution.

Remember: If it's not written down, it didn't happen.

Annotated Bibliography

Callanan, M.: Breaking the silence. *American Journal of Nursing,* 1994, January, 22–24.

Discusses support for the terminally ill patient through communication.

Crowther, D. J.: Metacommunication: A missed opportunity? *Journal of Psychosocial Nursing and Mental Health Services,* 1991, 29(4):13–16.

Presents communication as a multilevel phenomenon and discusses the importance of obtaining the transcending or underlying meaning when working with patients.

Fiesta, J.: Duty to communicate—"Doctor Notified." *Nursing Management,* 1994, 25(1):24–25.

Discusses the legalities of a nurse's responsibility and failure to communicate through reporting and charting.

Haselfeld, D.: Patient assessment: Conducting an effective interview. *AORN Journal,* 1990, 52(3):551–557.

Illustrates the importance of interviewing to the nursing process and provides guidelines for more effective interviewing techniques.

Oliver, S., and Redfern, S. J.: Interpersonal communication between nurses and elderly patients: Refinement of an observation schedule. *Journal of Advanced Nursing,* 1991, 16:30–38.

Research study focusing on the amount and type of nurse-patient interpersonal communication. Discusses the importance of touch as a means of communication.

Richter, J. M., Roberto, K. A., and Bottenberg, D. J.: Communicating with persons with Alzheimer's disease: Experiences of family and formal caregivers. *Archives of Psychiatric Nursing,* 9(5):279–285.

Examines communication processes of family members and formal caregivers for individuals with Alzheimer's disease and associated behavioral problems.

Stevenson, S.: Heading off violence with verbal de-escalation. *Journal of Psychosocial Nursing and Mental Health Services,* 1991, 29(9):6–15.

Presents therapeutic communication as a means to alter the course of the aggression cycle before the patient's behavior becomes violent.

Post-Test

True or False. Circle your choice.

T   F   1. The two basic forms of communication are verbal and nonverbal.

T   F   2. A common problem associated with verbal communication is the sending of messages one does not really mean.

T   F   3. Some authorities believe that nonverbal communication is the most accurate of all forms of communication.

T   F   4. In establishing a therapeutic relationship with a patient, the first step is to read his or her chart very carefully.

T   F   5. People communicate nonverbally via their behavior and their body posture.

T   F   6. Nonverbal clues may be a better indication of a patient's true feelings than what the patient actually says.

T   F   7. A patient who is highly anxious is usually a better listener than one who is relatively calm.

T   F   8. One should not offer a patient a choice if in reality he or she does not have a choice.

T   F   9. If a patient appears to be having difficulty making a decision, a staff member should make it for him or her.

T   F   10. The patient should be involved as much as possible in planning his or her own care and treatment plans.

Multiple Choice. Circle the letter or number you think represents the best answer.

1. The manner in which questions are asked can be improved by all of the following except:
   a. Listening before asking.
   b. Phrasing questions clearly and concisely.
   c. Asking only questions pertinent to the subject at hand.
   d. Phrasing questions so that a "yes" or "no" will suffice for the answer.

Post-Test

(continued)

2. If verbal communications are difficult, it is sometimes helpful and therapeutic to:
   a. Digress from focusing on the patient and the patient's problems and mention similar problems of your own.
   b. Ask the patient direct questions that require concrete answers.
   c. Ask several nonproductive questions that do not make the patient feel threatened.
   d. Engage in social activity with patients while they talk so that they will feel more comfortable.

3. The mental health worker's ability to interpret communication effectively is most dependent on:
   a. Sources available for validation of communication content.
   b. The immediacy with which the staff member attempts interpretation.
   c. The staff member's understanding of psychiatric terminology.
   d. How well the staff member listens and observes.

4. When observing behavior, the staff member should remember that behavioral symptoms:
   a. Have meaning.
   b. Are purposeful.
   c. Are multidetermined.
   d. All of the above.

5. Accurate recording of observations made in psychiatric settings includes:
   a. Employing psychiatric terminology whenever possible.
   b. Recording data as soon as possible.
   c. Expressing personal opinions and interpreting behavior.
   d. Using common, everyday descriptive language.
      (1) d only.
      (2) a and c.
      (3) b and d.
      (4) a, b, and c.
      (5) All of the above.

Post-Test

(continued)

6. The main purpose for record keeping (charting) in the psychiatric setting is to:
   a. Provide a subjective report of the patient's behavior.
   b. Provide an objective report of the patient's behavior.
   c. Provide a description of the patient's environment.
   d. Note behavioral signs of a specific illness.

7. If a patient becomes silent for a few seconds during an interaction, the staff member should probably:
   a. Interpret this as an indication that the patient is ready for the staff member to depart.
   b. Ask the patient a simple nonthreatening question to get the conversation going again.
   c. Remind the patient that you can help best if she or he shares her or his feelings with you.
   d. Remain with the patient and be quietly attentive.

8. The therapeutic relationship is enhanced when a staff member uses verbal and nonverbal communication to:
   a. Give attention and recognition to patients.
   b. Foster a patient's self-esteem.
   c. Indicate understanding.
   d. Communicate a feeling of acceptance and security.
      (1) d only.
      (2) b and c.
      (3) a and d.
      (4) a, b, and d.
      (5) All of the above.

9. Ms. Long, a social worker, approaches one of her patients and starts a conversation. The patient says, "I don't want to talk today." What response from Ms. Long would indicate that she understood and accepted her patient's behavior?
   a. "You say you don't want to talk?"
   b. "I'll sit here with you for a while."
   c. "There is no need for you to talk."
   d. "Why don't you want to talk today?"

Post-Test

(continued)

10. Mrs. Adams tells a staff member that she is feeling depressed about the recent death of her father. Which of the following responses would communicate understanding and acceptance?
    a. "I know just how you feel."
    b. "Everyone gets depressed when they lose a loved one."
    c. "This must be very difficult for you."
    d. "Try to think positive. He was ill only a short time and didn't have to suffer long."

11. Which of the following responses could prevent effective communication?
    a. "What you should do is. . . ."
    b. "In my opinion. . . ."
    c. "Try not to worry; everything will be all right."
    d. "Why did you do that?"
       (1) d only.
       (2) a, b, and d.
       (3) a, b, and c.
       (4) All of the above.

12. While communicating with a schizophrenic patient, the mental health worker should:
    a. Sit quietly and not encourage the patient to verbalize.
    b. Talk with the patient as one would with a normal person.
    c. Allow the patient to do all the talking.
    d. Use very simple, concrete language in speaking to the patient.

13. When talking to a patient for the first time, the staff member must realize:
    a. That hostile behavior in a patient indicates that the staff member's initial approach has been inadequate.
    b. That the case history should be read before talking with the patient.
    c. That the patient's physical appearance provides an accurate index as to whether he or she will be receptive.
    d. That the patient is a stranger to the staff member and the staff member is a stranger to the patient.

The Tools of the Nurse as a Person

OBJECTIVES: Student will be able to:

1. Answer the question "Are therapeutic persons born that way or do they learn to be therapeutic?"
2. Distinguish between the terms *genotype* and *phenotype.*
3. Identify the only truly therapeutic instrument for treating the mentally ill.
4. List 10 tools the nurse must develop to become therapeutically competent.

Not long ago, while addressing a group of students by invitation, one of the authors was asked whether there is such a thing as a therapeutic person and, if so, whether that means there is such a thing as a nontherapeutic person. The author's response was that there certainly are therapeutic persons, and, yes, there are nontherapeutic persons, and that sometimes there seem to be a lot more of the latter than the former in the world. A follow-up inquiry asked whether therapeutic persons were born that way or had to learn to be therapeutic. Being of the opinion that every person is a product of both genetic makeup (*genotype*) and the interaction of the environment with that genotype, the authors clearly believe that the resulting *phenotype* is significantly influenced by learning.

Current thinking suggests people can inherit certain tendencies or temperamental inclinations (personality predispositions) that may or may not show up in the phenotype (the product or result of the interaction between the genotype and the environment). Whether the genetic tendencies develop depends on the nature of people's experience in their environment. Thus, people who have the genetic tendency (genotype) to become fat may not become fat (phenotype) if they happen to develop a lifestyle that includes eating low-fat foods and getting plenty of exercise. Similarly, if a person's genotype includes an irritable, aggressive, abrasive predisposition, instead of a calm, accepting, nurturing predisposition, it may take a very intense and prolonged set of environmental learning experiences to produce an emotionally therapeutic person. Everyone knows a few of the first type—and that their environmental learning experiences were not nearly as intense and prolonged as they needed to be!

Whether you see yourself as genotypically suited to becoming a therapeutic person, it probably is true that, in mental health, the only truly therapeutic instrument *is* the person. Therefore, mental health nursing is most effective when the practitioner has developed a set of interpersonal relationship tools and a set of communication tools, keeps them sharp, and practices using them. So let's explore the therapeutic toolbox.

SELF-AWARENESS

Self-awareness means knowing about yourself—knowing whether you tend to overwhelm people with your opinions or whether you are quiet and reserved—and having some knowledge of why you are that way. It means seeing yourself as others see you; it means understanding how you react when you do not want to hear what someone is saying about you. It means knowing how, when, and why you distort issues and which issues bother you. Therapeutically, it is not a sin to have personal issues. It is a sin to be unaware of them so that you unconsciously inject them into your interactions with your patients. If you dislike authority, why? If you do not like to assume responsibility for your actions, why not? Do you maintain a balance between doing appropriately for others and having others do for you? How do you get your dependency needs met, your need for control, your need to love and be loved, your need for success and to feel good about yourself? You cannot help your patient gain insight if you have none yourself.

PERSONAL MENTAL HEALTH

Your own level of mental health is crucial. If you are depressed, chronically anxious, ritualistic, phobically incapacitated, pathologically guilty, preoccupied, angry, irritated, withdrawn, overly dependent, painfully shy, guarded, withdrawn, impulsive, angry, or distraught or have any of several other psychopathological manifestations (symptoms), your therapeutic effectiveness may be severely limited. Your tolerance, your judgment, your personal accessibility, and your relationship skills are diminished if you are not functioning in a mentally healthy manner. Patients are quick to recognize symptoms in staff, and they often bring them to your attention. If your personal mental health is impaired, please find a competent therapist and learn to function more effectively before attempting to rehabilitate someone else. Everyone experiences these symptoms occasionally. Only when they show up at inappropriate levels do difficulties arise.

RAPPORT

Rapport refers to the nature and quality of the relationship a staff member creates with a patient. Good rapport means you have successfully created a condition in which you and the patient feel comfortable with each other. The patient has a sense of your genuine interest and your warmth and acceptance. The ability to quickly build effective rapport with a patient is a necessary tool for therapeutic competence. Good rapport comes from being comfortable with yourself, which comes from effective use of the tools discussed in this chapter. It also comes from an ability to make others feel comfortable. Good eye contact, a calm voice, nonthreatening body language, an appropriate smile, and an easy, accepting attitude go a long way toward building rapport.

Add to those qualities a genuine interest in patients and what they have to say and a willingness to listen, be nonjudgmental, and be respectful of patients' worth as people, and you are nearly there. You must be careful not to be overly kind because patients may not trust such an approach. Be straightforward but genuinely concerned. *Always* be sensitive to the physical distance the patient needs to be comfortable. Few people like someone right in their faces. Each person has a physical distance at which she or he feels comfortable, and good observational skills and sensitive judgment are needed to find a distance that is comfortable for both you and the patient. One of the quickest ways to escalate scared, paranoid, angry, or resistant patients is to invade their physical comfort zone.

MODELING

Modeling refers to the idea that one person's behavior can influence the behavior of others. It happens daily in television ads, in the movies, and in everyday interactions. Often modeling occurs without the observer's being fully aware that it is happening. Have you ever found yourself doing something the way an admired friend does it?

Ideally, in mental health settings, the modeled behavior should be effective and appropriate and demonstrate to patients an alternative to some inappropriate or undesirable behavior they exhibit. A patient who responds angrily to something you have said may be expecting you to become angry also. If you refuse to become defensive and angry and, instead, remain calm, refuse to personalize the patient's comments, and keep paying attention to how the patient feels, you are modeling more appropriate behavior and showing the patient an alternative way to deal with being upset. The key here is to *show* patients new ways to behave, not *tell* them new ways to behave.

Suppose a patient asks you a question and you do not know how to respond. You could try to bluff your way through, make up something you hope will fly, leave the room, cry, get anxious, break out in a rash, tremble, say you have to go to the bathroom, or call your instructor—or you could simply say, "I don't know how to respond to that." It's honest, it will not get you or a patient in trouble, and it tells patients it is all right if they do not know how to respond sometimes either. You have modeled an appropriate response to uncertainty, which is something everyone needs to learn to do.

SELF-DISCLOSURE

Self-disclosure is probably one of the least understood and most often violated tools available to a person trying to be therapeutic. It refers to the idea of giving patients information about yourself. It can range from something as simple as giving your name to something as complex as being psychologically seduced into telling patients how you would handle their problems were you in their place (which should never be done by a beginner). Very limited self-disclosure is called for until you gain enough experience to know how to use it therapeutically. It can be therapeutic or quite antitherapeutic. The general idea from most studies reviewed by the authors indicates that self-disclosure is most effective when used to establish rapport and when the information is more about the caregiver's background and education and not about general likes and dislikes or views on subjects unrelated to the patient's difficulties or issues.

Interestingly, self-disclosure is sometimes misused by both patients and inexperienced caregivers. Inexperienced caregivers usually misuse self-disclosure because they are not skilled in developing therapeutic relationships or are unaware of how therapeutic relationships are different from social ones. Thus, they use self-disclosure that would be appropriate in social situations but not in therapeutic ones. Patients sometimes want to know more about a caregiver because the knowledge makes them feel closer and more in tune with the caregiver, a potentially good thing if handled appropriately. Sometimes, however, it makes them feel favored and more accepted by the caregiver and "one up" on those patients who have not been favored with such information. They use such information to establish their rank or status among other patients, and they sometimes are convinced that the information means they are more important to the caregiver than others are. Some patients may use personal information about the caregiver in social ways, and, as stated earlier, the nurse-patient relationship is never a social one.

Personal information about the caregiver can be used in other manipulative ways, too. Patients may use talking about the nurse or caregiver as a means of distracting the focus from themselves, avoiding self-disclosure about their own issues, or resisting dealing with feelings. If they are allowed to distract themselves from their own issues, they may lose an opportunity for real therapeutic benefit.

So, for the beginner, when the patient says, "What do you think I should do?" or "Tell me what you think about . . ." be prepared to say, "I could tell you that, but it's much more important what you think. Tell me how you see it." If the patient asks, "Do you have a boyfriend?" or "Where do you live?" be prepared to say, "It's kind of you to ask, but this is our time to talk about you and what brought you here. What do you think about. . . ?" If the patient persists with such questions after you use these or similar responses several times, it may be appropriate to say, "Mr. Jones, it is not appropriate for me to answer those kinds of questions. May we please concentrate on. . . ."

Students often ask that we be specific about certain issues related to self-disclosure. There may be exceptions to the recommendations, which are biased by social expectations and mores related to American culture. With that acknowledgment, our recommendations follow.

It is not a good idea to tell a patient your address or telephone number, whether you are married or have a boyfriend or have any personal problems, the make or kind of automobile you drive, the name of your pet, your father's occupation, or any one of a hundred other bits of personal information, even if the patient insists. When patients make such personal inquiries, you might respond by saying, "What makes you ask?" and then direct patients to a discussion oriented toward their own problems. You might also say, "This time is for you to talk about things that are important to you" or "It would be more helpful if you would talk about yourself." This point is especially important in the first few patient-staff contacts, when the patient may be unclear about the relationship and the purpose of the discussions. If all else fails, you may simply say that staff members are not permitted to discuss personal information.

Dating patients is also a very unwise practice, even after the patients have been discharged from the hospital, and should almost never be done. A nurse cannot be sure when a patient might need to return to the hospital, and it is difficult to mix personal and professional relationships. Therapeutic situations give power to the nurse or caregiver, and that power is abused when it is used or allowed to become a part of a social relationship. Those situations are called *dual relationships* and are generally considered unethical and, in some states, against the law if they involve sexual contact. If a patient's efforts to establish a social relationship persist, you might need to respond in the following manner: "I am sorry but it is hospital policy that staff members not see patients socially." A hospital is an impersonal object and a patient may ventilate anger toward it without causing any great harm. All of these boundary issues are discussed in some detail later in the chapter.

PERSONAL VALUES

People cannot escape their personal values. They are at the heart of human functioning. They will not be denied because they influence both our conscious and unconscious processes. Although they are learned, they are often *overlearned* and thus very resistant to challenge. That makes them one of the most important tools in the therapeutic toolbox. Their importance lies as much in their potential for nontherapeutic use as for their therapeutic use. People tend to base their judgments on their values because values tell people how to look at the world and provide points of view on all the issues they discuss.

What happens then, when people are faced with someone whose personal values are very different from theirs? It has been argued that Western culture is on a path to self-destruction because of its emphasis on individual rights and the individual's personal development. Typically, Western therapies seek to enhance the quality of the individual's life and strive to further an individual's efforts toward becoming independent from others. Therapists tend to see dependence as undesirable. What about you? Where do you stand on the importance of family, religion, sexual expression, capital punishment, abortion, cleanliness, pornography, adultery, child abuse, politics, and economic issues? Do not be deceived into believing your views of these things can be kept out of your interactions with patients. People cannot think independently of their values, which are part of the process of thinking. You

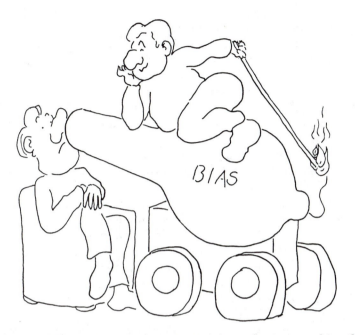

Figure 9–1. We can often see more clearly when others are pushing their biases on us than when we are pushing our bias on them. (From Bailey, D. S.: *You Are the Difference*. Gainesville, Ga.: Healthtree Press, 1987. Reprinted with permission.)

can, however, become as fully aware as possible of your values and thus know when they are influencing your relationship with patients. Unless you are aware of your values and of the need to keep your biases to yourself, you will unwittingly assume your values are best, both for you and for the patient. Personal values and biases unrelated to your therapeutic philosophy have no place in your interactions with patients (Fig. 9–1).

BOUNDARIES

Boundaries are the limits and responsibilities placed on those who assume the role of caregiver, and as such they define ethical practices. They are important because they tell caregivers how far they can go in doing certain things without risking harm to the patient or to themselves. Boundaries are lines nurses do not cross in the interest of preserving the patient's therapeutic interests.

Some boundaries are very clear, and others are not so clear. Becoming sexually involved with a patient is a very clear boundary that should never happen under any circumstances. This boundary was not always so clearly established as it is now, but in the last few years it has become absolute. The sensitivity to sexual harassment issues has forced more definition of what is and is not appropriate, and, clearly, sexual involvement with a patient is an abuse of the therapeutic relationship. Likewise, it is not appropriate to allow the therapeutic relationship to become a social relationship. As mentioned earlier, the power balance in such relationships may tend to place the patient in a "one-down" position and foster dependency and other nontherapeutic relationship dynamics (processes). The boundary between therapeutic and social relationships should not be violated.

Other boundaries involve not going beyond your training and expertise to do something in hopes that it will turn out all right. Do not misrepresent your credentials. If you are a student, say you are a student. It is far better to identify knowledge deficits than to have someone else discover them after harm has been done. Another boundary observed in mental health settings relates to patients' rights to have their problems dealt with privately. Therefore, caregivers must never violate any patient's right to that privacy. Some cases of protecting privacy are clear, such as never discussing patients or their difficulties outside the therapeutic setting. That includes not even discussing them with other students outside the learning environment. Other cases may not be so clear. What happens if a social acquaintance of yours is admitted to the treatment setting? In most cases, boundary violations would occur if you participated in that person's treatment in any way because your social relationship would be changed by the intimate knowledge you would gain from the treatment setting that you might never have known otherwise.

Another boundary relates to aggressive physical contact with patients. Although rare, sometimes a male patient is quite sexually inappropriate with a female student or nurse. Female patients are sometimes inappropriate with male staff, also. Sometimes patients slap you, spit at you, or call you socially unacceptable names. Sometimes they violate your comfort zone and try to intimidate you in terms of physical closeness. Is it ever acceptable for you to strike, push, or otherwise be physically aggressive with a patient? Although these occurrences are rare, you should be prepared to deal with them. Generally, the boundary is clear. Nurses do not become physically aggressive with patients. The major exception is if you believe your life is in danger. With appropriate use of the procedures you read in this book and observation of our Rules for Beginners (Table 9–1), you are unlikely to face such a situation.

Table 9–1. **Rules for Beginners**

1. Always know the patient's history. *Read the chart.*

2. Always tell the patient you are a student, assuming that you are.

3. Never allow a patient to tell you a secret with your agreement not to discuss the information with anyone else.

4. Try never to have discussions with patients in very private places—like the patient's room—where you cannot be seen by others.

5. Do not be concerned about saying to a patient, "I don't know what to say." If a patient asks you something you don't know, then say so. You may then offer to try to find someone who would know the answer, if appropriate.

6. Never try to *interpret the meaning* of behavior, dreams, verbalizations, or anything else.

7. Never tell patients how you would solve their problems.

8. Never give advice.

9. Never forget: What the patient has to say is important, not what you have to say.

10. Never promise a patient anything you are not *absolutely certain* you can do.

11. Never tell patients you want to be their friend.

12. Never dress seductively or behave seductively toward a patient. If you wonder if you are too seductively dressed, you are.

13. Never tell a patient your phone number, where you live, or that you will call them after hours.

14. Never forget: Talking or associating with a patient is first, last, and always a professional event, *never* a social event.

15. Never say anything without understanding why you are saying it.

16. Never give medicines for which you do not know the indications, contraindications, dosage range, side effects, and what to do in the case of an overdose.

17. Never attempt or assist in any therapeutic endeavor without identifying yourself as a student.

18. Never sign off on anything you did not personally do.

continued

Table 9–1. **Rules for Beginners** *continued*

19. Never break the confidence of patients by discussing anything about them with persons other than appropriate staff or instructors or in an appropriate learning environment.

20. Never try to cure patients by converting them to your religion.

21. Always, when in doubt, ask your instructor or other appropriate persons before proceeding.

The rules are lengthy but involve a lot of common sense and parallel much of what you already know about nursing. We tried to find ways of stating these principles in a more positive way, but students indicated they felt more comfortable with the structure of "the rules" as stated. Even if you violate the rules, nothing drastic may come of it, but when drastic situations occur, they almost always stem from violation of these rules. For that reason, follow them as closely as is appropriate for your situation. These are rules for beginners. As you gain experience, you may gradually modify some of them, even though experienced people usually readily agree with them. If your instructor wishes to modify or extend the rules, we would recommend to you the First Rule For Mentally Healthy and Smart Students: *Always do what your instructor says unless it contradicts legal or ethical restraints.*

CONFRONTATION

Confrontation is another technique that must be used with considerable care. In the therapeutic sense, confrontation means bringing some aspect of thinking, feeling, or behaving to the attention of the patient and asking the patient to deal with any differences in what the patient presents as being true and what appears to the caregiver to be true. In some cases, confrontation is carried out with the aim of immediately changing or modifying the behavior of the patient. Confronting a patient is probably best done after the caregiver is comfortable with most of the basic therapeutic tools presented in this chapter.

Therapeutic confrontation may be thought of as having three basic levels: The first is a mild and basically positive verbal confrontation that can easily be done by an inexperienced caregiver. For example, if a patient says, "I look so stupid in this dress," the caregiver might confront that by saying "You don't look stupid to me. What about the dress causes you to feel stupid?" A second level of confrontation involves interpretation of feelings created in the caregiver by the patient's behavior. If the patient makes repeated sexual references to the caregiver, the caregiver might respond, "Your remarks about my body make me feel very uncomfortable. Please don't make them anymore. If you do, I will call my supervisor." The third level of confrontation involves physical intervention. If a patient's behavior is becoming so uncontrolled that it is dangerous to the patient or others, the patient is confronted and, if necessary, physically restrained. This, too, is a rare event in most mental health settings and is usually done only by very experienced caregivers.

TOUCHING

Touching is another tool of great therapeutic potential but also one that holds many potential complications. In this society, touching is often associated with sexual intimacy, and that kind of touching has no place in mental health care. A difficulty is that, although the caregiver may have no sexual intention, the manner in which touching is interpreted by the patient is beyond the caregiver's control. An appropriate touch, however, appropriately interpreted by the patient, can sometimes communicate more than words ever could.

There is at least one other potential problem besides the possibility of being misunderstood. Touching is an invasion of personal space that may provoke a withdrawal response. Response to touch is so much governed by subcultural rules and expectations that it is probably a good idea to know the patient well or be very good at reading nonverbal cues before using touch as a therapeutic tool.

EMPATHY

The most single most important tool in therapeutic caregiving has been saved for last. Let's begin by understanding that empathy and sympathy are not the same. *Webster's New World Dictionary* defines *sympathy* as "pity or compassion felt for another's troubles, suffering, etc." and *empathy* as "the projection of one's own personality into the personality of another in order to understand the person better; ability to share in another's emotions, thoughts, or feelings." Sympathy, then, is passive; empathy is active. Empathy is to put yourself in the other person's shoes and see things from his or her point of view.

True empathy is not an easy thing to accomplish because it requires putting aside personal points of view. It requires learning to see other peoples' worlds the way they see them, not the way they seem to us. Truax and Carkhuff (1967) identified five levels of empathy, beginning with level I, in which the caregiver shows no awareness of how the patient is feeling or what the patient is thinking. In level II empathy, the caregiver is aware of what the patient is saying, but the understanding of what the patient is saying is inaccurate. In level III, the caregiver accurately reflects most surface-level behaviors and feelings but misses deeper feelings. The important thing in level III is that the patient can see that the caregiver is trying to understand and can feel positive about those efforts. This is the lowest level of empathy that is helpful to the patient.

In level IV, the caregiver is well enough in tune with what the patient is saying and feeling to be able to add to the patient's understanding of those feelings. This encourages the patient to go further into feelings and perceptions. In level V, the caregiver fully appreciates the thoughts and feelings of the patient and is able to respond from the patient's point of view. In doing so, the caregiver is able to help patients go deeper and deeper into feelings without concern because the caregiver truly understands, which enables patients to risk exploring their deepest fears.

The point of empathy is to let patients know that their feelings have been seen and understood. That sense of being understood is the thing that allows, and even encourages, patients to trust more and go further into self-understanding. If you are a beginner, level III is the goal to shoot for. Being empathetic requires paying very close attention to the patient, and just the fact that you are paying such close attention is likely to be helpful to the patient. As you become more adept, you can go further.

To show empathy for your patient, try the following:

1. Look at the patient. Keep good eye contact. Do not play with your hair, jiggle your legs, pick at your nails, or otherwise engage in distracting behavior. These are level I empathy behaviors.

2. Pay attention to your patient's nonverbal cues. Are you sitting too close for her or his comfort?

3. Try to look relaxed and comfortable. If you look and feel uncomfortable, chances are the patients will pick it up. If they do, and comment on it, just say something like "You noticed that I'm kind of new at this." This is a level III response. Do not say, "Yeah, you know how it is to be a student. I've been worried I might say the wrong thing. If you have children, I bet you know what I mean." This is a level II empathy response.

4. Respond to what the patient says by stating it back as a question:
   Patient: *"My son doesn't care what happens to me anymore."*
   Student: *"He doesn't care what happens to you anymore?"*

5. When you can understand the nature of the emotional pain being caused by the things the patient is saying, identify that.
   Patient: *"No. He hasn't even been to see me in over a year."*
   Student: *"He hasn't been to see you, and that's got you feeling really bad?"*

The response in item 4 is a level III response. It accurately reflected back to the patient what he had said. The response in item 5 is a level IV response because it interprets what the patient is saying and expresses understanding of how the patient must be feeling—a feeling that he has not yet expressed. This empathetic response allows the patient to move to a deeper discussion of feelings.

Once again, the key factor in demonstrating empathy is to pay attention, focus on the patient, on what he or she says, and on how it is said, and look for the unspoken feeling created by what is being said. The patient will appreciate the fact that you cared enough to listen.

▼ KEY POINTS ▼

Personal Tools Available to the Caregiver

1. Self-awareness: Knowing as much as possible about yourself and how you interact with other people.

2. Personal mental health: Important influence on your tolerance, judgment, ability to listen, and relationship skills.

3. Rapport: The nature and quality of the relationship you create with a patient. Good rapport means you and the patient feel comfortable with each other and share a sense of trust.

4. Modeling: Influencing the behavior of others by one's own behavior.

5. Self-disclosure: How much do you tell a patient about yourself, your interests, what you would do if you had their problems?

6. Personal values: People cannot think independently of their values. They are part of the *process* of thinking. Be aware of your values and know how they influence your relationships with patients. Your values represent your biases.

7. Boundaries: The limits and responsibilities people place on themselves when they assume the role of caregiver.

---

continued on page 188

Key Points continued

8. Confrontation: Bringing some aspect of thinking, feeling, or behaving to the attention of the patient and asking the patient to deal with it appropriately.

9. Touching: Physically touching a patient can be very therapeutic but holds many dangers. The caregiver must forever be aware of how the touch is given and how it is interpreted by the patient.

10. Empathy: The ability to share in another person's emotions, thoughts, and feelings. Five levels of empathy have been described.
   a. Reflects no awareness of how patients are feeling or what they are thinking.
   b. Caregiver knows what the patient is saying but the understanding of what is being said is inaccurate.
   c. Caregiver accurately reflects most surface-level behaviors and feelings but misses deeper feelings. However, patient knows caregiver is trying to understand and is comforted by that.
   d. Caregiver is well enough in tune with what the patient is saying and feeling to be able to add to the patient's understanding of those feelings.
   e. The caregiver fully appreciates the thoughts and feelings of the patient and is able to respond from the patient's point of view.

The key factor in empathy is to focus on patients, on what they say and on how they say it, and to look for the unspoken feeling created by what is being said.

Annotated Bibliography

Callaghan, P.: Organization and stress among mental nurses. *Nursing Times,* 1991, 87(34):50.

Investigates the effects of four occupational variables—role ambiguity, role overload, nonparticipation, and patients' psychopathology—on mental health nurses' reports of stress and job satisfaction.

Elfrink, V., and Lutz, E.: American Association of Colleges of Nursing essential values: National study of faculty perceptions, practices, and plans. *Journal of Professional Nursing,* 1991, 7(4):239–245.

Discusses the advantages of including values development opportunities in bachelor's-degree nursing education utilizing the seven professional values identified by the American Association of Colleges of Nursing.

Grainger, R. D.: Dealing with feelings: Beating burnout. *American Journal of Nursing,* 1992:15–17.

Provides examples highlighting behaviors that encourage burnout and behaviors that prevent burnout.

Kellet, J.: Caring about each other. *Nursing Standard,* 1991, 5(48):46.

Emphasizes the importance of a group support environment in nursing to counteract feelings of isolation and job-related stress.

Roberts, K. T., and Fitzgerald, L.: Serenity: Caring with perspective. *Scholarly Inquiry for Nursing Practice: An International Journal,* 1991, 5(2):127–146.

Presents a conceptual analysis of serenity to evaluate the usefulness of the concept to nursing practice and discusses the relationship of serenity to the concept of caring.

Thompson, J., and Brooks, S.: When a colleague commits suicide: How the staff reacts. *Journal of Psychosocial Nursing and Mental Health Services,* 1990, 28(10):6–11.

Examines some of the ways nurses deal with the suicide of a colleague and how the suicide affected their personal and professional lives.

Tout, L. R., and Shama, D. D.: A burnout instrument for hospice. *The Hospice Journal,* 1990, 6(4):31–130.

Presents an instrument to determine burnout in physical health and mental health practitioners and discusses validity and reliability studies as well as issues regarding possible application.

Tyler, P. A., Carroll, K., and Cunningham, S. E.: Stress and well-being in nurses: A comparison of the public and private sectors. *Journal of Nursing Studies,* 1991, 28(2):125–130.

Research study exploring the relationship between nursing stress and various aspects of self-reported health and well-being.

Reference

Truax, C. B., and Carkhuff, R. R.: *Toward Effective Counseling and Psychotherapy for Better or Worse.* Chicago: Aldine, 1967.

Post-Test

Matching. Match the skills in column B with the appropriate statement in column A.

Column A

1. Ability to share in others' emotions.

2. Sharing information about oneself with a patient.

3. To know oneself.

4. Bringing some aspect of thinking, feeling, or behaving to patient's attention.

5. Limits and responsibilities all caregivers must follow.

6. Building the relationship.

7. Shows patient alternate ways of handling situations.

Column B

A. Self-awareness

B. Rapport

C. Modeling

D. Self-disclosure

E. Boundaries

F. Confrontation

G. Empathy

True or False. Circle your choice.

T   F   1. According to the author, there is no such thing as a nontherapeutic person.

T   F   2. One's own level of mental health is unimportant when working with the mentally ill.

T   F   3. Patients can recognize symptoms of mental illness in staff members and often point them out to the staff member.

T   F   4. Establishing good rapport is not important in order to be therapeutically competent.

T   F   5. It is important to be aware of the physical distance a client needs in order to feel comfortable.

T   F   6. Modeling often occurs without the patient being fully aware that it is happening.

Post-Test

(continued)

T F 7. It is good to use self-disclosure when telling a patient what you would do in a given circumstance.

T F 8. Beginners should use self-disclosure a lot because it helps to build rapport with patients and helps cover up any nervousness on the part of the student.

T F 9. Caregivers should always answer personal questions that the patient asks of them so the patient does not feel rejected.

T F 10. It is not important to look at one's personal values when dealing with patients because they almost never influence an individual's work with the mentally ill.

T F 11. Becoming sexually involved with a patient is a boundary that should never be crossed.

T F 12. Sexual involvement with a patient is seen as an abuse of the therapeutic relationship.

T F 13. It is okay to strike a patient if he or she strikes you first.

T F 14. A potential problem with touching in a mental health setting is how the touch is interpreted by the patient.

T F 15. Empathy and sympathy are basically the same thing.

Multiple Choice. Circle the letter or number you think represents the best answer.

1. Self-awareness involves all of the following except:
   a. Knowing about yourself.
   b. Being able to see yourself as others see you.
   c. Denying that you have any personal issues.
   d. Knowing how you go about getting your needs met.
2. Rapport refers to:
   a. Being able to share in the emotions of others.
   b. Nature and quality of the relationship with a patient.
   c. Knowing yourself and how the patient perceives you.
   d. Being able to share personal information with the patient.

Post-Test

(continued)

3. Building good rapport with patients is important because:
   a. The patient feels more comfortable.
   b. It builds trust between the patient and the caregiver.
   c. The patient is able to sense genuine interest on the part of the caregiver.
   d. All of the above.

4. What traits assist caregivers in building rapport?
   a. Accepting attitude.
   b. Assertive personality.
   c. Calm voice, nonthreatening body language.
   d. Being overly kind.
      (1) a, c, and d.
      (2) a and c.
      (3) a, b, and d.
      (4) All of the above.

5. Self-disclosure:
   a. Helps to build rapport.
   b. Should be used often, especially by beginners who are nervous.
   c. Can be antitherapeutic if used incorrectly.
   d. Should be used to develop a more social relationship with patients.
      (1) a and c.
      (2) a and b.
      (3) a, b, and d.
      (4) a only.

6. Self-disclosure is most effective when the information shared by the caregiver:
   a. Is about caregiver's personal life.
   b. Mirrors patient's difficulties or issues.
   c. Is about caregiver's likes and dislikes.
   d. Is about caregiver's background and education.
      (1) b only.
      (2) b and d.
      (3) c and d.
      (4) a, c, and d.

Post-Test

(continued)

7. Beginners often misuse self-disclosure because:
   a. They like the patient and want to develop a social relationship with the patient.
   b. They are not skilled in developing therapeutic relationships.
   c. They are unaware of how therapeutic relationships differ from social relationships.
   d. They want the patient to feel more important than other patients.
      (1) b and c.
      (2) a, b, and d.
      (3) a and d.
      (4) All of the above.

8. A patient may take advantage of self-disclosure by a staff member:
   a. To establish rank with other patients.
   b. In order to try to develop a social relationship with the staff member.
   c. To distract attention from the patient's own issues.
   d. All of the above.
   e. Patients never take advantage of self-disclosure by a staff member.

9. Which of the following is not a basic level of confrontation?
   a. Positive verbal confrontation.
   b. Yelling at the patient when he repeats behaviors that he has been confronted on in the past.
   c. Interpretation of feelings created in the caregiver by patient's behavior.
   d. Physical intervention or restraint.

What level of empathy is being used in the examples given in questions 10 to 13?
   a. Level I
   b. Level II
   c. Level III
   d. Level IV
   e. Level V

Post-Test

(continued)

10. Patient: *I am really worried about my children. I have never been away from them for this long.*
    Student: *You're worried about your children because you've never been away from them this long?*

11. Patient: *I think my husband is having an affair.*
    Student: *(Blushes and continues to pick at nails.)*

12. Patient: *My family has disowned me since I've been in the hospital. They are ashamed to have a member of their family in a mental hospital.*
    Student: *It really hurts that your family has disowned you since you became ill?*

13. Patient: *It really hurts that my children don't come to visit me more often.*
    Student: *You know how children are. They never come around as much as parents feel they should.*

14. The most significant factor in demonstrating empathy is to:
    a. Make sure you identify the correct feeling.
    b. Maintain eye contact at all times.
    c. Pay attention and look for the unspoken feeling created by what is being said.
    d. None of the above.

Drug Therapy

OBJECTIVES: Student will be able to:

1. State the desired effects of major tranquilizers.

2. State the side effects of major tranquilizers.

3. List five of the most common major tranquilizers.

4. State the desired effects of minor tranquilizers.

5. State the side effects of minor tranquilizers.

6. List three important points to teach patients who are going home on medications.

7. Describe the goals of antidepressant therapy, sedative therapy, anticonvulsant therapy, and antiparkinson therapy.

8. List two specific nursing considerations each for major tranquilizers, minor tranquilizers, and antidepressants.

In the mid-1950s, the development of a group of drugs known as *phenothiazines* revolutionized the care of the mentally ill. It was first thought that these drugs might actually "cure" mental illness, which did not prove to be the case. However, these drugs did calm patients and decrease the severity of symptoms to the point that they could respond to other forms of therapy. Patients receiving phenothiazines became more aware of their surroundings, began to participate in daily activities, were more cooperative with hospital routines, and, of most importance, began to communicate. These drastic changes in patient behavior allowed the staff to begin to help patients establish interpersonal relationships and to cope more effectively with their environment.

Since this major breakthrough in drug therapy, many other drugs effective in the treatment of various psychiatric disorders have been developed. The two major classifications of the psychotropic drugs

(drugs active in decreasing symptoms of mental illness) are the tranquilizers, which are further divided into major and minor groups, and the antidepressants. This chapter also discusses anticonvulsants, sedatives, hypnotics, and antiparkinsons, which are also used in the treatment of psychiatric patients.

THE ROLE OF THE NURSE

Although this chapter focuses on the use of medication in the treatment of psychiatric patients, it also emphasizes the nurse's role in drug therapy. The nurse uses knowledge about medications, the patient, and the nurse's relationship with the patient in helping to evaluate and establish baselines to monitor the effectiveness of drug interventions. This requires all the skills nurses have in building a therapeutic relationship, plus assumption of the critical responsibility of consistently and knowledgeably administering and monitoring the effects, side effects, and overall response of the patient to the medication given. It also places the nurse in the important role of "teacher" to the patient. Because the nurse has the responsibility to help patients understand how to administer their own medications after discharge, this role cannot be underestimated or overlooked. It is critical to patients' health and safety.

Finally, there has been a significant increase in the number of elderly and debilitated patients requiring treatment, and the nurse has a special responsibility in assessing these patients' needs. When administering psychiatric drugs to the elderly and the debilitated, the nurse should put even greater emphasis on monitoring the effectiveness and side effects of medications. In addition, the nurse should not consider the average adult dose to be a safe dosage for these patients. Approximately one-third to one-half of the average adult dose is usually recommended.

MAJOR TRANQUILIZERS

The word *tranquilize* means "to make tranquil," that is, calm and basically free from agitation or disturbance. This definition describes exactly the effect tranquilizers are intended to have on disturbed patients. Drugs designated as major tranquilizers not only calm patients but also help to control severe agitation and reduce the frequency of hallucinations, delusions, thought disorders, and the type of withdrawal symptoms seen in catatonic schizophrenia. In other words, these drugs cause patients to exhibit more normal behavior. Several days of drug therapy may be necessary before the symptoms mentioned begin to subside, but during this time the patient usually becomes less fearful and hostile and less upset by any disturbance in sensory perceptions. As the patient's disturbed thinking and behavior improve, he or she becomes more receptive to psychotherapy and other forms of treatment.

The phenothiazine derivatives are the largest group of antipsychotic drugs. All the drugs in this group have essentially the same type of action on the body but vary according to strength and the type and severity of their side effects. Although rarely serious, phenothiazines produce several side effects that may cause discomfort. The patient should be observed carefully on a regular basis for the side effects listed in this section. Because early detection is important, all members of the treatment team ought to become thoroughly familiar with these major side effects.

Side Effects

Extrapyramidal Symptoms

There are three major types of extrapyramidal symptoms: (1) pseudoparkinsonism, with restlessness, masklike facial expression, drooling, and tremors; (2) akathisia, with inability to sit still, complaints of fatigue and weakness, and continuous movement of the hands, mouth, and body; and (3) dyskinesia, with lack of control over voluntary movements. For example, the patient might want to reach for something but be unable to do so. The patient may have a protruding tongue or a drooping head, and may become very frightened if stiffness of the neck and swallowing difficulties develop. Immediate action must be taken to combat extrapyramidal side effects, and administration of antiparkinson drugs usually produces a dramatic reduction in symptoms.

Autonomic Reactions

The autonomic reactions group of side effects includes dry mouth, constipation, excessive weight gain, and edema. Strict attention must be paid to patients' personal hygiene, and they should be informed of the possibility of these side effects and given suggestions as to how to combat them. Increasing a patient's intake of fluids, especially water, helps the dry mouth and also triggers the body's mechanism to reduce water retention, thus reducing the edema. Bethanechol (Urecholine) is also now being used to decrease mouth dryness. Because excessive weight gain is a potential problem, patients should be cautioned to decrease their intake of fattening foods and increase their intake of salads, fruits, and the like, which also helps to reduce constipation problems.

Postural Hypotension

Postural hypotension is a drop in blood pressure when a patient moves from lying flat in bed to a standing position. Symptoms include dizziness, heart pounding, and a "faint" feeling. Because patients could faint and injure themselves when first getting up, they should be cautioned to sit on the side of the bed first and dangle their feet a while before standing. Patients receiving a high dose of a phenothiazine drug should have their blood pressure checked on a regular basis. A patient given a large oral or IM dose of one of the phenothiazines should lie in bed afterward for about an hour.

Allergic Reactions

Allergic reactions are rare but serious. If the patient develops dermatosis, jaundice, or ulcerative lesions in the mouth or throat, the drug usually must be discontinued. Thus, if a patient complains of a sore throat or other signs of infection, the physician should be notified immediately.

Sedation

If a patient receiving phenothiazines is lethargic and wants to sleep a great deal, the dosage of medicine may be too high and need adjustment.

Decreased Sexual Interest

The possibility of decreased sexual interest needs to be explained so that the patient will know what is happening if sexual interest diminishes. Women patients may exhibit some of the signs and symptoms of pregnancy, such as absence of menstrual cycle, false-positive pregnancy tests, and weight gain. If the patient is checked further and there are no positive signs of pregnancy, she should be assured that the medication is the causative factor.

Photosensitivity

When photosensitivity occurs, the patient becomes especially sensitive to light, prone to sunburn, and may complain of visual problems. Therefore, lengthy periods of direct sunlight should be avoided, or protective clothing and glasses should be worn.

Other Side Effects

Patients on phenothiazines often experience blurred vision and drowsiness and should not drive or use dangerous equipment. They should be cautioned about taking other medications without their physicians' knowledge because phenothiazines may increase the action of other drugs, especially pain medications.

If any of these side effects causes the patient difficulty or serious hazards, the physician may try one of the following three remedies: (1) The drug dosage may be decreased; (2) if symptoms persist, the medication may be completely withdrawn for 24 hours and then restarted with a gradual buildup of the dosage; or (3) the drug may be changed to another phenothiazine derivative known to be less likely to produce the troublesome side effects.

Table 10–1 lists some of the major phenothiazine-type tranquilizers. Knowing these trade names will alert you to the fact that a patient is taking a phenothiazine drug and should be carefully observed for side effects (Table 10–2).

Patient Teaching

Because hospitals stays are shorter and shorter, an important responsibility of the nurse is to teach patients how to care for themselves at home. One of the most important aspects of caring for a patient on medication is to teach the patient all about the prescribed medication. Before you can teach the patient, you need to understand how the medication works, the expected action of the medication on the body, the importance of compliance with the treatment regimen, how to recognize if the medication is effective, and how to recognize side effects. After you have learned this information, you can then share it with patients so that they can administer the medicine appropriately at home.

It is important to teach patients the reason the antipsychotic medication is given: to reduce their symptoms of agitation and anxiety and to help control their behavior. Review with the patient that a thera-

Table 10–1. **Major Tranquilizers (Phenothiazine Derivatives); Antipsychotics (Major Tranquilizers, Neuroleptics, Antiemetics)**

Chemical Classification	Generic Name (Trade Name)	Route	Average Dosage for Daily Administration
Butyrophenone	Haloperidol (Haldol)	PO, IM	Oral dosage 0.5–5 mg 2–3 times/day; daily maximum 100 mg/day IM dosage (as lactate) 2.5 mg every 4–8 hours as needed IM dosage as decanoate: 10–15 times the daily oral dose administered IM at 4-week intervals
Dibenzoxazepine	Loxapine succinate (Loxitane)	PO, IM	Oral dosage 100 mg twice daily, increasing until psychosis controlled Average range 60–100 mg/day; not recommended to give over 250 mg/day IM dosage 12.5–50 mg every 4–6 hours as needed
Dihydroindolone	Molindone (Moban)	PO	Oral dosage 50–75 mg/day, increasing at approximately 3-day intervals, not to exceed 225 mg/day
Phenothiazines	Acetophenazine maleate (Tindal)	PO	Oral dosage 20 mg 3 times/day increasing to 60–120 mg/day (actively psychotic patients may require 400–600 mg/day)

Route	Drug	Dosage
IM, PO, IV, Suppository	Chlorpromazine (Thorazine)	Oral dosage 30–800 mg/day given at 4-hour intervals; average dosage 200 mg/day IM and IV average dosage 25 mg initially, repeated as needed, ranging from 100–1500 mg/day Rectal dosage 50–100 mg every 6–8 hours as needed
PO, IM, SC	Fluphenazine (Prolixin, Permitil, Prolixin Decanoate)	Oral dosage 0.5–10 mg/day at 6- to 8-hour intervals; range up to 40 mg/day IM dosage 2.5–10 mg/day at 6- to 8-hour intervals IM or SC Decanoate dosage 12.5 mg every 3 weeks
PO, IM	Mesoridazine besylate (Serentil)	Oral dosage 25–50 mg 3 times/day; maximum 100–400 mg/day IM dosage 25 mg initially; dosage ranging from 25–200 mg/day
PO, IM	Perphenazine (Trilafon)	Oral dosage for acute psychoses 4–16 mg 2–4 times/day; range 4–60 mg/day IM dosage 5 mg every 6 hours up to 30 mg/day
PO, IM, IV, Suppository	Prochlorperazine (Compazine)	Oral dosage 5–10 mg 3–4 times/day; maximum 40 mg/day; dosage may range to 150 mg for severely psychotic patients IM dosage 5–10 mg every 3–4 hours; maximum 40 mg/day IV dosage 2.5–10 mg; maximum 10 mg per dose and 40 mg/day Rectal dosage 25 mg twice per day

continued

Table 10–1. **Major Tranquilizers (Phenothiazine Derivatives); Antipsychotics (Major Tranquilizers, Neuroleptics, Antiemetics)** *continued*

Chemical Classification	Generic Name (Trade Name)	Route	Average Dosage for Daily Administration
Phenothiazines *continued*	Promazine (Sparine, Prozine)	PO, IM	Oral dosage for acute psychotic patient 10–200 mg every 4–6 hours, not to exceed 1000 mg/day; antiemetic dosage 25–50 mg every 4–6 hours as needed. IM dosage: initial dose 50–150 mg; average dose 10–200 mg every 4–6 hours as needed
	Thioridazine (Mellaril)	PO	Oral dosage for acute psychotic patient 50–100 mg 3 times/day initially, may increase to maximum of 800 mg in divided doses. Nonpsychotic patient: initial dose 25 mg 3 times/day; do not exceed 200 mg/day
	Triflupromazine hydrochloride (Vesprin)	PO, IM, IV	Oral dosage for acute psychotic patient 60 mg/day; maximum 150 mg/day; antiemetic 5–15 mg every 4 hours as needed up to 60 mg/day. IV dosage 1 mg as needed, up to maximum 3 mg/day

Trifluoperazine (Stelazine)	PO, IM	Oral dosage for acute psychotic patient 1–2 mg twice per day; do not exceed 40 mg/day; for nonpsychotic patient 1–2 mg twice per day; maximum 6 mg/day for maximum 12–14 weeks IM dosage 1–2 mg every 4–6 hours as needed; do not exceed 10 mg/day
Clozapine (Clozaril)	PO	Oral dosage 25 mg 1–2 times/day; may increase to 300–450 mg/day; psychotic patients may require 600–900 mg/day
Miscellaneous antipsychotic agent		
Thiothixene (Navane)	PO, IM	Oral dosage for acute psychotic patients 2 mg 3 times/day up to 20–30 mg/day; maximum 60 mg/day IM dosage 4 mg 2–4 times/day, maximum 16–20 mg/day

Table 10–2. **Major Tranquilizers (Potential for Side Effects)**

Drug (Most Commonly Used Trade Name)	Potential Sedation Factor	Potential for Extrapyramidal Side Effects
Haldol	Mild	High
Loxitane	Moderate	High
Moban	Mild	High
Tindal	Mild	Mild
Thorazine	High	High
Prolixin	Mild	High
Serentil	High	Mild
Trilafon	Mild	High
Compazine	High	Mild
Sparine	Mild	Mild
Mellaril	High	Mild
Vesprin	High	Mild
Stelazine	Mild	High
Clozaril	High	Mild
Navane	Mild	High

peutic response may take up to 3 weeks and that it is important to take the medication as the physician has ordered. The patient who misses a dose and remembers within an hour of the prescribed time should take the medicine. If it has been longer than 1 hour, the patient should wait until the next prescribed dose. However, remind the patient to take only a single dose, not a double dose, at the next scheduled time. Teach the patient to identify adverse side effects and to whom to report the side effects if they occur.

Teach the patient not to take over-the-counter drugs while on major tranquilizers, especially not antacids, which prevent or interfere with absorption.

Explain the importance of not reducing or stopping a drug when the drug has taken effect. Sometimes, when patients feel their symptoms less intensely, they tend to quit taking the drug. Patients should see their therapists before discontinuing usage.

MINOR TRANQUILIZERS

Tranquilizers reduce anxiety and the muscle tension associated with it. They are primarily useful in treating patients with psychoneurotic and psychosomatic disorders. In small doses, they are relatively safe and have few side effects. Unlike the major tranquilizers, however, some of the minor tranquilizers tend to be habit forming. If the drug is discontinued, the patient may experience severe withdrawal symptoms that may include even delirium and convulsions. They differ from barbiturates in that they produce a much lower level of drowsiness.

Side Effects

Patients are occasionally hypersensitive to the minor tranquilizers and may have rashes, chills, fever, nausea, and vomiting. These medications may also cause headaches, poor muscle coordination, some inability to concentrate, and dizziness. Patients taking these drugs should be cautioned against driving or performing any task that requires careful attention to detail and mental alertness. Excessive amounts of these drugs may lead to coma and death; however, death is much less likely to occur with an overdose of a minor tranquilizer than with an overdose of barbiturates. Table 10–3 lists many of the minor tranquilizers commonly used, and Table 10–4 cites their potential for side effects.

Patient Teaching

Provide patients with information about the specific drug. Include the medication's name, action, dose, the onset of effects, side effects, and interactions. Explain to patients that this drug is primarily to help them relax. While taking this drug, patients should continue to see their physicians because the drugs are habit forming and usually should not be taken for more than a few months. Patients should not discontinue the drug without consulting their physician.

Table 10–3. **Minor Tranquilizers**

Chemical Classification	Route	Generic Name (Trade Name)	Adult Dosage for Daily Administration
Antihistamine	PO, IM	Hydroxyzine (Anxanil, Atarax, Atozine, Durrax, E-Vista, Hydroxacen, HyPam, Hyzine-50, Neucalm, Quiess, Vamate, Vistacon, Vistaject-25, Vistaject-50, Vistaquel, Vistaril, Vistazine)	Antiemetic: IM 25–100 mg/4–6 hours as needed Antianxiety: 25–100 mg 4 times/day; do not exceed 500 mg/day Preoperative sedation: PO 50–100 mg; one time preoperative IM 20–100 mg
Benzodiazepines	PO	Alprazolam (Xanax)	0.25–0.5 mg 2–3 times/day; maximum 4 mg/day
	PO, IV	Lorazepam (Ativan)	Antiemetic: PO or IV 0.5–2 mg every 4–6 hours as needed Antianxiety: PO 1–10 mg/day usually in 2–3 divided doses; average dose 2–6 mg/day
	PO, IM, IV	Chlordiaxepoxide (Libritabs, Librium, Mitran, Reposans-10)	Anxiety: oral 15–100 mg divided in 3–4 doses/day; IM, IV 50–100 mg initially, followed by 25–50 mg 3–4 times/day as needed Preoperative: 50–100 mg prior to surgery
	PO	Clorazepate dipotassium (Gen-XENE, Tranxene)	7.5–15 mg 2–4 times/day or 11.25–22.5 mg in single dose at bedtime
	PO, IM, IV	Diazepam (Valium, Valrelease, Zetran)	PO 2–10 mg 2–4 times/day; IM, IV 2–10 mg; may repeat every 3–4 hours as needed

Route	Drug	Dosage
PO	Paroxetine (Paxil)	PO 20 mg once daily; give in A.M.; not to exceed 50 mg/day
PO	Oxazepam (Serax)	PO 10–30 mg 3–4 times/day
PO	Prazepam (Centrax)	PO 30 mg/day in divided doses not to exceed 60 mg/day
PO	Meprobamate (Equanil, Meprospan, Miltown, Neuramate)	PO 400 mg 3–4 times/day; do not exceed 2400 mg/day
PO	Clonazepam (Klonopin)	PO initial dose should not exceed 1.5 mg administered in 3 divided doses; average maintenance 0.5–20 mg/day, should not exceed 20 mg/day
PO	Buspirone (BuSpar)	PO 15 mg/day in 3 doses; may increase to maximum 60 mg/day
PO	Halazepam (Paxipam)	PO 20–40 mg 3 times/day; dosage has not been established for patients under 18 years of age
IM, IV	Midazolam hydrochloride (Versed)	IM usual average dose 5 mg 1 hour preprocedure IV 150–350 µg/kg; give over 5- to 30-second periods

Table 10–4. **Minor Tranquilizers: Potential for Side Effects**

Drug Name Generic (Most Commonly Used Trade Name)	Potential Sedation Effect	Possible Side Effects
Hydroxyzine (Atarax)	Moderate	Mild
Alprazolam (Xanax)	Mild	Mild
Lorazepam (Ativan)	Mild	Mild
Chlordiazepoxide (Librium)	Moderate	Moderate
Clorazepate dipotassium (Tranxene)	Mild	Mild
Diazepam (Valium)	Moderate	Moderate
Paroxetine (Paxil)	Mild	Mild
Oxazepam (Serax)	Moderate	Mild
Prazepam (Centrax)	Mild	Mild
Meprobamate (Equanil)	Mild	Mild
Clonazepam (Klonopin)	Mild	Mild
Buspirone (BuSpar)	Moderate	Mild
Halazepam (Paxipam)	Moderate	Moderate
Midazolam hydrochloride (Versed)	High	High

Explain to patients the importance of taking the drug as prescribed and to not to take more of it or take it more often or longer than prescribed. Teach patients not to take this drug with other medicines such as pain medications, sleeping pills, over-the-counter antihistamines, or any other drugs that cause drowsiness or with alcohol.

A patient who forgets a dose and remembers within an hour of the scheduled time should take it. After 1 hour, the patient should skip that dose and resume taking the medication at the next scheduled time. The patient should not double the dose.

Explain that this drug may make patients feel dizzy, drowsy, or sleepy. They must be certain they are sufficiently alert to participate in any activities requiring alertness, such as driving a car or operating mechanical or electrical equipment.

ANTIDEPRESSANTS

Two types of antidepressants have been prescribed for several decades: monoamine oxidase (MAO) inhibitors and tricyclics. However, several types of new antidepressants have been introduced recently, despite the fact that little is known about the specific action of these drugs. Antidepressants work biochemically to elevate patients' mood. They also help to decrease patients' preoccupation with feelings of worthlessness, inadequacy, and hopelessness.

MAO Inhibitors

Because MAO inhibitors tend to produce a number of severe side effects, authorities in psychiatry are questioning their value. Many of these side effects have led to fatalities or to prolonged and serious medical problems. Because these drugs are primarily used to treat depressed patients who often have suicidal tendencies, another drawback occurs. From 1 to 2 weeks of drug therapy are necessary before MAO inhibitors effect behavior change. The suicidal patient needs faster-acting medicine.

Hypertensive (high blood pressure) crises have occurred after patients receiving MAO inhibitors have consumed certain foods such as cheese, bananas, and avocados or beverages such as beer and Chianti. Patients taking MAO inhibitors must also avoid certain other drugs used for relieving colds, hay fever, and nausea. Hypertensive crises may cause severe headaches and intracranial bleeding. Nausea and vomiting, chills and fever, neck stiffness, sensitivity to light, chest pain, and heart arrhythmias may also occur. When any of these symptoms appear, they should be reported immediately, and the drug therapy should be discontinued by the physician.

If the patient suffers from any severe major medical problem and especially if there is a history of impaired kidney function, MAO inhibitors are contraindicated. In addition, MAO inhibitors should not be mixed with other MAO inhibitors and should not be given if the patient is taking alcohol, barbiturates, or morphinelike drugs because they potentiate the action of these drugs. The MAO inhibitors include isocarboxazid (Marplan), phenelzine (Nardil), and tranylcypromine (Parnate).

Cyclic Antidepressants

Cyclic antidepressants are used to elevate the patient's mood and stimulate the patient's activity level. Like the MAO inhibitors, drugs in this

Table 10–5. **Drugs Commonly Used for Depression**

Chemical Classification	Route	Generic Name (Trade Name)	Adult Average Dose for Daily Administration
Bicyclics	PO	Fluoxetine hydrochloride (Prozac)	PO 20 mg/day in A.M.; may be increased over several weeks to a maximum of 80 mg/day in divided doses not to exceed 20 mg/dose
	PO	Trazodone (Desyrel)	PO 50 mg 3 times/day; do not exceed 400 mg/day
Monoamine Oxidase (MAO) inhibitors	PO	Isocarboxazid (Marplan)	PO 10 mg 3 times/day; do not exceed 60 mg/day
	PO	Phenelzine sulfate (Nardil)	PO 15 mg 3 times/day; do not exceed 90 mg/day
	PO	Tranylcypromine sulfate (Parnate)	PO 10 mg twice a day; do not exceed 60 mg/day
Tetracyclics	PO	Maprotiline hydrochloride (Ludiomil)	PO 75 mg/day; do not exceed 225 mg/day
Tricyclics	PO, IM	Amitriptyline hydrochloride (Elavil, Endep, Enovil)	PO 30–100 mg/day at bedtime; may give up to 300 mg/day in divided doses IM 20–30 mg 4 times/day
	PO	Amoxapine (Asendin)	PO 25 mg 2–3 times/day; may increase to 300 mg/day
	PO	Desipramine hydrochloride (Norpramin, Pertofrane)	PO 25 mg 3 times/day; may increase to 300 mg/day

	PO	Doxepin hydrochloride (Adapin, Sinequan)	PO 30–150 mg/day at bedtime; should not exceed 300 mg/day
	PO	Imipramine (Janimine, Tofranil, Tofranil PM)	PO 25 mg 3–4 times/day or total dose at bedtime, not to exceed 300 mg/day
	PO	Nortriptyline hydrochloride (Aventyl, Pamelor)	PO 25 mg 3–4 times/day; do not exceed 150 mg/day
	PO	Protriptyline hydrochloride (Vivactil)	PO 15 mg 3–4 times/day; do not exceed 80 mg/day
	PO	Trimipramine maleate (Surmontil)	PO 50–150 mg/day at bedtime, not to exceed 200 mg/day
Tricyclics	PO	Clomipramine hydrochloride (Anafranil)	PO 25 mg/day; may increase to maximum 250 mg/day
	PO	Sertraline hydrochloride (Zoloft)	PO 50 mg/day single dose; may increase to maximum 200 mg/day
	PO	Bupropion (Wellbutrin)	PO 100 mg 3 times/day; may increase to maximum 450 mg/day
Other	PO	Venlafaxine hydrochloride (Effexor)	PO 75 mg/day given in 2–3 divided doses; may increase to maximum 225 mg/day; however, severely depressed patients may require 375 mg/day given in divided doses

group tend to take 1 to 4 weeks of therapy before significant changes occur in the patient's outlook. Antidepressants are sometimes given in large doses in the afternoon or evening because their sedating effect may facilitate the patient's ability to sleep. Because these drugs sometimes excite patients rather than sedate them, patients must be observed closely for individual reactions.

Common side effects include dry mouth, fatigue, weakness, blurring of vision, constipation, parkinsonian syndrome, and increased perspiration. Most, if not all, of these symptoms can be controlled by lowering the dosage of the medication. Table 10–5 lists some commonly used antidepressants, and Table 10–6 cites their potential for side effects.

Patient Teaching

Provide information to patients about the specific drug. Include the medication's name, action, dose, onset of the effects, and possible side effects. It is particularly important to caution patients to be alert to certain food and drug interactions while using these drugs. For MAO inhibitors, teach patients:

1. Do not take with excessive caffeine or foods containing tyramine or tryptophan, such as bananas. (If possible, have a dietitian visit the patient to provide a full explanation of the food-drug interaction.) Do not take with over-the-counter drugs and many other prescription drugs, such as insulin and oral antidiabetic medications.
2. Do not take with sleeping pills.
3. Do not take with alcohol.
4. The medication may require 2 to 3 weeks to reach therapeutic effectiveness.

For cyclic antidepressants:

1. Explain to patients that maximum therapeutic effectiveness may not occur for 2 to 3 weeks.
2. Help patients' families understand that potential for suicide sometimes increases when the patients' mood elevates enough for them to have enough energy to carry out the process.
3. Teach patients the importance of good oral hygiene because of the drugs' drying effect on the mouth, as well as the importance of a high-fiber diet to counteract the constipating effects of the drugs.

Table 10–6. **Drugs Commonly Used for Depression (Potential for Side Effects)**

Generic Name (Most Commonly Used Brand Name)	Sedative Effects	Potential Anticholinergic Effects
Fluoxetine hydrochloride (Prozac)	Mild	Mild
Trazodone (Desyrel)	Mild	Mild
Isocarboxazid (Marplan)	Mild	Mild
Phenelzine sulfate (Nardil)	Moderate	Moderate
Tranylcypromine sulfate (Parnate)	Moderate	Moderate
Maprotiline hydrochloride (Ludiomil)	Mild	Mild
Amitriptyline hydrochloride (Elavil)	High	High
Amoxapine (Asendin)	Moderate	High
Desipramine hydrochloride (Norpramin)	Mild	Mild
Doxepin hydrochloride (Adapin, Sinequan)	High	Moderate
Imipramine (Tofranil)	Moderate	Moderate
Nortriptyline hydrochloride (Aventyl)	Moderate	Moderate
Protriptyline hydrochloride (Vivactil)	Moderate	Moderate
Trimipramine maleate (Surmontil)	High	Moderate
Clomipramine hydrochloride (Anafranil)	High	High
Sertraline hydrochloride (Zoloft)	Mild	Mild
Bupropion (Wellbutrin)	Moderate	Moderate
Venlafaxine hydrochloride (Effexor)	Mild	Mild

The nurse should teach patients to take these medications with food or after a meal to decrease gastric irritation and, as with major tranquilizers and other medications, stress the importance of taking the medication as prescribed. Explain to the patient the importance of reporting the use of this medication before any type of surgery, including dental surgery.

SEDATIVES AND HYPNOTICS

The barbiturate hypnotics, nonbarbiturate hypnotics, and other sedatives are considered similar in effect to the minor tranquilizers in that they act to reduce anxiety. A main difference in their action is that these drugs, more than the tranquilizers, tend to cause the patient to be sleepier. Barbiturates, however, are much more dangerous because an overdose, whether accidental or planned, can cause death. The barbiturates are also highly addictive and greatly potentiate the action of drugs such as alcoholic beverages and narcotics. Because these drugs, along with the minor tranquilizers, are often used by depressed patients, observe the patient closely for suicidal intentions. When suicidal potential exists, only small amounts of these drugs should be given in order to avoid the deliberate taking of a massive overdose (especially if the patient is an outpatient). It may even be necessary to check the hospitalized patient's mouth carefully to make sure the medication has been swallowed and is not being saved until enough is collected to constitute a deadly overdose. Never leave the medication with a patient to take when the patient is "ready."

Compared with barbiturate hypnotics, the nonbarbiturate hypnotics have less toxic effects if an overdose occurs, are less habit forming, and result in fewer hangovers. They are also less likely to cause "paradoxic excitement" (i.e., rather than calm) in patients who have unusual reactions to drugs. Patients can also develop tolerance or allergic reactions to barbiturates, which makes these drugs ineffective. In that case, nonbarbiturate hypnotics can be safely substituted.

After administration of these drugs, patients should be observed closely for any reactions. If they fall into a deep sleep, they should not be awakened for the next dose. If a patient seems unusually nonresponsive, the next dose of medication should be withheld and the patient's physician notified at once. Elderly patients, especially those with cerebral vascular disease, may react to sedatives and hypnotics in a manner opposite to the desired effect. They may become excited, confused, and try to get up. Maintaining safety may require staying with the patient, talking in a quiet, calm manner, repeating the patient's name, and telling the patient where she or he is, in order to reorient the patient to the environment.

Barbiturates and sedatives, when abused, can cause a certain degree of euphoria; therefore, a patient with a history of alcoholism or drug abuse who is taking any of these drugs over a long period should be carefully observed. Staff members might help the patient learn to handle nervousness with alternative methods, such as listening to music, taking a warm bath at bedtime, or developing a hobby in order to help the patient gradually give up sedatives and tranquilizers. Table 10–7 lists frequently used sedatives and hypnotics.

ANTICONVULSANTS

Anticonvulsants are used to treat various kinds of convulsive seizures. Phenobarbital and phenytoin (Dilantin) are the most commonly used of all anticonvulsant drugs. Phenobarbital often has to be given in doses so large that it produces sleepiness and lethargy. Dilantin is not a hypnotic and is often used in conjunction with phenobarbital in order to allow better control of seizures with fewer sedative side effects. However, Dilantin may cause gastric irritation, dizziness, nausea and vomiting, blurred vision, nervousness, and excessive growth of gum tissue and hair, especially facial hair. Some patients are particularly sensitive to the drug and develop skin rashes, dermatitis, and fever, and some may have difficulty breathing. Such serious side effects as hallucinations, psychosis, hepatitis, and systemic lupus erythematosus have been reported due to Dilantin therapy.

ANTIPARKINSONS

The three antiparkinson drugs frequently used in treating psychiatric patients are diphenhydramine (Benadryl), benztropine (Cogentin), and trihexyphenidyl (Artane). The drugs are used to combat the parkinson-like side effects often produced when the patient is receiving tranquilizers or other antipsychotic drugs. They reduce muscle rigidity, excessive drooling, and sweating. If the dosage is too high, the patient may have difficulty voiding, blurred vision, and dry mouth. Sucking on hard candies is one way patients can avoid oral discomfort.

OTHER DRUGS

Some other drugs are used quite often in the treatment of psychiatric patients and, therefore, are included here.

Flurothyl (Indoklon).
    This drug is a central nervous system stimulant administered by inhalation and used instead of electroconvulsive therapy (ECT) to produce convulsions in depressed patients. Its use for this purpose is not widespread.

Table 10–7. Sedatives and Hypnotics

Chemical Classification	Generic Name (Trade Name)	Route	Adult Average Dose for Daily Administration
Barbiturates	Phenobarbital (Barbita, Luminal, Solfoton)	PO, IM, IV, SC	Sedative PO or IM 30–120 mg/day in 2–3 divided doses Hypnotic PO, IM, IV, SC 100–300 mg at bedtime
	Pentobarbital (Nembutal)	PO, IM, IV, Suppository	PO hypnotic 100–200 mg at bedtime or 20 mg 3–4 times/day IM 150–200 mg IV initial 100 mg; may repeat up to 500 mg Rectal 100–200 mg at bedtime
	Secobarbital sodium (Seconal)	PO, IM, IV	Hypnotic: Oral, IM 100–100 mg at bedtime IV 50–250 mg at bedtime Sedation: Oral 20–40 mg 2–3 times/day
	Amobarbital (Amytal)	PO, IM, IV	PO for insomnia 60–200 mg at bedtime; PO for sedation 30–50 mg/2–3 times a day IM, IV 60–200 mg; do not exceed 500 mg IM or 1000 mg IV
	Butabarbital (Butalan, Buticaps, Butisol sodium)	PO	PO sedative 15–30 mg 3–4 times/day PO hypnotic 50–100 mg at bedtime

PO, IM, IV	Phenobarbital (Luminal sodium)	PO 100–200 mg at bedtime IM, IV 30–120 mg/day in 2–3 divided doses
PO	Estazolam (Prosom)	PO 1 mg at bedtime; may increase to 2 mg
PO	Flurazepam hydrochloride (Dalmane)	PO 15–30 mg at bedtime
PO	Quazepam (Doral)	PO 7.5–15 mg at bedtime
PO	Temazepam (Restoril)	PO 15–30 mg at bedtime
PO	Triazolam (Halcion)	PO 0.125–0.25 mg at bedtime
PO	Chloral hydrate (Aquachloral, Supprettes, Noctec)	Sedation 250–1000 mg/day in 3–4 doses Hypnotic 500–1000 mg at bedtime or prior to a procedure
PO	Ethchlorvynol (Placidyl)	PO 500–1000 mg at bedtime
PO	Glutethimide (Doriden)	PO 250–500 mg at bedtime

Lithium carbonate.
This drug is used in the treatment of manic-depressive psychoses because it is effective in decreasing the manic patient's excessive motor activity, talking, and unstable behavior by acting on the patient's brain metabolism. Patients should be observed for the following signs of lithium intoxication: nausea, vomiting, diarrhea, sudden loss of appetite, drowsiness, muscle weakness, and poor motor coordination. If these symptoms occur, discontinuation of the drug is required. Knowing that this drug acts on brain metabolism and seeing it drastically improve patient behavior lead many authorities to believe that many psychiatric disorders may be due to faulty metabolism and thus may someday be curable through drug therapy.

Methohexital (Brevital).
This rapid-acting, ultra-short-acting barbiturate is administered IV; it is used to induce light surgical anesthesia before ECT treatments.

Succinylcholine (Anectine).
This drug is used to produce skeletal muscle relaxation prior to ECT treatment.

GENERAL CONSIDERATIONS

Drug therapy is not a cure for mental illness; at best, it is only an adjunct to psychotherapy and other treatment methodologies. It is important, however, because it allows many patients to control symptoms to such a degree that they can function as effective members of society. Just as diabetics may be required to take insulin for the rest of their lives in order to survive, many mentally ill patients must take psychotropic drugs on a long-term basis.

Because many of these drugs are relatively new, these patients should be watched for unexpected side effects and complications. Families are usually interested in patients' progress and should be actively involved in the care plan. Patients should assume the responsibility for taking their own medications at home and should learn the correct amount and frequency of doses from the staff. The staff should also explain to the patient that many of the medications taken are effective because a certain amount of the drug (blood level) is constantly in one's system. Skipping a dose or stopping the medication lowers the blood level, and the medication may become ineffective. Many patients stop taking their medications as soon as they feel better because they believe they are cured. Unfortunately, they fail to realize that the medication has brought about much of their improvement and that a relapse will occur if they stop taking their prescribed drugs.

Patients and their families should be well informed concerning possible side effects and know to report them to the staff as soon as they appear. Most patients will cooperate about taking medication if they know how it will help and why it is being given.

SPECIFIC NURSING CONSIDERATIONS

Major Tranquilizers

1. Responses are highly individualized, and finding the lowest effective dose for the patient is important. In addition, many signs and symptoms are dose-related.
2. Bed rails may be needed for the first few days of therapy because of the hypotensive reactions, drowsiness, and dizziness that may occur in initial attempts to stabilize a dosage.
3. Phenothiazine drugs are not stable when mixed with other medications. Do not mix unless approved by the pharmacist.
4. When giving phenothiazines IM, inject them deeply and slowly to prevent tissue irritation and avoid injection into the subcutaneous tissue.
5. Urinary retention and constipation may occur. Record intake and output.
6. Upon discharge, explain the following to the patient:
   a. Importance of taking medication as ordered to maintain a therapeutic blood level.
   b. Tolerance can develop, but most medications do not produce physical dependence.
   c. Refrain from activities requiring mental alertness and coordination until reevaluation by the physician.
   d. If in liquid form, medication is sensitive to light and must be kept out of direct sunlight.
   e. Medication may turn urine pink to reddish brown.
   f. Patients should carry identification indicating they are receiving phenothiazine medication.
   g. A physician should be consulted if the patient becomes pregnant or intends to become pregnant.
   h. Teach patients that if they miss a dose, to take the dose as soon as possible. More than 1 hour past the dose time, patients should skip the dose and take the next scheduled dose.

    i. Teach patients that they should not take more of the medicine than prescribed nor take it more often than prescribed.

    j. Remind patients to keep follow-up appointments as recommended by their physician. The primary reason is to allow the physician to monitor possible side effects and to gauge the effectiveness of medications.

    k. Stress that patients should not stop taking medications without consulting their physician.

    l. Make *certain* that the patient understands not to drink alcoholic beverages or take other CNS depressants while taking major tranquilizers.

    m. Stress to patients the importance of not sharing their medications with family members or friends. The medicine was prescribed by their physician only after considering that particular patient's medical condition. That same medication might be harmful to someone else.

Minor Tranquilizers

1. Unlike major tranquilizers, the possibility of physical and psychological dependence is always present.

2. Alcohol should be avoided by patients who are taking these drugs, which augment the depressant effects of alcohol.

3. In prolonged chlordiazepoxide (Librium) therapy, periodic blood cell counts and liver function tests are recommended.

4. Prepare IM Librium immediately before administration and dispose of unused portion.

5. Intravenous diazepam (Valium) cannot be mixed with other drugs or any type of solution. It therefore cannot be added to IV fluids. Administer IV Valium slowly, taking at least 1 minute for each 5 mg (1 mL).

6. After prolonged administration of Valium or Librium, withdrawal symptoms may occur.

7. Upon discharge, make the following directives clear to the patient:

    a. Take the medication only as directed by the physician. Do not take more than prescribed or more often than prescribed.

    b. Even if the patient thinks the medicine is not working, the dosage should not be increased without talking to the physician.

    c. Patients who are taking a medication on a regularly scheduled basis and miss a dose should take the dose as soon as possible.

More than 1 hour past the dose time, the dose should be skipped, and the next scheduled dose should be taken.
d. Report side effects to the physician.
e. After stopping this medication, the body may take up to 3 weeks to adjust. During that time the patient may experience minor withdrawal symptoms.
f. Never share medications with family or friends. The medication might be harmful to another person with different medical problems or who is taking other medications.

Antidepressants

1. Instruct patients which foods to avoid when taking MAO inhibitors.
2. Warn patients against mixing medications with over-the-counter items such as cough syrup.
3. Monitor effectiveness of the drug as evidenced by patients' renewed interest in themselves and their surroundings. Therapeutic response is very variable, occurring sometime from 2 days to 2 months.
4. When patients begin to show renewed interest, evaluate and supervise patients because the risk of suicide increases when the medication helps patients feel strong enough to carry out suicidal plans.
5. Patients may require assistance in getting in the upright position during the initial stage of therapy because of orthostatic hypotension.
6. Upon discharge, make the following directives clear to the patient:
   a. Notify physician of any plans to become pregnant.
   b. Take the medication only as directed by the physician. Do not take more than prescribed or more often than prescribed.
   c. Even if the medicine does not seem to be working, do not increase the dosage without talking to the physician.
   d. Patients who are taking a medication on a regularly scheduled basis and miss a dose should take the dose as soon as possible. More than 1 hour past the dose time, the dose should be skipped and the next scheduled dose taken.
   e. Report side effects to the physician.
   f. Never share medications with family or friends. The medication might be harmful to another person with different medical problems or who is taking other medications.
   g. If the medication causes stomach upset, take it with food.

   h. Stress to patients that it may take 3 to 4 weeks for them to feel the benefit of the medication.
   i. This medicine may cause drowsiness. Patients should determine their response to this medication before driving or doing anything else requiring mental alertness.
   j. Patients should get up slowly because dizziness, fainting, or light-headedness may occur upon rising.

Sedatives and Hypnotics

1. Barbiturates, especially short-acting ones, may cause dependence: if this occurs, withdrawal may be very serious.
2. Patients should be informed that taking these drugs with each other or with alcohol may be fatal and should be completely avoided.
3. Barbiturates significantly reduce the effectiveness of oral anticoagulants, and these drugs should not be given together.
4. Discourage patients from mixing these drugs with any over-the-counter drugs, especially drugs such as antihistamines, which can give additive central nervous system depression.
5. Caution patients against abruptly discontinuing these drugs because withdrawal symptoms may occur.
6. Encourage patients to try relaxation exercises or other means of decreasing stress before using these drugs, which are habit forming.
7. Upon discharge, make the following directives clear to the patient:
   a. Notify the physician of any plans to become pregnant.
   b. Take the medication only as directed by the physician. Do not take more than prescribed or more often than prescribed.
   c. Even if the medicine does not seem to be working, do not increase the dosage without talking to the physician.
   d. Patients who are taking a medication on a regularly scheduled basis and miss a dose should take the dose as soon as possible. More than 1 hour past the dose time, the dose should be skipped and the next scheduled dose taken.
   e. Report side effects to the physician.
   f. Never share medications with family or friends. The medication might be harmful to another person with different medical problems or who is taking other medications.
   g. This medicine may cause drowsiness. Patients should

determine their response to this medication before driving or doing anything else requiring mental alertness.

h. Patients should get up slowly because dizziness, fainting, or light-headedness may occur upon rising.

i. Patients who are discharged with a prescription for sleeping pills should not leave the pill bottle at the bedside to avoid accidental overdose. Patients who think they may have taken an overdose must call an emergency number such as 911 and get immediate help; overdose may lead to death.

j. Birth control pills containing estrogen may not work effectively for women who are taking barbiturates. Other means of birth control should be used.

k. Be aware that long-term use may cause dependence. Dependence may be recognized by a strong desire for the drug or a need to increase the dosage for the desired effect.

Anticonvulsants

1. Include patients and their families in health teaching on use of the medication as a part of the therapeutic regimen.

2. Upon discharge, make the following directives clear to the patient:

   a. To avoid gastrointestinal problems, take medication with fluids or food.

   b. Continue under medical supervision and do the scheduled laboratory testing to monitor blood levels. Toxicity may develop without proper follow-up.

   c. Be aware of conditions that lower the seizure threshold, such as fever and low blood sugar.

   d. Notify the physician of any plans to become pregnant.

   e. Take the medication only as directed by the physician. Do not take more than prescribed or more often than prescribed.

   f. Even if the medicine does not seem to be working, do not increase the dosage without talking to the physician.

   g. Patients who are taking this medication only once a day and miss a dose should take the dose as soon as possible unless it is the following day. In that case, skip the missed dose and take the next dose as scheduled. Never double the dose. Patients who are taking the medication more than once a day who miss a dose should take the missed dose as soon as possible unless the next dose is within 4 hours. In that case, skip the missed dose and take the next scheduled dose.

    h. Report side effects to the physician. Do not change brands of anticonvulsant medication without consulting the physician.

    i. Never share medications with family or friends. The medication might be harmful to another person with different medical problems or who is taking other medications.

    j. Birth control pills containing estrogen may not work effectively for women who are taking anticonvulsants. Other means of birth control should be used.

    k. Do not take antacids within 4 hours of taking an anticonvulsant because they reduce the anticonvulsant's effectiveness.

Antiparkinsons

1. It sometimes takes 2 or 3 days for these medications to reach therapeutic effectiveness.
2. Monitor intake and output because oliguria can interfere with the excretion of these drugs.
3. Most antiparkinson drugs should be given after meals.
4. Upon discharge, make the following directives clear to the patient:

    a. Notify the physician of any plans to become pregnant.

    b. Take the medication only as directed by the physician. Do not take more than prescribed or more often than prescribed.

    c. Even if the medicine does not seem to be working, do not increase the dosage without talking to the physician.

    d. Patients who are taking an antiparkinson medication on a regularly scheduled basis and miss a dose should take the dose as soon as possible unless it is within 2 hours of the next scheduled dose.

    e. Report side effects to the physician.

    f. Never share medications with family or friends. The medication might be harmful to another person with different medical problems or who is taking other medications.

    g. This medicine may cause drowsiness. Patients should know their response to this medication before driving or doing anything else requiring mental alertness.

    h. This medication may reduce patients' tolerance to heat because they sweat less. Therefore, use caution not to become overheated.

    This chapter does not have a summary of key points as found in other chapters. Instead, the drug tables serve to summarize the pharmacological content of this chapter.

Annotated Bibliography

Carey, N., Jones, S. L., and O'Toole, A. W.: Do you feel powerless when a patient refuses medication? *Journal of Psychosocial Nursing and Mental Health Services,* 1990, 28(10):19–25.

Explores the issue of the right of patients to refuse medication and the nurse's feelings of powerlessness when this occurs.

Chapman, T.: The nurse's role in neuroleptic medications. *Journal of Psychosocial Nursing and Mental Health Services,* 1991, 29(6):6–8.

Relates the possible side effects of neuroleptic medications and explores the issue of whether the drawbacks to the medication outweigh the benefits.

Chatterton, R. Clozaril: An Australian experience. *Journal of Psychosocial Nursing,* 1995, 33(4):24–27.

Discusses the reintroduction of clozaril, an antipsychotic medication, and its possible side effects.

Dauner, A., and Blair, D. T.: Akathisia: When treatment creates a problem. *Journal of Psychosocial Nursing and Mental Health Services,* 1990, 28(10):13–18.

Explores the symptoms and dangers of akathisia, an extrapyramidal symptom that is a side effect of antipsychotic medications.

Gamage, C. A., and Plant, L. D.: Fluoxetine, electroconvulsive therapy, and prolonged seizures. *Journal of Psychosocial Nursing,* 1995, 33(2):24–26.

This study concludes that patients who had ECT after 14 days' absence from Prozac had no prolonged seizure activity.

Long, K., and Long, R.: Treating obsessive-compulsive disorder. *Nurse Practitioner,* 1995, 6(3):136–137.

Discusses using serotonin-reuptake inhibitors as a treatment for obsessive-compulsive disorder.

Lund, V. E., and Frank, D. I.: Helping the medicine go down: Nurses' and patients' perceptions about medication compliance. *Journal of Psychosocial Nursing and Mental Health Services,* 1991, 29(7):6–9.

Research study on the perceptions of psychiatric patients as compared with the perceptions of nurses on medication compliance.

Natvig, D.: The role of the interdisciplinary team in using psychotropic drugs. *Journal of Psychosocial Nursing and Mental Health Services,* 1991, 29(10):3–8.

Addresses the effectiveness of the team approach in the use of psychotropic drugs as a treatment plan.

Sachdev, P. S.: Psychoactive drug use in an institution for intellectually handicapped persons. *The Medical Journal of Australia,* 1991, 155:75–79.

Research study examining the use of psychoactive drugs for the treatment of long-stay developmentally disabled patients in an institution.

Scahill, L., and Lynch, C. A.: Tricyclic antidepressants: Cardiac effects and clinical implications. *Journal of Child and Psychiatric Nursing,* 1994, 7(1):37–39.

Reviews cardiac effects of tricyclic antidepressants when they are used with children.

Taylor, D.: Following serotonin pathways in the central nervous system. *Nursing,* 1995, 25(4):36.

Discusses the biologic mechanisms of serotonin.

Wilkerson, L.: A collaborative model: Ambulatory pharmacotherapy for chronic psychiatric patients. *Journal of Psychosocial Nursing and Mental Health Services,* 1991, 29(12):26–29.

Discusses the use of the medication clinic and medication group to shift the responsibility for medication management to the patient and family through education and participation.

References

Deglin, J. H., and Vallerand, A. H.: *Davis's Drug Guide for Nurses* (ed. 5). Philadelphia: F. A. Davis Co., 1997.
Lacy, C., Armstrong, L., Lipsey, R., and Lance, L.: *Drug Information Handbook* (ed. 2). Hudson, Ohio: Lexi-Comp, 1994–95.

Post-Test

Matching. Match the letter of the appropriate item in column B with the descriptive statements in column A.

Column A	Column B
1. Helps control severe agitation.	A. Antidepressants
	B. Lithium
2. Helps elevate the patient's mood.	C. Major tranquilizers
3. Combats parkinson-like side effects.	D. Indoklon
	E. Antiparkinson
4. Used in treatment of manic depressives.	F. Anectine
5. Produces skeletal muscle relaxation prior to ECT.	

Matching. Match the letter of the appropriate item in column B with the drugs in column A. (Letters in column B may be used more than once.)

Column A	Column B
1. Valium	A. Major tranquilizer
	B. Antiparkinson
2. Tofranil	C. Anticonvulsant
3. Dalmane	D. Antidepressant
	E. Minor tranquilizer
4. Vistaril	F. Sedative-hypnotic
5. Cogentin	
6. Compazine	
7. Dilantin	
8. Aventyl	
9. Mellaril	

Post-Test

(continued)

True or False. Circle your choice.

T   F   1. Phenothiazines are a cure for mental illness.

T   F   2. The phenothiazine derivatives are the largest group of antipsychotic drugs.

T   F   3. Increased sexual interest is a major problem with patients who are receiving phenothiazines.

T   F   4. One of the main difficulties in using minor tranquilizers is that they tend to be habit forming.

T   F   5. An MAO inhibitor is usually given with another MAO inhibitor to achieve the desired effect.

T   F   6. Patients no longer need to take their medication when they feel better.

Short Answers. Answer the following questions as briefly and specifically as possible.

1. What effect might one expect the tranquilizers to have on a patient?

_____

_____

_____

2. If a patient is having an autonomic reaction to a medication, what is the nursing responsibility?

_____

_____

3. What are the two categories of antidepressants?

_____

_____

4. What are the common side effects to watch for in a patient receiving a tricyclic antidepressant?

_____

_____

Post-Test

(continued)

Multiple Choice. Circle the number or letter you think represents the best answer.

1. Which side effects are characteristic of lithium carbonate?
   a. Diarrhea.
   b. Nausea and vomiting.
   c. Excessive thirst.
   d. Muscle weakness and motor incoordination.
   e. Loss of appetite.
      (1) b and d.
      (2) a, b, and c.
      (3) a, d, and e.
      (4) All of the above.

2. Parkinson-like symptoms that occur as a side effect of the phenothiazine drugs can best be controlled by:
   a. Mellaril.
   b. Colace.
   c. Artane.
   d. Cogentin.
   e. Compazine.
      (1) a only.
      (2) b and e.
      (3) c and e.
      (4) b and d.
      (5) c and d.

3. Jaundice, photosensitivity, and parkinsonian syndrome may occur in patients receiving:
   a. Valium.
   b. Elavil.
   c. Miltown.
   d. Thorazine.

4. Which of the following are true of extrapyramidal symptoms?
   a. They may appear after a single dose of the phenothiazines.
   b. They may appear after prolonged administration of the phenothiazines.
   c. They indicate that the phenothiazines are affecting the deeper brain centers.

Post-Test

(continued)

   d. They are not controllable.
   e. They are fatal.
     (1) a, d, and e.
     (2) a, b, and c.
     (3) a and d.
     (4) b and c.
     (5) a and c.

5. The time required to reach an effective blood level of antidepressant medication is:
   a. 24 hours.
   b. 2 days.
   c. 2 weeks.
   d. 30 days.

6. Side effects from antipsychotic agents such as Thorazine include:
   a. Extrapyramidal symptoms.
   b. Mental confusion.
   c. Hypotension.
   d. Habituation.
   e. Dryness of the mouth.
     (1) a, b, and c.
     (2) a, c, and d.
     (3) a, b, and d.
     (4) a, c, and e.
     (5) All of these.

7. In administering medications on a psychiatric service, one should:
   a. Check identification by reading the identification bracelet.
   b. Carry only one drug at a time on a tray.
   c. Mix poorly accepted medications in food or drink.
   d. Inspect the mouth of the patient who is likely or suspected to hoard medications to be sure the medications are swallowed.
     (1) a and b.
     (2) a and d.
     (3) a, c, and d.
     (4) All of the above.

Electroconvulsive Therapy

OBJECTIVES: Student will be able to:

1. Describe two theories about why ECT works.
2. List diagnostic tests necessary before administering ECT.
3. List general guidelines for caring for the patient before ECT.
4. List general guidelines for caring for the patient after ECT.

This chapter discusses the technique of electroconvulsive shock therapy, sometimes called ECT or EST. This controversial treatment was introduced by Ugo Cerletti and Lucio Bini of Rome in the late 1930s. Physicians have continued to refine this technique and now administer muscle relaxants and anesthesia prior to the treatment to reduce the violent aspects of the patient's convulsion. Fractures and contusions often occurred before such medications were used. When treatments include muscle relaxants and anesthesia, only a slight tremor in the patient's hands and feet, lasting approximately 1 to 2 minutes, is visible. Patients do not remember treatment activities, and the only pain they experience is an occasional post-ECT headache.

Although no one is certain why ECT works, two theories are frequently offered: One suggests that ECT breaks up neural patterns or memory traces in the brain and thus permits patients to forget, or at least think less about, the painful aspects of their life experiences. The other suggests that patients who receive ECT treatments perceive them as a form of punishment and thus improve after treatment because they feel they have been punished for unacceptable thoughts or actions. This latter theory gains much of its support from the fact that ECT seems to work most effectively with depressed patients. As previously discussed, depressed patients frequently have severe guilt feelings. Perhaps ECT reduces guilt by causing the patients to feel that they have "paid" for all their sins. Nevertheless, these explanations are only theories about why ECT is effective, and the authors know of no conclusive research demonstrating that either theory is anything more than educated speculation.

Although ECT treatments are done on a routine basis in many hospitals, the procedure is potentially dangerous and administering it requires a great deal of care. All of the following tests or procedures should be completed, prior to the first treatment, for any patient scheduled for ECT:

1. A thorough physical examination including:
   a. Blood chemistry or biochemical profile to determine any unsuspected conditions that require treatment prior to the ECT.
   b. A complete blood count (CBC) to identify any infection.
   c. A urinalysis to check the specific gravity and look for dehydration or the presence of blood cells indicating a urinary tract infection.
2. A thorough mental status examination.
3. An electrocardiogram (ECG) because ECT places a great deal of strain on a patient's heart and also to rule out heart disease, hypertension, and lung disease.
4. Chest and lumbosacral (spinal) x-ray films, along with routine blood studies, to determine if any abnormalities exist.
5. An electroencephalogram (EEG) to determine whether abnormal electrical activities are already occurring in the patient's brain. If organic brain disease is possible, a complete skull x-ray series and a brain scan are also completed.

If any significant abnormality is discovered, the physician will likely choose another treatment method. However, in some cases (e.g., chronic suicidal patients), a physician may decide that the need for the treatment outweighs the potential risks involved.

The 1985 National Institute of Mental Health Consensus Panel on ECT also recommended that ECT be limited primarily to treating depressed patients. Depressed patients, patients with involutional melancholia, and manic-depressive patients seem to be most effectively treated with ECT. These same patients are most likely to experience significant guilt feelings and to be anxious and worried. Because they may have heard inaccurate and terrifying stories about ECT and because their physician has reviewed the real dangers, these patients are often extremely anxious about ECT treatments. They require considerable support and encouragement from the staff. They are likely to need to spend a good bit of time just talking about the procedure to openly explore their anxieties and feelings with a staff member who is familiar with the procedure and who can be friendly, informative, supportive, and attentive. Pre-ECT care and support are a vital aspect of the total treatment procedure.

Some questions frequently asked by persons who are to receive ECT treatments follow. The answers given are by no means the only appropriate answers. A nurse's answers may also vary in order to comply with the rules and procedures of a particular institution.

Will I feel any pain?

The only discomfort you might feel would be from the shot that will be given to you immediately prior to the treatment. You will not feel the electricity, and you will not remember anything that happens. You may feel some muscle stiffness for a few hours after the treatment, but usually a warm bath and a little exercise will make you feel much better. Some patients have a post-ECT headache that lasts for a few hours.

Will I die?

No. There is some risk associated with any treatment procedure, but this treatment is safe because we take a great deal of care to be sure that you are able to tolerate the treatment.

Is there a possibility that I could be electrocuted?

It is not possible for you to be electrocuted. The machines used produce only a very small amount of electrical current that is not enough to electrocute you.

How many treatments will I have to take?

The number of treatments you will receive will depend on what your physician thinks is best and on the progress you make after each treatment. Usually 8 to 12 treatments are used.

Will I lose my memory?

People usually do not remember the treatment itself and may be confused for a few hours or even a few days after ECT treatments; however, there is rarely any permanent memory loss, and you will probably remember everything you want to remember within a few days to a few weeks after treatment.

Will my mind be ruined?

No. Most people are able to do things as well or better than they could before the treatment. Immediately following the treatments you may be confused, but the confusion will usually go away within a short period of time.

PROCEDURAL GUIDELINES

The major tasks that need to be accomplished when a patient is to receive ECT follow. These are general guidelines and the particular policies and procedures of each institution must be taken into account.

Pretreatment

1. At some point prior to the ECT treatment, the physician should discuss the patient's health status with the patient and explain the ECT procedure and its risks. The explanation should include diagnosis, prognosis, complete explanation for the procedure, purpose and benefits, risks involved, and all alternative treatments that are available. After being informed, the patient is asked to sign a permit or consent form. The purpose is to ensure that patients understand all ramifications of their choices. In addition, this permit somewhat helps the nurse and physician in the event a legal suit is filed in which the patient or family claims the procedure was unnecessary or unexplained.

   Adult patients and married children under the legal age may sign their own permits. Adult guardians must sign a permit for children under the legal age. However, seldom is ECT the treatment of choice for children.

   This permit must be witnessed and dated and is part of the patient's legal record. It accompanies the patient to the surgical suite or treatment room where the treatment will be performed.

2. Prior to treatment, patients must have certain diagnostic tests to ensure that they are sufficiently physiologically stable to handle the ECT treatment. Nurses should have an understanding of the tests and the normal and abnormal values so that the physician can be notified prior to the scheduled treatment if any test results do not fall within the normal range.

3. The patient has to be without food or water (NPO) for at least 8 hours before treatment. This requirement should be carefully explained to the patient. If the patient is at all confused, disoriented, or noncompliant, monitoring may be necessary to ensure that the patient remains NPO. Sometimes patients who are ambivalent about receiving ECT express their ambivalence in efforts to sabotage the NPO rule and thus delay the onset of treatments. This problem likely means the patient has not been properly emotionally prepared for the treatments.

Because many ECTs are done on an outpatient basis, family assistance is needed to help the patient maintain the NPO status. In addition, ECTs have a cumulative effect, and the patient who is receiving a series of treatments frequently becomes progressively confused and cannot be relied on not to eat or drink during the NPO period.

4. Patients should be given ample opportunity to ask questions and express their anxieties. They are likely to be quite anxious and upset prior to treatment and may ask the same questions several times. Members of the treatment team must be supportive during this period and patiently answer any questions a patient might ask, regardless of how many times the question is repeated.

5. Just prior to the treatment, ask the patient to void. Any discomfort and embarrassment the patient might experience from becoming incontinent during the treatment is thus reduced. All watches, rings, hairpins, jewelry, and the like should be removed from the patient and placed in a valuables envelope. Such items may cause burns or be lost during or after the treatment procedure. Post-ECT confusion prevents many patients from remembering what they did with their valuables. Care should be taken to protect their valuables and to reassure them that they are not lost.

6. All objects that are removable should be taken from the mouth (e.g. chewing gum, bridges, dentures) to prevent the patient from aspirating these items during the treatment. Contact lenses should be removed also.

7. Pre-ECT medication is administered by the member of the treatment team responsible for that particular task. This medication must be the accurate amount and given as close to the time specified by the order as possible. The patient may complain of a dry mouth.

Treatment

1. To make sure it is available and functioning properly, all equipment to be used during the treatment, including the ECT machine, oxygen equipment, emergency cart, and any emergency trays that might be necessary in case of complications, should be carefully checked. The patient should be accompanied to the treatment room and asked to lie on the stretcher or operating table where the treatment is to be given. The safety straps should be secured. The straps should be snug enough to keep the patient from falling from the table but loose enough to allow for slight

movement when the seizure occurs. Some institutions may require the patient to wear a hospital gown during this procedure.

2. The patient's temporal area, where the surfaces of the electrodes will be placed, should be cleaned prior to treatment. Treatments may be administered by applying electrodes to either one or both temporal areas, depending upon the physician's choice of technique. Because cleansing solutions may vary, check the institution's procedures manual for specific instructions. Usually a special paste is applied to the skin of the temporal area in order to keep the electrodes from burning the skin on which the electrical activity occurs. After the treatment, this paste should be removed with warm water to keep it from caking on the patient's hair and skin.

3. After the operative medication is administered, an airway of some type is generally put into the patient's mouth in order to ensure that the patient will continue to have an open airway.

4. A physician should administer the shock. As soon as the electrical current hits the brain, the patient has a grand mal type of seizure. Thanks to the use of muscle relaxants and anesthesia, the seizures are generally very mild. However, two healthcare workers should be present to help hold the patient on the stretcher or table if the need arises. Care should be taken not to constrict patients' movements any more than is necessary to ensure that they do not hurt themselves by hitting themselves or by falling off the table.

5. After the patient has regained consciousness and the physician has determined that the patient is having no difficulty breathing, the patient should be removed to a recovery area. Someone should stay with patients at all times until they are fully conscious.

Post-Treatment

1. After the patient has regained consciousness and is able to stand and move about, a warm bath or mild exercise may relieve soreness in muscles and joints. Patients should also be given a light breakfast such as coffee, juice, and toast because they were NPO several hours prior to treatment. Many physicians routinely request that 10 grains of aspirin be given to their patients as soon as they are fully recovered to relieve post-ECT headaches.

2. Patients may be confused after ECT treatments and thus require a great deal of supervision, assistance, and reassurance. Answer any questions, and be as supportive and attentive as possible.

3. Sometimes, even after one or more treatments, patients may be very uncertain of themselves and may develop or retain anxieties about ECT treatment. In such cases, continual reassurance, support, and attentiveness are necessary to help patients deal with their anxieties about ECT treatments.

4. Because ECTs are frequently done on an outpatient basis, the patient's family must understand that constant attendance may be necessary, possibly for several weeks, depending upon the number of ECTs administered and the patient's level of confusion. The patient should not drive an automobile and may even need assistance initially with activities of daily living such as dressing and grooming. However, this inability is temporary, and the confusion should begin to clear within weeks.

▼ KEY POINTS ▼

1. One theory of ECT suggests that it works by breaking up neural patterns or memory traces in the brain and thus permits the patient to forget or at least think less about the painful aspects of life experiences. A second theory suggests that patients who receive ECT treatments perceive them as a form of punishment and thus improve after treatment because they feel they have been punished for unacceptable thoughts or actions.

2. Because the procedure is potentially dangerous if not done properly, all of the following tests should be completed on any patient scheduled for ECT prior to the first treatment:
   a. A thorough physical examination.
   b. A thorough mental examination.
   c. An ECG because ECT places a great deal of strain on a patient's heart.
   d. Chest and lumbosacral (spinal) x-ray films, along with routine blood studies, are usually obtained.
   e. An EEG to check for any abnormal electrical activities already occurring in the patient's brain. If organic brain disease is possible, a complete skull x-ray film series is also completed, along with a brain scan.

3. Depressed patients, patients with involutional melancholia, and manic-depressive patients seem to be those most effectively treated with ECT.

---

continued on page 238

Key Points continued

4. Patients receiving ECT require considerable support and encouragement from the staff, including an opportunity to openly explore their anxieties and feelings with a staff member who is familiar with the procedure and can be friendly, informative, supportive, and attentive.

5. Pretreatment procedural guidelines
    a. At some point prior to the ECT treatment, written, informed consent must be obtained from the patient.
    b. Several hours before the ECT treatment, the patient's chart should be checked to see that pretreatment procedures have been completed.
    c. The patient needs to be without food or water for at least 8 hours before treatment.
    d. Patients should be given ample opportunity to ask questions and express their anxieties.
    e. Just prior to the treatment, ask the patient to void.
    f. All hairpins, jewelry, and the like should be removed from the patient and placed in a valuables envelope.
    g. All objects that are removable should be taken from the mouth; contact lenses should be removed also.
    h. Pre-ECT medication is administered.

6. Post-treatment procedural guidelines
    a. After regaining consciousness, the patient should be given a warm bath or mild exercise. Patients should also be given a light breakfast and may receive 10 grains of aspirin as soon as they are fully recovered.
    b. Patients may be confused after ECT treatments and thus require a great deal of supervision, assistance, and reassurance.
    c. If the patients develop or retain anxieties about having ECT treatment, continual reassurance, support, and attentiveness are necessary to help them deal with their anxieties about ECT treatments.

Annotated Bibliography

DeVane, C. L., Lim, C., Carson, S., Tingle, D., Hackett, L., and Ware, M.:
  Effect of electroconvulsive therapy on serum concentration of alpha-1-acid
  glycoprotein. *Journal of Biological Psychiatry,* 1991, 30:116–120.

Research study examining the effect of ECT on alpha-1-acid glycoprotein and the
potential effect this may have on patients receiving both ECT and cyclic
antidepressants for treatment of depression.

Douyon, R., Serby, M., Klutchko, B., and Rotrosen, J.: ECT and Parkinson's
  disease revisited: A "naturalistic" study. *American Journal of Psychiatry,*
  1989, 146(11):1451–1455.

Research study examining the possible therapeutic effects of ECT on Parkinson's
disease.

Gamage, C. A., and Plant, L. D.: Fluoxetine, electroconvulsive therapy, and
  prolonged seizures. *Journal of Psychosocial Nursing,* 1995, 33(2):24–26.

Discusses the absence of prolonged seizures when the patient abstains from the
use of Prozac 14 days prior to having ECT.

Hertzman, M.: ECT and neuroleptics as primary treatment for schizophrenia.
  Journal of Biological Psychiatry, 1992, 31:217–220.

Discusses the advantages of ECT as a treatment for schizophrenia and its use in
conjunction with neuroleptics.

Krystal, A., Weiner, R., Coffey, C., Smith, P., Arias, R., and Moffett, E.: EEG
  evidence of more "intense" seizure activity with bilateral ECT. *Journal of
  Biological Psychiatry,* 1992, 31:617–621.

Research study testing the ability to separate unilateral and bilateral ECT seizures
in order to better characterize seizure generalization, which may be an important
factor in the determination of adequacy.

Scott, A., Gow, S., Garden, W., Shering, P., and Whalley, L.: Repeated ECT
  and prolactin release in depressed patients. *Journal of Biological
  Psychiatry,* 1992, 31:613–616.

Research study testing prolactin release over a course of ECT in depressed
patients who were not receiving neuroleptic drugs in order to evaluate whether
prolactin release lessens over the course of ECT treatment.

Post-Test

True or False. Circle your choice.

T   F   1. ECT is a simple procedure with no risks involved.

T   F   2. Legal consent from the patient is not necessary before ECT is administered.

T   F   3. It is necessary for the patient to go without food or water for 8 hours before an ECT treatment.

T   F   4. When the electric current reaches the brain, the patient has a petit mal type of seizure.

T   F   5. After an ECT treatment, a patient may be confused and need a great deal of supervision, assistance, and reassurance.

T   F   6. If a patient seems very embarrassed to remove his dentures before an ECT treatment, it is all right for the patient to leave the dentures in.

Short Answer. Answer the following questions as briefly and specifically as possible.

1. Give two commonly expressed theories as to why ECT is effective.

_____

_____

_____

2. Why is an ECG completed before the patient receives ECT treatment?

_____

_____

_____

3. Which psychiatric diagnostic category seems to show the best improvement after receiving ECT?

_____

_____

Post-Test

(continued)

4. Why is it necessary to remove dentures and bridges from the patient's mouth prior to ECT?

_____

_____

_____

Multiple Choice. Circle the letter or number you think represents the best answer.

1. Mrs. Jones is a patient who is scheduled for shock treatment. Miss Smith, a student nurse, becomes very anxious and is unable to help with the treatment. What mental mechanism is at work?
   a. Identification
   b. Denial
   c. Regression
   d. Suppression

2. Which of the following physical complications never occurs as a result of ECT?
   a. Dislocated jaw
   b. Compression fractures
   c. Respiratory arrest
   d. Electrocution
   e. Cardiac arrest

3. ECT is most effective in the treatment of:
   a. Depression.
   b. Neuroses.
   c. Catatonic schizophrenia.
   d. Personality disorders.
      (1) a and b.
      (2) a and c.
      (3) b and c.
      (4) All of the above.

Post-Test

(continued)

4. An appropriate approach to patients complaining of amnesia following ECT is to:
   a. Explain that forgetting is the usual reaction, which will clear up after the treatments are finished.
   b. Help them remember those things they have forgotten.
   c. Tell them that the amnesia will subside in a few hours.
   d. Tell them that the amnesia is selective and that they will not forget important things.

5. If Mr. Brown is treated with ECT, the nurse should:
   a. Take measures to prevent physical injury, especially fractures.
   b. Provide a secure pretreatment and post-treatment environment.
   c. Monitor vital signs.
   d. Remain with the patient during his confused state.
   e. Assure the patient that he will not notice any memory loss.
      (1) a and c.
      (2) c, d, and e.
      (3) a, b, c, and d.
      (4) All of the above.

Other Therapies

OBJECTIVES: Student will be able to:

1. List and briefly define *talk therapies.*
2. Define *behavior modification.*
3. List several advantages and disadvantages of behavior modification.
4. State at least 10 principles of cognitive therapy.
5. Define *auxiliary therapies.*

TALK THERAPIES

Psychotherapy, as talk therapy is generally called, can be done either on an individual basis or in groups and may be under the direction of a physician, clinical psychologist, or other therapist. The aim of the therapy is the same, that is, to help patients gain understanding and insight into their problems so they can learn to deal with them more effectively. Psychotherapy may be used in conjunction with drug therapy, electroconvulsive shock therapy (although not if a patient becomes confused during treatment), art therapy, recreational therapy, and occupational therapy. Frequently, a combination of two or more types of therapy is used and often yields the best results.

Although there is a great deal of argument about the relative effectiveness of various types of talk psychotherapies and, for that matter, many other forms of mental health therapy, it is probable that three things are necessary for an improvement in the patient's ability to cope with the stresses of life. First, the patient must want to get better. Second, the patient must come to a better understanding of the cause of his or her problems and in turn learn methods or techniques for dealing more effectively with them. Third, if therapy is to be successful, the patient must have an environment in which it is possible for change to take place. So many times we see promising beginnings negated when the patient returns to an environment that either does not support the patient's attempts to change or actively discourages such changes. For example, a young woman who was hospitalized for depression discovered the courage to face the fact that she had married her husband to escape an abusive home environment and not because she loved him. When she tried to discuss that issue with her husband, he immediately demanded that she leave the hospital and took her to the "preacher," who told her that she needed only to trust God and pray for Him to make her love her husband and He would. She is still depressed and has made several suicide attempts.

As in the previous case, the third task is often the most difficult to accomplish. In the hospital, most treatment teams are successful in creating a therapeutic environment in which desirable changes can occur. However, when the patient goes home to a nonsupportive environment, it often happens that the best insight and the best treatment available are insufficient to overcome the adverse effects of the environment. In such cases, family therapy is advisable; otherwise, it is quite probable that the patient will have to return for further treatment and, even then, the patient's issues may never be resolved without family treatment.

A form of psychotherapy known as *cognitive behavior therapy* is currently the leading talk therapy. Although a number of leading practitioners work in the cognitive therapy arena (Albert Ellis, Robert Glasser, Aaron Beck, Maxie Maultsby, and Arnold Lazarus, to name a few), generally, cognitive behavior therapy advocates maintain that people can use their cognitive or thinking capacity to deal with problems and issues and, ultimately, to change their behavior. They believe that distortions in thinking account for much of the psychological misery people experience and that helping them to "think straight" and to correct the distortions in their thinking will allow them to redirect their lives and become much more functional in their behaviors. Although there are variations on this theme among the advocates of cognitive behavior therapy, almost all, in some fashion, appreciate that *thinking* leads to *feelings* and feelings lead to *behavior*. If a person is feeling anxious, depressed, and so forth, the individual should examine his or her thinking to find the distortions leading to the negative feelings. Thus, straightening out one's thinking is a primary goal of cognitive therapy. The following represent some of the kinds of thinking or cognitive disturbances with which cognitive therapy is concerned:

Probability overestimation is a form of distorted thinking in which the individual inappropriately assumes that an event is more likely than it actually is, for example, "If my son takes that trip, I *know* he will be killed." This thinking style is guaranteed to keep the individual perpetually anxious.

All-or-none thinking is black or white and leaves little room for more rational approaches. For example, the belief that "I *must* be loved by Alice Jones and no one else will do," unrealistically eliminates approximately 3 billion other women inhabiting the earth and severely restricts one's choices. Yet many people commit suicide every year because they hold such an irrational belief.

Fortune-telling suggests that one might irrationally believe that "because I failed to land that new account, and should have, my boss will hate me forever."

Negating or disqualifying the positive involves being unable to accept positive things said about oneself and bringing up a negative trait in response to any attempt at highlighting a positive trait. As Freeman and Greenwood (1987) put it, this distorted form of thinking is "constantly snatching defeat from the jaws of victory."

Catastrophizing represents "the sky is falling, the sky is falling" mentality in which a person can never be happy and feel good because any minute something bad is going to happen. This cognitive distortion lies at the heart of many of the problems of the anxious patients you will see in your work.

Magnification or minimization occurs when people enlarge or magnify their bad points while minimizing their good points and maximizing the good points of others. Or, conversely, they may magnify their good points and minimize or ignore their liabilities while also minimizing the good points of others. In the first case, those people will likely feel depressed and miserable themselves. In the second case, they may make those around them feel miserable and depressed.

Emotional reasoning involves a thinking distortion in which a person interprets feelings as evidence of the truth of his or her state of being. The logic is that "if I feel depressed, things must really be hopeless and helpless" or "I feel inadequate so I must be useless."

Phonyism is a perception that praise and acceptance are undeserved because people feel they did not do their absolute best or did not perform the task well enough and are thus insufficiently worthy of praise and acceptance. They may become anxious or depressed because they are certain they will be discovered to be phony. Then, of course, they will be deservedly scorned.

Overgeneralization refers to an inappropriate conclusion that is based on a single or random event. If someone fails the first test in nursing school and believes that means he or she is not smart enough to be in the program or is incapable of doing the work, the individual may drop out of the program. A more rational thought might be, "Wow!

This is going to be harder than I thought. Guess I'm going to have to study harder."

Selective abstraction occurs when someone selects from a situation a few points or instances that support a particular view. The person then proceeds to ignore any evidence that does not support his or her view. (Politicians are masters of this distortion.) An anxious person can almost always find something to be anxious about, especially if he or she largely ignores data suggesting no need for anxiety.

Should / must / ought statements are usually intended to motivate people to behave in a certain manner. The primary motivational impetus comes from the guilt, shame, and doubt created when the person does not do as prescribed. The problem is that guilt, shame, and doubt decrease motivation and produce anger and resentment, even when the individual complies with the directive should/must/ought. When these feelings are internalized rather than appropriately confronted, the individual will likely become depressed or anxious.

Personalization involves taking issues unrelated to oneself and applying them anyway. At the extreme of this distortion the behavior is labeled paranoid or delusional. However, the distortion can be much more subtle. For example, if a woman enters a room in which several people are present and her ear catches the phrase "She is the most stupid . . ." while she simultaneously observes that a member of the group, laughing, glanced up at her, she may conclude that they were talking about her. This distortion occurs even more subtly when, for example, a supervisor is talking to a group of people about problems in the workplace and someone assumes the supervisor is blaming him or her for the problems.

In summary, cognitive behavior therapy is not intended to "cure" patients but rather to increase their ability to respond to their issues with straight thinking. Straight thinking leads to more functional behavior, which will allow the person to become emotionally healthy. Cognitive behavior therapy is usually not used with psychotic patients or patients with low intellectual ability.

As a member of a treatment team, an individual needs to support and reinforce the efforts of the team members who are responsible for individual or group psychotherapy. The skills and techniques presented in the chapter on communicating with patients should be helpful in developing support skills for the talk therapies.

BEHAVIOR THERAPY

Behavior therapy is a term used to specify a particular kind of treatment wherein no claim is made to do anything other than change or modify the behavior of the patient. For this reason, it has been called simplistic by many of its critics.

Essentially, behavior therapy consists of deciding which behaviors exhibited by a particular patient are desirable and which are undesirable and then trying to increase the frequency of the desirable behaviors and eliminate or decrease the frequency of the undesirable behaviors. This method of treatment has been particularly effective in the treatment of children and persons with compromised intellectual ability.

As one might imagine, behavior therapy has advocates and critics. The movie *A Clockwork Orange* presented both the capabilities of behavior therapy as well as some of the drawbacks. In this movie, a young sociopathic man (one who engages in extremely antisocial acts and who demonstrates no remorse for immoral, unethical, or illegal acts) was conditioned, using behavior therapy techniques, against responding to anything in a hostile or sexual way. He had been a very hostile young man who had beaten and mugged several persons and sexually assaulted several others. After he was conditioned to not react to any stimulus in a hostile or sexual manner, he was returned to his community. Of course, being unable to respond in a hostile manner, his former enemies and even his friends quickly began to take advantage of him. In the end, he was taken back and deconditioned because of the public uproar over the treatment he had received. Members of his community considered the conditioning technique to be barbaric and inhumane. This scenario points out that just because a particular technique works, it may not be fully used because of social pressures and unforeseen consequences.

Basically, conditioning operates on the idea that people will behave in ways that get them what they want; that is, certain actions are rewarded and are thus likely to recur. People respond in this manner every day of their lives. For example, you are reading this book because you wish to gain more knowledge about the subject matter. It may be that you need this knowledge to obtain a degree, to get a better job, to be a better mental health worker, or simply because you are curious about the treatment of the mentally ill. You would not be reading this book if it would not help in some way to get you something you want. Factory workers who work 40 hours a week at jobs they find boring usually do so because working at the factory gets them the money they need to obtain other satisfactions in life. Such conditioning factors operate in our lives in other ways. If a 4-year-old realizes that, to get mother's attention, he must lie on the floor and kick his heels and scream at the top of his voice, he will engage in that type of behavior whenever he wants his mother's attention. The same is true for the young woman who goes to medical school not because she wants to be a doctor, but because it gains her the approval she so desperately wants and needs from her parents. Sometimes an individual engages in self-destructive behavior to gain some apparently superficial end; yet that end has a great deal of meaning to that individual. The idea, again, is that people behave in ways that get them what they want, although they may not always be aware of or attend to the long-term consequences of the behavior or may not even be aware that their behavior often appears inappropriate to others.

In behavior therapy, an effort is made to ascertain which behaviors exhibited by an individual are desirable and which are undesirable and then to selectively reward the desirable behaviors and ignore the undesirable behaviors. This is done to increase the desirable behaviors and decrease the undesirable behaviors. Little attention is paid to the causes of the behavior or to the dynamics of the behavior in the traditional psychotherapeutic sense. A behaviorist does not ask why a patient is hostile because hostility is not a concept the patient is willing to deal with. Rather, the behaviorist asks which specific *behaviors* does he or she wish the patient to engage in. The behaviorist wants to know which *behaviors* make the patient appear hostile. The therapist argues that the patient seems hostile only because he or she is engaging in certain behaviors and that if the patient ceases to engage in those behaviors, he or she will not be called hostile.

Although rather astonishing behavioral changes can be made in a relatively short time, this method of treatment has definite limitations. For one, a great deal of control is required over the patient's behavior. The environment must be controllable in a way that prevents unwanted reinforcement or reward of certain behaviors and ensures reward of desired behaviors. There is also the problem of maintaining the frequency of the desired behaviors once the patient leaves the controlled environment and the systematic application of reinforcement is no longer possible.

AUXILIARY THERAPIES

(Occupational Therapy, Art Therapy, Recreational Therapy, Adventure Therapy, Music Therapy)

It has been said that humans are social creatures and, therefore, must respond to a wide range of social and interpersonal situations. To successfully meet the demands of today's complex and ever-changing society, people must indeed possess a good capacity for flexibility. By and large, mentally ill patients have developed maladaptive and, thus, inflexible ways of responding to their environments that result in varying degrees of loss of social adaptability. Their range of interests and activities becomes quite constricted and they may or may not lose contact with reality. Many patients experience personality disorganization ranging from mild to severe.

To assist mentally ill patients in their attempts to once again interact effectively with others, occupational, art, recreational, adventure, and music therapists provide a wide range of activities. These activities require patients to become involved in something outside themselves, thus affording them less time to dwell on their problems. These activities also require interaction with the therapist and possibly with one or more other patients in the treatment program. If patients are given interesting and challenging projects at a level of difficulty that is appropriate for them, they benefit from participation. By having to collect their thoughts, organize their actions, and use their own initiative, they can be led to become active once again in their own lives as well as in the lives of their families and friends. Hopefully, the successful completion of projects will enhance the patient's self-concept and afford them a sense of pride or accomplishment that often has been lacking for some time. Success also encourages patients to respond to their environment and the people in it in a healthier fashion.

Not all patients are delighted about the opportunity to participate in such therapeutic activities. Often they prefer to remain in their rooms or to engage in some solitary activity. It is important that they be gently, but firmly, encouraged to participate in therapeutic activities. If patients receive repeated invitations to join the group and are not rejected when they refuse to participate, they may later become more willing to join in group activities. Frequently, patients do not wish to participate because they have experienced so many failures that they are certain they will fail again. Their anxieties should be taken into account and an effort made to understand them. As is generally the case with mentally ill persons, a great deal of understanding, reassurance, and patience is required to help the individual feel comfortable enough to engage in any new activity.

It is always important to be certain that once patients agree to participate, they are not expected to engage in some activity that is likely to cause them to be humiliated in front of others or in which they are likely to fail. Activities must be carefully selected and expectations kept in line with the patients' capabilities. If at all possible, conferences between the members of the treatment team, including those from auxiliary therapies, should be held to discuss the patient's progress, treatment goals, capabilities, and needs.

Perhaps the most important thing to keep in mind regarding therapeutic activities is that these auxiliary therapies should provide the patient with an opportunity to relax, engage in something enjoyable, and provide a break in the regular therapeutic routine. It should be a time of fun for the patient, and the patient should be encouraged to participate as freely and as spontaneously as possible.

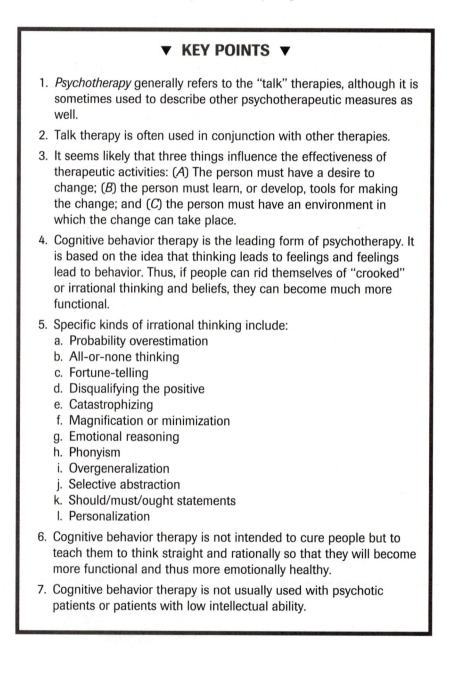

▼ KEY POINTS ▼

1. *Psychotherapy* generally refers to the "talk" therapies, although it is sometimes used to describe other psychotherapeutic measures as well.

2. Talk therapy is often used in conjunction with other therapies.

3. It seems likely that three things influence the effectiveness of therapeutic activities: (*A*) The person must have a desire to change; (*B*) the person must learn, or develop, tools for making the change; and (*C*) the person must have an environment in which the change can take place.

4. Cognitive behavior therapy is the leading form of psychotherapy. It is based on the idea that thinking leads to feelings and feelings lead to behavior. Thus, if people can rid themselves of "crooked" or irrational thinking and beliefs, they can become much more functional.

5. Specific kinds of irrational thinking include:
   a. Probability overestimation
   b. All-or-none thinking
   c. Fortune-telling
   d. Disqualifying the positive
   e. Catastrophizing
   f. Magnification or minimization
   g. Emotional reasoning
   h. Phonyism
   i. Overgeneralization
   j. Selective abstraction
   k. Should/must/ought statements
   l. Personalization

6. Cognitive behavior therapy is not intended to cure people but to teach them to think straight and rationally so that they will become more functional and thus more emotionally healthy.

7. Cognitive behavior therapy is not usually used with psychotic patients or patients with low intellectual ability.

Key Points continued

8. Behavior therapy is a form of treatment in which no claim is made for changing anything except the patient's behavior.

9. The essential aim of behavior therapy is to increase desirable behavior and decrease undesirable behavior. Behavior therapy is especially helpful in working with children and intellectually compromised people.

10. In behavior therapy, little or no attention is paid to the cause of the behavior in the tradition of psychoanalytic and other therapies that treat behavior as symptomatic of past learning or traumatic experiences.

11. A major obstacle in behavior therapy is the amount of control one must have over the patient to ensure that reinforcements are properly administered and that unwanted reinforcement does not occur.

12. Auxiliary therapies include occupational therapy, art therapy, recreational therapy, adventure therapy, and music therapy.

13. The major focus of auxiliary therapies is to help the patient regain the social flexibility and adaptability to maintain relationships.

14. Not all patients are delighted with the opportunity to participate in auxiliary therapeutic activities. However, staff support for such activities can go a long way toward encouraging patient participation.

15. Because many patients have a self-perceived history of failure, auxiliary therapy tasks must be chosen with care. Expectations must be kept in line with the patient's ability, and great care must be exercised to ensure that patients do not feel humiliated or demeaned by tasks they are asked to do.

Annotated Bibliography

Beutler, L. E., and Harwood, M. T.: Prescriptive psychotherapies. *Applied & Preventive Psychology,* 1995, 4:89–100.

Reviews research as a means to establish a base for effective tailored therapy for individual needs.

Bond, M.: Setting up groups: A practical guide. *Nursing Standard,* 1991, 5(48):47–51.

Describes the concepts and methods used in establishing two distinct types of support groups.

Bowers, J. J.: Therapy through art: Facilitating treatment of sexual abuse. *Journal of Psychosocial Nursing and Mental Health Services,* 1992, 30(6):15–24.

Presents the use of art therapy to help sexually abused patients access traumatic memories. Includes a case study.

Buxman, K.: Humor in therapy for the mentally ill. *Journal of Psychosocial Nursing and Mental Health Services,* 1991, 29(12):15–18.

Discusses the use of humor in a psychiatric setting to promote communication and social interaction and to relieve tension and anxieties in patients.

Erbs-Palmer, V. K.: Incorporating psychiatric rehabilitation principles into mental health nursing. *Journal of Psychosocial Nursing,* 1995, 8(3):36–44.

Discusses the differences between a rehabilitation approach and a treatment approach.

Forisha, B., Grothaus, K., and Luscombe, R.: Dinner conversation: Meal therapy to differentiate eating behavior from family process. *Journal of Psychosocial Nursing and Mental Health Services,* 1990, 28(11):12–16.

Discusses the use of meal therapy in patients with eating disorders to evaluate family dynamics and to work through the meanings that family members have evolved into a system.

Glaister, J. A.: The art of therapeutic drawing: Helping chronic trauma survivors. *Journal of Psychosocial Nursing and Mental Health Services,* 1992, 30(5):9–17.

Describes the use of therapeutic drawing in working with severely traumatized patients. Provides case examples and an explanation of the patient's attempts at expression in the drawing.

Hamer, B. A.: Music therapy: Harmony for change. *Journal of Psychosocial Nursing and Mental Health Services,* 1991, 29(12):5–7.

Discusses the successful use of music therapy to strengthen ego, increase socialization, decrease psychotic symptoms, and increase activity in low-functioning patients.

Hundley, J.: Pet project: The use of pet facilitated therapy among the chronically mentally ill. *Journal of Psychosocial Nursing and Mental Health Services,* 1991, 29(6):23–26.

Discusses the benefits of using pets in therapy and offers information on implementing a pet-facilitated therapy in an inpatient setting.

Kreidler, M. C., and Carlson, R. E.: Breaking the incest cycle: The group as a surrogate family. *Journal of Psychosocial Nursing and Mental Health Services,* 1991, 29(4):28–32.

Examines the use of the group to help incest survivors work on healing issues and deal with unresolved family issues.

McFarlane, A. C.: Individual psychotherapy for post-traumatic stress disorder. *Psychiatric Clinics of North America,* 1994, 17(2):393–408.

Explains the need for a conceptual model and the way in which that model can be incorporated as a tool to offset the subsets of symptoms in post-traumatic stress disorder.

Robbin, R., Vaicunas, J., and Akers, J.: The behavioral, cognitive, and sociocultural perspectives. In Bootzin, R. R., Acocella, J. R., and Alloy, L. B. (eds.): *Abnormal Psychology: Current Perspectives,* 6th ed. New York: McGraw-Hill, 1993, pp. 60–81.

Discusses the founding fathers' theories in behavioral, cognitive, and sociocultural perspectives.

Zerhusen, J. D., Boyle, K., and Wilson, W.: Out of darkness: Group cognitive therapy for depressed elderly. *Journal of Psychosocial Nursing and Mental Health Services,* 1991, 29(9):16–21.

Research study examines the benefits of nurses facilitating cognitive group therapy with nursing home residents suffering from depression.

Reference

Freeman, A., and Greenwood, V.: *Cognitive Therapy.* New York: Human Sciences Press, 1987, p. 25.

Post-Test

True or False. Circle your choice.

T   F   1. Basically, behavior modification uses the idea that people behave in ways that get them what they want.

T   F   2. Mentally ill patients to a large extent have lost their social adaptability because of their maladaptive ways of responding to their environment.

T   F   3. It is the mental health worker's responsibility to see that all patients participate in every activity and not allow excuses from anyone.

T   F   4. Occupational therapy is an important measure in the treatment of the psychiatric patient because it offers a means for the individual to achieve a feeling of accomplishment.

T   F   5. If you were using behavior modification with a patient with poor table manners, you would just accept these manners without comment.

T   F   6. Behavior modification is especially helpful in the treatment of children and mentally retarded persons.

T   F   7. Cognitive behavior therapy is the leading talk therapy in the mental health field at this time.

Short Answer. Answer the following as briefly and specifically as possible.

1. What three elements are essential for an improvement in a patient's ability to cope with life's stresses?

a. _____

b. _____

c. _____

2. Which of the previous three tasks is the most difficult to accomplish?

_____

_____

Post-Test

(continued)

3. What is the primary purpose of psychotherapy?

_____

_____

_____

4. List at least seven kinds of cognitive distortions that cognitive therapists look for when treating patients.

a. _____ e. _____

b. _____ f. _____

c. _____ g. _____

d. _____

Multiple Choice. Circle the letter or number you think represents the best answer.

1. Which of the following will be most likely to get Mr. Cartwright, a patient on a behavior modification ward, to change his eating habits:
   a. Accept his table manners without comment.
   b. Urge him to eat as the other patients do.
   c. Offer him a reward for each improvement in his table manners.
   d. Point out to him that his eating habits distress the other patients.

2. Limits should be set:
   a. To help the patient reduce his anxiety.
   b. To help the patient learn to control his behavior.
   c. To establish the authority of the staff over the patient.
   d. To punish inappropriate behavior.
   e. To protect people and property from injury.
     (1) a, b, and e.
     (2) a, b, and c.
     (3) b, d, and e.
     (4) All of these.

3. Steps and techniques involved in setting limits are:
   a. Identify the need for the limit.
   b. Help the patient to understand the need for the limit.

Post-Test

(continued)

   c. Allow the patient to verbalize his feelings about the limit.
   d. Consistency.
   e. Evaluate the limit frequently.
      (1) a, c, and e.
      (2) b, c, and d.
      (3) a, b, and d.
      (4) All of these.

4. Which of the following are advantages of group therapy?
   a. Gives the therapists a chance to supply authoritative answers to problems common to the group.
   b. Provides for the resolution of problems through group discussion and discovery of possible solutions.
   c. Gives the mentally dull an opportunity to reason and form judgments through group interaction.
   d. Allows the therapist to interact with several patients at one time so that all have access to professional counseling.

5. Occupational therapy is an important measure in the treatment of the psychiatric patient because it primarily:
   a. Offers the poor patient an opportunity to partially pay for care by selling items he or she makes.
   b. Provides an opportunity to keep the patient active.
   c. Offers a means for the individual to achieve a feeling of accomplishment.
   d. Offers an opportunity to observe the patient.

6. A therapeutic health-promoting environment for patients (milieu therapy) provides for:
   a. A testing ground for new patterns of behavior.
   b. Acceptance as an individual.
   c. Unconditional acceptance of behavior.
   d. Protection from self-injury.
   e. A continuous appraisal of the patient's needs.
      (1) b only.
      (2) b and c.
      (3) a, b, and d.
      (4) All of the above.

Post-Test

(continued)

7. Which of the following are true about psychotherapy?
   a. The aim of psychotherapy is to help the patient learn new patterns of behavior.
   b. Psychotherapy refers to a certain type of relationship between one or more patients and a therapist.
   c. In family psychotherapy, the therapist treats only the neurotic or psychotic family member.
   d. Group therapy, psychoanalysis, and counseling are three common types of psychotherapy.
      (1) b only.
      (2) b and c.
      (3) a, b, and d.
      (4) All of the above.

Therapeutic Approaches to Specific Populations

PART

IV

Care for Aggressive Patients

OBJECTIVES: Student will be able to:

1. Describe effective techniques for dealing with:
   a. Verbally aggressive patients.
   b. Violent, agitated, or physically destructive patients.
   c. Demanding patients.
   d. Uncooperative patients.
   e. Sexually aggressive patients.
2. Address issues such as lying and stealing, which may involve more than one patient.
3. List appropriate responses to intimidating or physically abusive behavior.

Several groups of behaviors are commonly associated with the aggressive patient. Included are verbally abusive behavior, agitated or destructive behavior, demanding behavior, lying and stealing behavior, fighting behavior, arguing behavior, irritating behavior, and, finally, uncooperative behavior. It is important to keep in mind that, although patients behave in an aggressive manner for various reasons, management of the behavior is generally the same. The specific behaviors usually associated with the aggressive patient are presented individually and discussed in some detail in this chapter.

VERBALLY ABUSIVE BEHAVIOR

Patients usually become verbally abusive because of frustrating circumstances beyond their control. They then displace the anger and frustration to family, other patients, or staff members. Many verbally abusive patients have developed this pattern of behavior in response to their belief that they are going to be rejected. In an attempt to reject before they can be rejected, they become hostile to others. Thus, others respond to their hostility in a like manner and a vicious, self-defeating cycle begins. This pattern is often referred to as a self-fulfilling prophecy because the patient expects rejection, behaves as though he or she has already been rejected and thus is, in fact, rejected because of angry or defensive behavior. To break this cycle, it is imperative that staff members not respond to a patient's verbal aggression in a punitive, hostile, or rejecting manner.

Therapeutic treatment for verbally aggressive patients often hinges on the ability of staff members to recognize that, in most cases, these patients do not mean anything personal by their abusive remarks. They are simply displacing their frustration and anger from the object or situation creating those feelings to the staff member. The ability to express negative feelings can be a healthy sign. It may also indicate that patients feel that the staff member is capable of accepting the abuse and can deal with it in an effective manner. It also may mean that patients feel comfortable enough to express their frustrations because they know that, if they lose control of themselves, the staff will take nonpunitive steps to help them regain control. These patients need to be accepted as they are and staff members must try to understand the patient's words from the patient's point of view. When limits must be set, it is important that the limits be on the patient's actions and behaviors, not on the patient's feelings. The verbal expression of aggression is an important outlet for the frustrations and tensions that these patients feel.

A key to managing these types of patients is to teach them to find more socially acceptable ways of expressing their frustrations. Sometimes it is difficult to discourage a particular behavior without appearing to be rejecting, and sometimes the behavior may be so aggressive that it cannot be tolerated. In such cases, it may be necessary to actually tell a patient that, although staff members still accept and care about him or her as a person, they are not willing to accept the individual's verbally abusive behavior. Judgmental, moralistic, or disparaging remarks about the patient's behavior typically only make matters worse.

Staff members should be careful to not let patients draw them into arguments. Anytime a staff member argues with a patient, the patient wins. Aside from the fact that the patient will feel that he or she is "one up" on staff members who lose their tempers, such staff members provide inappropriate role models for the patient. In many instances, patients are not able to use good judgment or act in a rational manner. Staff members, however, are expected to show good judgment, restraint, and socially appropriate behavior at all times. One of the most important therapeutic tools that staff members have is their own behavior. If a staff member provides an acceptable behavioral model, patients are likely to benefit by identifying with the staff member and patterning their behavior accordingly.

Because verbally abusive patients are quite upsetting to other patients, staff members must remain calm and controlled when patients have emotional outbursts. If possible, a staff member should accompany such patients to their rooms or to a more isolated area. There the staff member can reassure and calm the patient while allowing the patient time to regain control. Many patients are later embarrassed by their outburst and may resent the staff for having permitted them to engage in behaviors that make them look bad in front of fellow patients. Staff members should not press patients for an explanation of their behavior when they are upset. It is usually more effective to give them time to calm down so that they can discuss their situation in a more rational manner.

When patients become so upset that they have difficulty regaining control, they should be given their prn (*pro re nata,* "as needed") medications. The dosage should not be enough to heavily sedate the patient but enough to permit resumption of the ability to relate to staff members who are trying to help. When the patient is calm, a staff member can explore the kinds of responses the patient would likely have encountered if the same behavior had occurred in everyday life situations. The staff member then has the opportunity to help the patient consider other ways of dealing with the feelings that caused the emotional outburst and the aggressive behavior. By discussing the negative results of previous outbursts, the patient may gain insight about the need for changing his or her behavior.

Finally, staff members should analyze their own response to these patients. If they have any negative or hostile feelings toward a particular patient, they should try to find effective ways of coping with those feelings. It is sometimes helpful to discuss such feelings with a fellow staff member or supervisor. Psychiatric patients are sensitive to the attitudes of others and a staff member's negative feelings may cause a patient to become even more abusive because he or she feels rejected.

VIOLENT, AGITATED, OR PHYSICALLY DESTRUCTIVE BEHAVIOR

There are probably few places that the old adage "an ounce of prevention is worth a pound of cure" applies more than in dealing with patients who are violent, agitated, or physically destructive. Violence usually occurs only when a patient feels threatened and unable to do anything else. Perhaps the single most important factor in dealing with such patients is to learn to recognize danger signals or behaviors that indicate the patient is about to become agitated or violent. When conditions are likely to lead to the patient's becoming upset and combative, it is usually wise to use the patient's prn medications and to try to remove the patient to an area in which violent behavior could be more easily handled. Frequently, when patients are isolated with only one staff member, they are less prone to be physically assaultive because the patient is not stimulated by other patients who are becoming upset and milling around. Patients usually calm down much more quickly when they do not have an audience.

Once such patients are in a quiet area and have been given appropriate prn medication, they should be encouraged to talk about their anger and to discuss the reasons they became violent. As with verbally abusive patients, it is also important to explore alternative ways of expressing patients' anger and hostility and to help them explore similar kinds of behavior or incidents that might have occurred in the past.

Perhaps one of the most detrimental approaches to patients who become upset and potentially combative is to try to "manhandle" them or physically coerce them without giving them an opportunity to accompany a single individual to a quieter, more secluded place. *Frequently, when patients are very upset, the simple act of a staff member's taking their arm or touching them is sufficient to cause them to lose control completely.* Therefore, it is probably best never to touch patients who are agitated or out of control until all other approaches have failed. Threatening patients with various forms of punishment such as shots, seclusion room lockup, bed restraints, or other such punitive acts will further increase their agitation. If a staff member can approach potentially combative patients in a nonthreatening, calm, reassuring manner and if the staff member does not appear to be afraid of such patients, the staff member will likely be able to relate to them in an effective manner. Arguing with agitated patients or otherwise irritating them will practically ensure these patients' loss of control. One should try to reduce a patient's perception of threat—not increase it.

It is frequently helpful with patients who tend to be physically abusive or combative to explain to them very clearly and directly the expected behaviors and then to verbally praise and support patients who make an effort to engage in those behaviors. It is especially important that staff members be consistent in their expectations of patients and in reinforcement of the expected behaviors. If patients are told that a particular consequence will follow a particular behavior, then it is of utmost importance that the behavior be dealt with that way. Otherwise, patients cannot learn to trust the staff and may be tempted to engage in certain undesirable behaviors just to see if they can get away with them. At the very least, patients may feel unprotected and unsafe and as though the staff may not actually be in control of the unit if appropriate consequences are not administered.

Another important way of helping patients learn to deal with their physically abusive or combative behavior is to have them understand the inappropriateness of the behavior and to confront them with it. This should never take place at the height of a patient's agitation but rather after the patient has had time to calm down and can be fairly rational in looking at his or her behavior.

If all efforts to calm violent or destructive patients fail, it is necessary to physically control their behavior. This procedure is called a "takedown." A takedown is undertaken only to protect the patient himself or herself, other patients, staff members, or property. Even in these cases, only the minimum force needed to control the patient should be used. Staff members should use force carefully but as quickly and efficiently as possible. If a patient has become violent, first remove all other patients and unnecessary staff members from the area. Then collect enough staff members so that there is no doubt about the outcome of the confrontation. Sometimes this further agitates the patient, but it is necessary to ensure the proper outcome. At least five people are needed: one for each arm and leg and one to give general assistance. One person should be in charge and receive instant response from the other staff members. Pillows, towels, or a blanket may be wrapped around staff members' arms to reduce blows and avoid injury from thrown objects. From that point, the proper procedure is to get the patient off his or her feet and, as gently as possible, placed face down on the floor. Every effort should be made to accomplish this without injuring the patient. Some authorities suggest using the patient's clothing for restraint; others suggest, when using the patient's limbs for restraint, grasping near the major joints to reduce the patient's leverage and thus the likelihood of severe injury to staff.

When the patient is under staff control, the person in charge should decide whether to give a prn medication and whether mechanical restraints are necessary. If mechanical restraints are used, care must be taken to see that they are not unnecessarily uncomfortable. They should be removed as soon as the patient regains control, and the patient should be told that this will happen. Other patients who might have been involved should be reassured and given an opportunity to express their feelings about the incident. The staff should then discuss the incident and try to find ways of preventing future recurrences. In most states it is also necessary to have a physician's or psychologist's order to apply physical restraints. When possible, get the order before initiating the takedown. If the takedown occurs in an emergency situation, then call the attending doctor immediately after completing the procedure.

DEMANDING BEHAVIOR

One of the most difficult patients to deal with is the passive, whiny patient who constantly seeks a particular staff member's attention and who demands support and reassurance from that person. Such patients often become annoying in their demands because nothing the staff member does is enough. First they want their shaving kit, and then they want their toothpaste, and then they want their shoe polish, and then they want their medicine, and then they want to talk, and then they want to make a telephone call, and on and on. Frequently, such patients seek to control all of a particular staff member's time, unconsciously or irrationally believing the amount of time spent with the staff member is an indication of their worth as a person. In other words, such patients' feelings of worth are directly related to the amount of contact they are able to establish with the staff. Usually, a staff member finds it impossible to attend to all assigned duties if constantly required to deal with a demanding patient. It is more helpful to both the staff member and the patient if a structured program can be developed in which the patient is guaranteed access to the staff member at certain times and the staff member makes frequent but brief contacts with the patient at times that are convenient for the staff member. In this way the staff member takes the initiative for the contacts, which encourages the patient to be more adaptable in delaying immediate gratification of his or her dependency needs.

Sometimes the most effective thing a staff member can do is to ignore the patient who makes constant demands. It is important, however, that the staff member not show annoyance or anger toward the patient. It may be necessary at times to confront such patients with the fact that their behavior is inappropriate and to help them understand that they must learn other ways of meeting their needs. Frequently patients do not recognize that they are unrealistically demanding and that their behavior affects other people. Verbal reinforcement should be given to patients when they show independent activity and when they can meet their need for attention in acceptable ways.

LYING AND STEALING BEHAVIOR

Managing patients who lie and steal is among the most frustrating of all mental health tasks because it is difficult to simultaneously play the roles of policeman and therapist. Frequently, it is difficult to ascertain whether a patient is actually guilty of lying or stealing. When confronted with such behaviors, patients are likely to become quite agitated and upset.

These behaviors are troublesome because they often involve other patients. For example, one patient may steal from other patients, which irritates and upsets the other patients, or a patient may lie about a patient or staff member to another patient, upsetting and irritating that patient.

If a staff member is certain that Mr. Smith lied or stole something, it is probably best, after discussing the behavior with the treatment team or at least with the charge nurse, to simply confront Mr. Smith with the behavior rather than asking whether the behavior occurred. Asking about the occurrence gives him more opportunity to get into trouble because he feels compelled to deny the behavior. Mr. Smith may later feel resentful that the staff member caused him to further compound his lies when the staff member was already aware of the truth.

In confronting the patient with lying or stealing behavior, it is important to be as nonpunitive and as accepting of the patient as possible while rejecting the *inappropriate behavior*. If the patient is aware that other patients and staff members know that the patient has a problem with lying or stealing, the patient may be encouraged to stop the behavior. It is also important to ask the patient to restore any property that may have been taken and to explore with the patient the reasons for the lying or stealing behavior. Frequently, it is important to discuss with patients the inappropriateness of such behaviors and the potential consequences of such behaviors outside the treatment center. Patients should be encouraged to verbalize appropriate behaviors and to explore the effect these behaviors have on their feelings about themselves. It is important to confront patients at a time when other patients cannot observe the confrontation. Such confrontations should not be humiliating to patients. Staff behavior that is judgmental or moralistic is inappropriate, and reasoning with patients on religious grounds is usually not an effective means of dealing with lying or stealing behavior.

ANTAGONISTIC, INTIMIDATING, OR PHYSICALLY ABUSIVE BEHAVIOR

As in dealing with patients who are likely to become physically abusive, one of the most important things in preventing fights among patients is to recognize potential situations or conditions that are likely to cause tempers to flare. It is also important to recognize personality conflicts among certain patients. Those who have conflicts might be kept busy doing things that will not bring them into frequent contact. Further, the staff should not permit patients who are likely to have conflicts to engage in activities that might cause their basic personality differences to be exaggerated or that put them into competition with each other.

If a fight does occur, it is important to separate the participants and to refrain from taking sides unless a staff member has observed blatant aggression by one of the patients. The same is true for verbal arguments between patients. If patients are actually involved in a physical fight, it is important to separate them so that each can be dealt with independently. If at all possible, remove them to separate areas and away from any audience. If sufficient staffpower is not available to physically separate the patients, then a staff member might attempt to distract them in some way. When appropriate, humor, a request for help with some task requiring skill the patient possesses, immediate dispatch to the lab for tests, or some other distraction may be used. After the patients have calmed down, it might help to have a therapeutic confrontation, letting the two sit down with a staff member and discuss what upsets them about each other. It is sometimes helpful to explore the patients' feelings about themselves as well as their feelings about the other patient. The staff member might then be able to help both patients understand their conflict and to suggest alternative ways of dealing with their feelings about each other. Sometimes patients who have been antagonistic toward each other become good friends once they understand their differences and the reasons for their behavior.

One of the most effective ways to help avoid fighting and arguing is to plan a program of activities that will not permit the patients so much free time that they become bored. Group therapy or community meetings may be used to settle disagreements before they reach the stage of serious arguments and fights. Again, it is important that staff members provide good role modeling for the patients. Role playing is also sometimes helpful. A staff member may play the part of one of the patients when dealing with patients who have been separated after a serious argument or fight. The staff member would then respond in a manner that would be appropriate if the staff member were actually the other patient. Sometimes it helps to have patients switch roles with each other after they have had time to calm down.

Perhaps one of the most serious staff errors is to ignore or to accept disruptive behavior from a patient who is known to be annoying or upsetting to other patients. It is also important to remember that a staff member should not intervene in a constructive argument that is being appropriately handled by the patients.

UNCOOPERATIVE BEHAVIOR

With an uncooperative patient, it is important to be aware of the patient's diagnosis because, in some cases, a patient is significantly psychologically regressed and is not being intentionally uncooperative. In other cases, a patient is uncooperative for what seems to him or her a legitimate reason. Some of these reasons include fear of hospitalization, of medications, or of unusual treatments such as electroconvulsive shock treatments. Sometimes patients are uncooperative because they think they may fail or that they may look foolish. One of the least constructive steps is to approach such patients in a threatening manner and to threaten them with punishment if they do not obey orders or if they do not do what is asked of them. The patients' reasons for being uncooperative should be explored. The staff member should be reassuring and use a kind, but firm, approach. If a staff member calmly explains the reason patients are being asked to follow directions, they will usually comply. It is almost always detrimental to try to force a patient to do something. Try to not have an audience when asking a patient to do something. An audience often makes a patient feel he or she must resist for the benefit of the audience, particularly if the patient has established himself or herself as a "black sheep" among the other patients. Because a little humor goes a long way with patients, it can be used to avoid authoritative "orders" that may cause argumentative patient behaviors that sometimes lead to more serious conflicts. A staff member with a smiling face who approaches a patient and says, "This little pill is demanding to be swallowed immediately" may get more cooperation than a staff member with a serious face who says, "You have to take this medication right now."

It is sometimes necessary to make patients' privileges dependent on cooperation with the staff. Within reason, patients must learn to live in accordance with unit policy and regulations. Whenever possible, however, patients should be given a choice of alternatives. Giving patients a choice permits them to maintain a feeling of independence, lets them remain responsible for their behavior, and reduces resentment toward compliance. When patients do not have a choice in the behavior requested, do not play verbal games with them. For example, if Mr. Smith must take a certain medication, do not ask him if he would like to take his medicine. Asking that question leaves the questioner open to a confrontation because Mr. Smith can simply say, "No, I don't want to take my medication." In such situations, it is better to say, "Mr. Smith, it's time to take your medicine. Would you rather have it with water or juice?"

Mentally ill patients often test limits set by staff members. Highly manipulative patients especially need to know that the staff is in charge of the unit and that inappropriate behavior will not gain extra attention or special privileges for them. They need to know that they are expected to participate in ward activities, work assignments, and therapeutic activities. If patients refuse to comply or are uncooperative, it is important that they not be rejected by staff members. Such patients should not be made to feel that the staff has a personal dislike for them or that the staff is annoyed or angry with them. Instead, the staff should stress that the patient is liked and accepted but that the uncooperative behavior is not acceptable.

Although it is important to be firm in gaining patients' cooperation with the behaviors expected of them, it is also important to recognize that occasionally a patient has a legitimate reason for not cooperating; understanding is necessary when patients balk for an appropriate reason.

SEXUALLY AGGRESSIVE BEHAVIOR

Patients who are sexually aggressive seem to be especially upsetting to many mental health workers. Sometimes this is related to the staff members' moral beliefs. However, personal beliefs must be set aside when treating patients who are mentally ill. Although it is not necessary to condone sexual misconduct, it is vitally important that a noncondemnatory, nonjudgmental approach be used with patients who are sexually acting-out. Some staff members may be frightened of sexually aggressive patients and may fear for their own personal safety. Good unit management requires that such feelings be considered in setting staffing patterns and even in deciding whether a particular patient is appropriate for the unit. Staff members also must use good judgment in not being alone with patients with known sexually acting-out tendencies.

Mentally ill patients have the same basic sexual needs as healthy individuals, but they often find that appropriate outlets (husband or wife, or boyfriend or girlfriend) for these needs are far removed, especially when the patient has been hospitalized for a significant period. In some cases, patients feel too unattractive, too insecure, or too inadequate to find someone with whom they might develop an intimate relationship that might lead to appropriate sexual activity. In other cases, patients have such poor interpersonal relationship skills that they alienate appropriate sexual partners. The sexual frustration such patients feel often causes them to engage in inappropriate sexual activities such as fleeting sexual relationships with other patients or sexual advances toward staff members. Staff members must discuss with these patients the inappropriateness of their actions, set limits on their acting out, and try to arrange for appropriate outlets.

Very often, the simple arrangement of a weekend pass for a married person eliminates inappropriate behavior. Other patients, especially adolescents, have not yet learned to handle their affectionate and sexual feelings in socially acceptable ways. With adolescents and other patients who have sexual problems, it is important that staff members be firm but supportive when inappropriate behavior occurs. If the behavior cannot be therapeutically ignored, the patient should be confronted and encouraged to discuss the behavior. If it is possible, the behavior might be temporarily ignored until the staff has an opportunity to discuss the behavior and plan the patient's care accordingly.

Motivational considerations other than sexual attraction may need evaluation. Sexual behavior may be exhibited by a patient as a way of getting a staff member's attention or as a way of embarrassing a staff member who has caused a patient to feel slighted in some way. It may also be a way of testing limits and seeking reassurance that inappropriate behavior will be controlled by the staff. Finally, one must consider that such behavior is motivated by a patient's fear of rejection. Thus, the patient tries to provoke anger in an attempt to confirm rejection and reduce the anxiety of unconfirmed rejection.

Staff members must be careful that their warm, friendly, accepting attitudes toward patients do not become seductive. If Mr. Smith does mistake Miss Jones' warmth and acceptance for love or sexual feelings, he may begin to act out sexually toward her. If this occurs, Miss Jones should try to remain calm and say, "Mr. Smith, I like you as a person but it makes me uncomfortable when you say you love me or when you try to touch me." If the behavior persists, Miss Jones should first be sure that her behavior toward the patient is not subtly encouraging him and then firmly tell him, "Mr. Smith, I have tried to be nice about this but you won't let me. Your behavior is inappropriate and must stop." If the patient persists further, Miss Jones should ask her supervisor to assign someone else to work with the patient.

Patients do not often act out sexually toward staff members but when they do, the behavior must be dealt with firmly and with the patient's being able to perceive as little as possible of the staff member's anxiety.

▼ KEY POINTS ▼

1. Patients who are verbally abusive often are so because they become overly frustrated and displace their frustration from the cause to some convenient person or situation.

continued on page 272

Key Points continued

2. A self-fulfilling prophecy occurs when a patient expects some particular outcome (such as being rejected) and, because of that expectation, begins to act (angrily and defensively) as though the outcome had already occurred. In doing so, the anticipated outcome, rejection, is almost sure to follow.

3. Handling verbally aggressive behavior therapeutically requires that staff members not personalize the patient's statements and that staff set limits on the patient's actions and behaviors, not on the patient's feelings.

4. Verbal expression of anger and hostility can be an important outlet for such feelings and should probably not be discouraged by staff unless it further agitates the patient or other patients on the unit.

5. Judgmental, disparaging, or moralistic remarks to an upset patient will usually only make matters worse.

6. Anytime a staff member argues with a patient, the patient wins. Staff members are expected to show good judgment, restraint, and socially appropriate behaviors at all times.

7. When patients have emotional outbursts, it is imperative that staff members remain calm and collected.

8. As quickly as possible, remove verbally or physically aggressive patients to a private area in which they will not have an audience.

9. When patients are having trouble regaining control, it is appropriate, and sometimes required, that they be given prn medications to prevent escalation.

10. With violent, agitated, or physically destructive patients, "an ounce of prevention is worth a pound of cure."

11. Perhaps the single most important element in dealing with violent, agitated, or destructive patients is to be aware of danger signals or behaviors that indicate that a patient's anger is escalating.

12. With angry, violent patients, be very aware of the need to give them physical and emotional space. Do not permit an audience that might stimulate or further agitate the patient; move other patients and unnecessary staff away from the area. Do not threaten the patient with consequences if they do not calm down. Threatening behavior of any kind usually only escalates the problem.

Key Points continued

13. Do not try to force angry or violent patients and do not try to touch them unless a takedown becomes necessary. Then make certain you have overwhelming odds so that the outcome is never in doubt.

14. Once such patients are calm, discuss with them the feelings that caused the loss of control and discuss more socially appropriate ways of dealing with those feelings.

15. Overly demanding patients often believe that the more time they are able to spend with staff, the greater their personal worth. It may become necessary to structure time with such patients and to explore their feelings about getting dependency needs met.

16. Lying or stealing behavior on the part of patients is often frustrating because it is difficult to play the roles of policeman and therapist simultaneously.

17. While confronting patients who lie or steal, it is important to reject the *behavior,* not the patient.

18. In dealing with antagonistic, intimidating, or physically abusive behavior, prevention is again a key factor. Do not place patients with personality conflicts in a competitive situation.

19. If patients become involved in a fight, separate them if possible, refrain from taking sides, and do not permit an audience for which they must "show off." Then, when they calm down, discuss other ways of dealing with their frustration and conflict.

20. Distraction techniques should be used when possible. Using humor, requesting help with some task, sending the patient for lab tests, or other such techniques may help to distract a patient from his or her anger.

21. One of the most serious errors made by staff members is to ignore or to accept from a patient behavior that is known to be annoying or upsetting to other patients.

22. Be sure to know an uncooperative patient's diagnosis. Regressed patients usually are not being intentionally uncooperative.

23. Sometimes patients are uncooperative because they are afraid of a procedure or technique or are afraid of failing or looking foolish.

continued on page 274

Key Points continued

24. It is almost always detrimental to try to force patients to do anything, and one should not try to gain compliance by threatening patients with punishment.

25. One technique for gaining compliance is simply to explain to a patient why you want him to follow your request. Another is to approach a patient with choices, such as, "Would you rather take your medicine with water or orange juice?" In difficult cases, it is sometimes helpful to make patients' privileges contingent on cooperation with the staff.

26. Be aware that, although patients sometimes test limits with the staff, patients sometimes balk at compliance for a good reason.

27. When dealing with sexually aggressive patients, it is important to be nonjudgmental and noncondemning.

28. Sometimes moral beliefs or feelings of threat to personal safety create staff anxiety in dealing with sexually aggressive patients.

29. Mentally ill patients generally have the same sexual needs as the mentally healthy. However, outlets for sexual needs may be limited and thus more sexual acting out may be seen among psychiatric patients.

30. Patients sometimes act out sexually as a way of gaining a staff member's attention or as a way of embarrassing a staff member whom they feel has embarrassed them. It may also be a way of testing limits and gaining reassurance that acting-out behavior will be appropriately managed by the staff.

31. Staff members must be careful that their warm, friendly, accepting attitudes toward patients do not become seductive.

32. Sexual acting out by patients is rare, but when it occurs it must be managed quickly and effectively by the staff. It is important that staff learn to deal with such situations with as little anxiety as possible.

Annotated Bibliography

Beck, C. K., and Shue, V. M.: Interventions for treating disruptive behavior in demented elderly people. *Nursing Clinics Of North America,* 1994, 29(1):143–155.

Discusses behavioral techniques, multimodal approaches, environmental modifications, and group programs for disruptive patients.

Blair, D. T.: Assaultive behavior: Does provocation begin in the front office? *Journal of Psychosocial Nursing and Mental Health Services,* 1991, 29(5):21–26.

Explains how factors such as involuntary admission, dementia or organic brain disorder, staff attitude, denial of the possibility of assault, and the educational level of the staff can all contribute to an assaultive episode.

Blumenreich, P., Lippmann, S., and Bacani-Oropilla, T.: Violent patients: Are you prepared to deal with them? *Postgraduate Medicine,* 1991, 90(2):201–206.

Presents information on the signs of impending aggression, methods for healthcare workers to prevent or minimize the chance of attack, use of seclusion or restraint, and intervention methods for dealing with violent patients.

Cahill, C. D., Stuart, G. W., Laraia, M. T., and Arana, G. W.: Inpatient management of violent behavior: Nursing prevention and intervention. *Issues in Mental Health Nursing,* 1991, 12:239–252.

Discusses the critical role of psychiatric nurses in inpatient settings in the management of potentially violent patients.

Harris, D., and Morrison, E. F.: Managing violence without coercion. *Archives of Psychiatric Nursing,* 1995, 9(4):203–210.

Proposes emphasizing negotiation and collaboration rather than control for managing violent patients. Discusses a critical analysis of the historical and traditional methods of managing violence.

Martin, K. H.: Improving staff safety through an aggression management program. *Archives of Psychiatric Nursing,* 1995, 9(4):211–215.

Examines the effectiveness of an aggression management program and subsequent aggression-related staff injuries.

Murray, M. G., and Snyder, C.: When staff are assaulted: A nursing consultation support service. *Journal of Psychosocial Nursing and Mental Health Services,* 1991, 29(7):24–29.

Discusses work with violent patients and nursing support services for those who have been assaulted.

Stevenson, S.: Heading off violence with verbal de-escalation. *Journal of Psychosocial Nursing and Mental Health Services,* 1991, 29(9):6–10.

Presents therapeutic communication as a means to alter the course of the aggression cycle before the patient's behavior becomes violent.

Weinrich, S., Edbert, C., Eleazer, G. P., and Haddock, K. S.: Agitation: Measurement, management, and intervention research. *Archives of Psychiatric Nursing,* 1995, 9(5):251–260.

Summarizes literature that is related to the measurement, management, and interventions for agitation as well as identifies a nursing agenda for research conducted in this area.

Post-Test

True or False. Circle your choice.

T   F   1. The key to managing aggressive patients is to teach them to find more socially acceptable ways of expressing their frustrations.

T   F   2. It is appropriate and necessary for a staff member to argue with a patient if the staff member is right and the patient is definitely wrong.

T   F   3. A staff member's own behavior is often his or her most therapeutic tool.

T   F   4. Staff members should not press patients for an explanation of why they behaved in a certain manner.

T   F   5. A patient usually becomes violent only when he or she feels threatened and unable to react in another manner.

T   F   6. Generally, touching agitated patients tends to have a calming effect on them.

T   F   7. Sometimes the most effective approach a staff member can have toward a patient who makes continuous demands is to ignore him or her.

T   F   8. It is often necessary to physically force patients to comply with rules when they are resistant.

T   F   9. An effective approach for dealing with a hostile patient is to accept his or her feelings without indicating approval, disapproval, or value judgment.

Multiple Choice. Circle the number or letter you think represents the best answer.

1. In dealing with a hostile patient, the staff member should:
   a. Understand that hostility is the result of a basic character defect.
   b. Be aware of his or her own reactions to the expressed hostility.
   c. Avoid reacting defensively toward the patient.
   d. Set limits on the patient's behavior.

Post-Test

(continued)

    (1) a and b.
    (2) b and c.
    (3) b, c, and d.
    (4) All the above.

2. Effective approaches for dealing with hostility include:
   a. Recognizing the patient's feelings of hostility.
   b. Allowing the patient to set the pace in the establishment of staff-patient relationships.
   c. Accepting his or her feelings without indicating approval, disapproval, or value judgment.
   d. Conveying to the patient that it is wrong to feel hostile.
   e. Planning approaches to meet the patient's individual needs.
      (1) a, b, and c.
      (2) b, d, and e.
      (3) a, c, and e.
      (4) a, b, c, and e.

Situation. Mrs. Jones tells you in a loud, angry tone of voice that she is very irritated by the incompetence of the medical and nursing staff. You say, "You sound angry." Mrs. Jones says, "Wouldn't you be angry if you had to fight for everything you get?" The next two questions apply to this situation.

3. What would be your most supportive response to Mrs. Jones?
   a. "Yes, I guess I would."
   b. "Tell me about the things that are irritating you and making you feel angry."
   c. "The doctor and nurses are trying to help you. Please cooperate."
   d. "You'll have to learn to control your anger."

4. What would be your most nonsupportive response to Mrs. Jones?
   a. "Yes, I guess I would."
   b. "Tell me about the things that are irritating you and making you feel angry."
   c. "The doctor and nurses are trying to help you. Please cooperate."
   d. "You'll have to learn to control your anger."

Post-Test

(continued)

5. Mrs. White, a staff member, has been talking to a patient and, as she gets up to leave, the patient puts his arms around her and tries to kiss her. She should:
   a. Kick him in the groin.
   b. Tell him his behavior is inappropriate.
   c. Tell him that she is going to tell his wife if he does not stop.
   d. Tell him that his behavior makes her uncomfortable and ask him to stop.

Short Answer. Answer the following as briefly and specifically as possible.

1. If a staff member is certain that a patient has stolen an article from another patient, how should the staff member handle the situation?

_____

_____

_____

2. What is one of the most effective ways to keep patients from fighting and arguing?

_____

_____

_____

3. When does a patient usually resort to physical violence?

_____

_____

_____

4. Why is it a good idea to try to isolate a patient who appears to be becoming physically destructive?

_____

_____

_____

Care for Anxious Patients

OBJECTIVES: Student will be able to:

1. Differentiate between behavioral manifestations of anxiety in a healthy person and those behaviors in a mentally ill patient.

2. State an understanding of the purpose of anxious behaviors exhibited by patients.

3. Identify two reasons anxious patients have difficulty making a decision.

4. Report at least one major difficulty with anxiolytic medication.

5. Explain why talking helps to reduce anxiety in patients.

6. Identify three cognitive behaviors that are problems for anxious patients.

7. State the reason it is important to ask an agitated patient why he or she wants to engage in a particular behavior.

8. State when it is best to not be too friendly with an agitated patient.

9. List techniques used in working with patients exhibiting compulsive behaviors.

10. Identify useful and appropriate responses to patients exhibiting phobic behaviors.

We have already talked about the fear and anxiety felt by many patients. Constant, excessive worry and a high level of physical tension are hallmarks of anxious patients, and many have specific phobias. A large number of patients show restless, somewhat agitated behavior while others show compulsive, ritualistic behavior. They have many "what if" concerns and a vague feeling that something bad is going to happen. (For a review of symptoms, see Chapter 5.) In contrast, in mentally healthy persons, anxiety is usually limited to very brief periods, its source is apparent, and the person takes action to correct the problem causing the anxiety.

In practically all cases, the behavior associated with the anxious patient is aimed at reducing the subjective feeling of anxiety that the patient experiences. Anxiety tells the patient and the staff that something needs to be done and often initiates the "fight or flight" stress response in the patient. Another difficulty is that patients are often so anxious that they cannot make a decision. This may occur because a patient sees so many possible solutions that no single solution seems appropriate or "best" and the patient does not want to decide among the alternatives for fear of making the wrong choice. It may also be that the patient cannot find even one acceptable solution. Thus, no action is taken and the anxiety continues.

This chapter discusses many behaviors that might be expected from such patients and explores ways of managing those behaviors. It should be understood that drug therapy is often used in conjunction with the behavior management techniques presented here. Drug therapy is aimed at the physiological components of anxiety, whereas psychotherapy is aimed at the cognitive components of the anxiety. One concern with anxiolytic medications is that many are addictive, requiring that the patient be carefully withdrawn from them when the medications are discontinued after extended use.

Anxiety is, in many ways, a disorder of control. Thus anxious patients are often upset by new and unfamiliar surroundings. In these situations, patients become more frightened, agitated, and sometimes more withdrawn when they do not know what is expected of them or how they should behave. Uncertainty and conflict, often arising out of a fear of loss of control, are the primary causes of anxiety. Therefore, it is important that new patients who are anxious, worried, or upset be introduced to the unit by carefully explaining what is expected of them, where they will sleep, how they will get meals, when the doctor will come, and what they should do if they need help. These patients frequently need someone to talk to them to reassure them and simply to provide company. They may have many questions, some of which will be repeated more than once. These questions should always be answered carefully and fully, and patients should be reassured that someone will be available to help if they need anything.

On an open unit, anxious patients can frequently be seen moving about, searching for someone to talk with about their fears. It is important that staff members take time to talk to such patients and try to help them understand and recognize their fears. Patients can usually be helped to calm down by gradually easing them off the subject of a particular fear or worry and then getting them to talk about things that do not arouse anxiety or fear and thus are not upsetting to them.

It sometimes happens that highly anxious patients are afraid of other patients on the unit. It may be helpful to introduce such patients to other patients and to encourage them to talk with some of those patients. It is sometimes helpful to point out that all the patients are there for the same reason, to receive help for their difficulties, and that the staff is there to see that they all receive whatever help they need. Try to avoid situations in which one patient is made to express a view or opinion that may conflict with other patients' views.

Frequently, an anxious patient becomes upset over something that has a great deal of importance to that particular patient but that may be of little or no importance to other patients or to staff members. In such cases, the patient may benefit from some specific concession made to permit the patient to decrease his or her anxiety or fear by engaging in a particular calming behavior. For example, it is frequently the case that, when a patient is about to go on leave or is about to be discharged, the patient is quite afraid that no one will come to pick him or her up and may want to call a family member for reassurance that someone is coming. The patient might be quite relieved, and thus calmer, if allowed to call the family.

Cognitive therapists often address the anxious patient's tendency to catastrophize, to overvalue certain aspects of a situation, or to overestimate the probability of some event. They teach patients to realistically evaluate the probability of the event and to recognize their tendency to make a catastrophe out of something that is highly improbable. This is usually accomplished not by directly challenging patients' assumptions, for example, but rather by asking questions that point out the overestimation of the likelihood of an event. If a patient says, "I feel like I'm going to die!" the therapist might respond by saying, "I can see you're frightened. What is it you think will cause your death?" The therapist will then proceed through a number of questions that lead the patient to understand that he or she has catastrophized the situation, overestimated the probability of the occurrence, and has based his or her assumptions on beliefs that are irrational. The therapist will then help the patient supplant the irrational beliefs with rational ones.

Relaxation techniques are also often used to treat anxious patients, as is visual imagery training, systematic desensitization, and flooding. *Systematic desensitization* is a technique using the inherent properties of response gradients. That is, someone is exposed to a feared stimulus at a great distance until it can be tolerated; then, in small steps, the individual is exposed to the same stimulus at decreasing intervals, bringing him or her closer and closer to the feared stimulus.

Flooding is a technique in which the patient is saturated with exposure to the stimulus and learns to not fear the stimulus because, even with saturation, the patient experiences no harm from the exposure. The use of such techniques requires careful consideration and should be conducted only by persons specifically trained in their use.

RESTLESS, AGITATED BEHAVIOR

Patients who are restless are frequently reassured and calmed by having a mental health team member take them for a brief walk or by simply taking them to a quiet place and sitting down to talk with them. Usually, if agitated or restless patients are allowed to speak their mind, they are able to settle down more quickly and to feel reassured. Unless patients are allowed to speak their mind and express the things that are troubling them, a great deal of unnecessary angry and frustrated acting out may occur. For example, in one case three attendants were used to restrain a female patient who was caught trying to enter another patient's room. Because no one thought to ask why the patient wanted to go into the other patient's room, she was simply told that she could go into her own room but not into the other patient's room. After a great deal of acting-out behavior and after the patient had been restrained by the attendants, a nurse asked the girl why she wanted to go into the other patient's room. The patient explained that she had dropped her ring and it had rolled under the door. When the ring was retrieved, the patient calmed down and was released. The problem could have been prevented in the first place by simply asking the patient why she wanted to go into the room.

If patients are allowed to discuss their anxieties and feelings, sometimes referred to as *ventilation,* much of the emotional pressure they feel seems to be relieved. This is particularly the case at bedtime for patients with anxieties. It is usually not a good policy to insist that patients go to bed whether they are sleepy or not. Frequently, patients who are forced to go to bed become quite agitated and restless and are much more likely to act out than if they are taken to a quiet area in which they will not disturb patients who may be trying to sleep. These agitated patients typically do much better when they are allowed to stay up for a while to discuss their feelings with a staff member. As soon as the patients calm down, they may then be returned to their rooms and encouraged to try to sleep. Other patients may be able to go to sleep without leaving their rooms if a mental health team member simply comes and sits with them or if they are allowed to leave a light on. Sometimes patients will agree to go to bed if they are given some small favor such as a glass of juice, a drink of water, a cup of decaffeinated coffee, or simply a chance to walk around for a few minutes. Some prn medication should also be considered for such patients.

Occasionally, patients seem to become more anxious if staff members or other patients are friendly and supportive of them. In these circumstances, it is best to maintain a businesslike manner. Such patients need time to accept the idea that others can like them and be interested in them without expecting something in return.

COMPULSIVE BEHAVIOR

One form of anxious behavior that is sometimes difficult to control is *compulsive behavior,* which may or may not include *ritualism.* Patients engage in ritualistic behaviors in an effort to "prevent" something bad that they fear will happen. To a lesser degree, many people engage in similar behaviors when they follow superstitions such as "Don't walk under a ladder," "Breaking a mirror means 7 years of bad luck," or "It's bad luck if a black cat crosses the road in front of you." The major problem with compulsive behaviors is that they significantly inhibit a patient's ability to lead a normal life. Some patients carry their ritualistic behaviors to such extremes that they create significant physical problems. One of the most common ritualistic behaviors is that of hand-washing. Some patients have been known to wash their hands more than 100 times a day and continue to wash them despite the fact that their hands are cracked and bleeding from the soap, water, and scrubbing. Some cannot leave the house without checking numerous times to be certain the door is locked. Such patients should never be approached in a demanding and threatening way because such behavior only increases the patient's insecurity and anxiety, thus creating more need for the ritualistic behavior.

Sometimes it is possible to talk with patients about their compulsive or ritualistic behavior and to encourage them to try other ways of controlling their anxiety. Sometimes it is possible to help patients begin to reduce a ritual by leaving off one of the components of the ritual, the next day leaving off another component, and the following day leaving off yet another component until the ritualistic behavior is eliminated or stopped. By reducing the compulsive behavior a little at a time, the patient is permitted to adjust to the new conditions slowly rather than have to suddenly deal with all the anxieties that the ritual helped to control. Conversely, many behavior therapists believe that the only effective way to manage such behaviors is to reach 100 percent elimination of the behavior immediately. Those therapists use behavior logs, enviromental reminders, and even physical restraint devices to prevent the patient from engaging in the ritualistic or compulsive behavior.

Such treatment techniques should never be used except as part of an overall treatment plan directed, integrated, and controlled by a therapist skilled in those techniques.

It is never helpful to be critical of a patient's ritualistic behavior. It is important to remember that, although the behavior may be quite silly to an observer, it has a very real meaning to the patient. Most important is to allow patients to know that they and their problems are accepted by the staff members. This usually does more to relieve patients' anxiety than reassurance that "everything is going to be all right." The patient does not think things are going to be all right and feels rejected if that is all he or she is offered in the way of reassurance. Instead of saying, "Don't worry so much" to a patient, say, "I can see that you are upset about this. Why don't we talk about it?" Other reassuring statements include, "You seem to feel hurt about Mrs. Jones' saying she hates you. Let's talk about it" or "Let's talk about why you believe people don't like you" or "I've noticed you always wring your hands and seem upset when your mother calls." Such statements give patients an opportunity to talk if they want to. It is not useful to insist that they talk when they obviously do not want to. More often than not, however, patients like to talk and a staff member who listens well will be highly valued by patients. The information you gain from listening to patients may provide valuable clues to the treatment team and should always be reported to them.

PHOBIC BEHAVIOR

Phobic patients have specific fears or anxieties and may become quite upset, frightened, or agitated when confronted with the phobic or feared object. Frequently these patients seek reassurance by asking repeatedly whether someone will be able to help, whether they are going crazy, and whether they will be able to recover from their illness. Perhaps the best reply to such requests for reassurance is to simply tell the patient that you will be happy to talk about problems any time you are free. The patient may also be told that talking about problems is often the best way to begin solving them. Although phobic behaviors will likely need specific and advanced behavioral, cognitive, and pharmacological intervention, listening to the patient's concerns will go a long way toward helping the patient feel accepted despite his or her fears and phobias.

In summary, while managing anxious patients, it is most important that staff members remain calm and restrained. Anxious patients frequently try to provoke anxiety in staff members. If they are successful, they feel their own anxiety is justified. If they are not successful, they tend to be reassured. When anxious patients perceive uncertainty or conflict among staff members or other patients, they are likely to respond by becoming even more anxious themselves.

▼ KEY POINTS ▼

1. Constant, excessive worry, and a high level of physical tension are hallmarks of anxious patients, and many have specific phobias.

2. The behavior associated with the anxious patient is usually aimed at reducing the subjective feeling of anxiety that the patient is experiencing.

3. When anxious patients perceive uncertainty or conflict among staff members or other patients, they are likely to respond by becoming even more anxious themselves.

4. Patients cannot make decisions because they see so many possible solutions that no single solution seems appropriate and they fear making the wrong choice.

5. Drug therapy is aimed at the physiological components of anxiety, whereas psychotherapy is aimed at the cognitive components of the anxiety.

6. Anxious patients are often upset by new and unfamiliar surroundings.

7. Uncertainty and conflict, often arising out of a fear of loss of control, are the primary causes of anxiety.

8. It is important that staff members take time to talk to anxious patients to help them understand their fears and to get them to talk about things that do not arouse their anxiety.

9. It may be helpful to introduce highly anxious patients to other patients on the unit and to encourage them to talk with one another.

10. Frequently, anxious patients become upset over something that has a great deal of importance to them but that may be of little or no importance to other patients or staff members. Even so, they must be afforded an opportunity to discuss those issues.

11. Anxious patients tend to catastrophize, to overvalue certain aspects of a situation, or to overestimate the probability of some event.

---

continued on page 286

Key Points continued

12. In addition to medication, relaxation techniques are also often used to treat anxious patients, as is visual imagery training, systematic desensitization, and, sometimes, flooding.

13. Patients who are restless are frequently reassured and calmed by having a mental health team member take them for a brief walk or to a quiet place to sit and talk.

14. Unless patients are allowed to say what is on their minds and to express the things that are troubling them, a great deal of unnecessary anger and frustration may result.

15. If patients are allowed to discuss their anxieties and feelings, much of the emotional pressure they feel seems to be relieved.

16. Frequently, anxious patients who are forced to go to bed become quite agitated and restless. Such patients seem to do much better when they are allowed to stay up for a while to discuss their feelings with a staff member.

17. Sometimes patients will agree to go to bed if they are given some small favor such as a glass of juice, a chance to walk around for a few minutes, or a short conversation with a staff member.

18. Occasionally, patients seem to become more anxious if staff members or other patients are friendly and supportive of them. In these circumstances, it is best to maintain a businesslike manner.

19. Compulsive behavior is a manifestation of anxiety that is difficult to control and sometimes includes behavioral rituals.

20. The major problem with compulsive behaviors is that they significantly inhibit a patient's ability to lead a normal life.

21. Patients displaying extreme ritualistic behaviors should never be approached in a demanding and threatening way. Such behavior only increases the patient's insecurity and anxiety.

22. For many compulsive or ritualistic behaviors it is possible to talk with patients about their behavior and encourage them to try other ways of controlling their anxiety.

23. By trying to reduce the compulsive behavior a little at a time, the patient is permitted to adjust to the new conditions slowly rather than to suddenly have to deal with all the anxieties that the ritual helped control.

24. It is never helpful to be critical of a patient's ritualistic behavior; it has a very real meaning to the patient.

Key Points continued

25. Patients will feel rejected if "everything is going to be all right" is all they are offered as reassurance. Patients must know that they and their problems are accepted by the staff.

26. Patients like to talk, and a staff member who listens well will be highly valued by patients. The information may provide valuable clues to the treatment team and should always be reported to them.

27. Phobic patients have specific fears or anxieties and may become quite upset, frightened, or agitated when confronted with the phobic or feared object.

28. Help the patient understand that talking about fears or phobias is often the best way to begin solving them.

29. Straightforward, realistic reassurance that patients are safe and secure may be needed.

30. Providing information and education about the nature and process of phobic reaction often has a calming effect on patients.

31. Encourage patients to work with their primary therapist to resolve the phobic reactions.

Annotated Bibliography

Barth, F. D.: Obsessional thinking as "paradoxical action." *Bulletin of the Menninger Clinic,* 1990, 54:499–511.

Offers an integration of theoretical approaches to obsessive-compulsive neurosis and attempts to explain the resistance frequently encountered with patients, using Schafer's theory of obsessional thinking as a paradoxical or conflictual action.

Benham, E.: Coping strategies: A psychoeducational approach to post-traumatic symptomatology. *Journal of Psychosocial Nursing,* 1995, 33(6):30–35.

Discusses self-destructive coping behaviors and ways to encourage healthy coping behaviors as well as giving helpful interventional tips.

McFarlane, A. C.: Individual psychotherapy for post-traumatic stress disorder. *Psychiatric Clinics of North America,* 1994, 17(2):393–408.

Compares a conceptual model with other schools of therapy for the treatment of post-traumatic stress disorder.

Simoni, P. S.: Obsessive-compulsive disorder: The effect of research on nursing care. *Journal of Psychosocial Nursing and Mental Health Services,* 1991, 29(4):19–23.

Expresses the importance of paying close attention to behaviors, feelings, and cognitions when treating patients with obsessive-compulsive disorder.

Turner, D. M.: Panic disorder: A personal and nursing perspective. *Journal of Psychosocial Nursing,* 1995, 33(4):5–8.

Discusses biologic etiology for panic disorder and implications for nurses treating patients with the disorder.

Wesner, R. B.: Alcohol use and abuse secondary to anxiety. *Psychiatric Clinics of North America,* 1990, 13(4):699–713.

Discusses the prevalence and complications of using alcohol to overcome feelings of anxiety. Offers case examples and treatment plans.

Whitley, G. G.: Ritualistic behavior: Breaking the cycle. *Journal of Psychosocial Nursing and Mental Health Services,* 1991, 29(10):31–35.

Explores biologic theories of causation and the use of behavior and medication therapy as treatments of choice.

Post-Test

True or False. Circle your choice.

T   F   1. Anxious patients are frequently upset by new and unfamiliar surroundings.

T   F   2. Phobias are unusual in truly anxious patients.

T   F   3. An anxious patient's ritualistic behavior is aimed at reducing his or her objective feelings of anxiety.

T   F   4. Uncertainty and conflict are the primary causes of anxiety.

T   F   5. An anxious patient should be encouraged to not talk about his or her fears because they are unrealistic.

T   F   6. An agitated, restless patient should not be allowed to say what is on his or her mind because it may upset other patients.

T   F   7. It is a good policy to insist that patients go to bed whether or not they are sleepy.

T   F   8. Sometimes a friendly, supportive staff member can cause a patient to become more upset and anxious.

T   F   9. Excessive handwashing is a sign of anxiety.

T   F   10. The most effective way to discourage ritualistic behavior is to gently criticize the behavior to the patient. By your doing so, the patient will recognize that the behavior is not helping and that it makes him or her look bad in front of others.

Multiple Choice. Circle the letter or number you think represents the best answer.

1. An anxious patient:
   a. Feels threatened by unknown danger.
   b. Is unable to concentrate.
   c. Displays indecision.

Post-Test

(continued)

    d. May make many demands for attention.
      (1) a and c.
      (2) b and d.
      (3) a, b, and c.
      (4) All of the above.

2. The characteristic that distinguishes fear from anxiety is that fear:
    a. Usually has a specific object.
    b. Evokes a milder degree of emotion.
    c. Persists over a longer period of time.
    d. Occurs in the absence of real danger.

3. Which of the following are characteristic of anxiety?
    a. Feeling of helplessness.
    b. Reaction to evident danger.
    c. Reaction to future danger.
    d. Many attempts to alleviate by use of defense mechanisms.
    e. Leads to a neurosis if not halted.
      (1) a, b, and d.
      (2) a, c, and e.
      (3) a, c, d, and e.
      (4) c, d, and e.
      (5) All of the above.

4. The individual suffering from normal anxiety:
    a. Is able to focus on what is happening.
    b. Is able to recognize and face the threat realistically.
    c. Sometimes uses mental mechanisms for relief.
    d. Hears voices.
      (1) a only.
      (2) a and c.
      (3) a, b, and c.
      (4) All of the above.

5. Reassurance can be given to the anxious patient by:
    a. Remaining calm and confident with the patient.
    b. Guessing the patient's worries and getting him or her to talk.
    c. Giving correct information when the patient needs it.
    d. Remaining with the patient.
      (1) a only.

Post-Test

(continued)

(2) a, c, and d.
(3) c and d.
(4) b, c, and d.

6. A characteristic of anxiety is:
   a. Feeling of helplessness.
   b. Anticipation of pleasure.
   c. Decrease in muscular tension.
   d. Relationship to specific objects.

Situation. Mary Jane, age 18, an honor student at Haven College, is admitted to the hospital during exam week in a state of extreme anxiety. She tells the staff member that if she flunks out she will not be able to go to medical school as her parents want her to. The next two questions apply to this situation.

7. As Mary and the staff member enter the dayroom, Mary tries to break away and appears terrified of the group of patients. The staff member should take the following action:
   a. Gently steer Mary to her own room and stay with her.
   b. Call for the orderly to drag Mary away forcibly.
   c. Talk quietly and calmly to Mary as they proceed to her room.
   d. Warn Mary that she will be put in restraints if she does not behave.
      (1) a only.
      (2) b only.
      (3) a and c.
      (4) b and d.

8. The next day Mary is calmer. She tells the staff member how disappointed her parents will be if she flunks. The staff member:
   a. Tells Mary her parents will love her, anyway.
   b. Allows Mary to explore her feelings about this.
   c. Advises Mary to study hard so she can pass.
   d. Ignores the remark.

9. When a patient has an anxiety attack at night and refuses to remain in his or her room because of fear, you should:
   a. Explain that there is nothing to be afraid of.

Post-Test

(continued)

    b. Let him or her sit out in the hall by the nurse's station.
    c. Leave a light burning in the patient's room.
    d. Place him or her in a seclusion room.

10. Which of the following responses is most appropriate in relation to a patient who is pacing the halls, wringing his or her hands, and crying?
    a. "You seem all upset right now, but I'm sure you won't feel this way much longer."
    b. "Sit here a minute and I'll get your nerve medicine."
    c. "I'll stay with you; perhaps I can help."
    d. "Sit down a minute; you'll feel better in a little while."

11. The primary defense mechanism used against anxiety is:
    a. Reaction formation.
    b. Denial.
    c. Suppression.
    d. Compensation.
    e. Repression.

Care for Suspicious Patients

OBJECTIVES: Student will be able to:

1. Describe behaviors common to the suspicious patient.
2. Explain why suspicious patients are often rejected by patients, family, and, sometimes, staff.
3. State the expected response when paranoid patients are challenged.
4. Identify the reason paranoid patients often try to get staff on their "side."
5. List the major defense mechanisms used by paranoid patients.
6. State the best response to a paranoid patient who says, "You better not touch me!"
7. Respond appropriately when a paranoid patient criticizes a staff member, rule, or unit policy.
8. List effective ways of managing suspicious behaviors.

In addition to the fearfulness and distrustfulness shown by the suspicious or paranoid patient, this type of patient tends to be quarrelsome and aloof. Such behaviors often evoke a great deal of anger in other patients and staff members. This leads to rejection of the patient, causing him or her to respond with hostility and confirming the patient's negative expectations about interpersonal relationships. Such patients, therefore, feel ill at ease in interpersonal relationships and tend to interpret minor oversights as significant personal rejections. In fact, they often find slights or injustices where none exist. They are likely to overreact to seemingly insignificant occurrences and are often unable to control their feelings and their behaviors in situations appropriately requiring restraint and understanding. Such patients are frequently overly concerned with fairness and with being certain that they are being treated as everyone else is treated.

Projection is the major defense mechanism used by paranoid patients. People without significant mental illness sometimes resent in others that which they fear in themselves, and they may or may not have much insight into that tendency. However, without realizing it, paranoid patients project their own hostility and aggressive impulses onto other people. The projection causes these patients to perceive hostility and rejection from others. Thus, the patients become fearful, agitated, and overly concerned about their rights. Because they see themselves as the focal point of everyone's behavior, they interpret anything that happens in their environment as having special meaning for them. Another point to remember in understanding paranoid patients is that they frequently show good ego strength; that is, they appear to be capable people who feel no need to rely on anyone but themselves. They tend to be opinionated, stubborn, and defensive and react with hostility when their opinions are challenged.

Dealing with the suspicious or paranoid patient requires a considerable amount of diplomacy. It is not in the best interest of the patient or the staff member to argue. In an argument, paranoid patients may perceive that they must defend their position and will feel quite self-righteous about venting their hostility, anger, and frustration. They tend to believe they are defending their position for the benefit of mankind or for some other lofty or grandiose cause, thus justifying their unreasonable anger.

Paranoid patients sometimes put much effort into trying to win staff members to their side because they see staff members as authority figures. If they succeed, they feel their position is justified. Again, a great deal of tact and preparation is needed to effectively manage this situation. If a staff member tells a patient that he or she does not agree with the patient's position, that staff member is inviting an argument that he or she will almost always lose. The staff member will lose because such patients usually have an extreme, narrowly focused, and unrelenting commitment to their position, and reasoning, by definition, is lost on the irrational patient. On the other hand, making an appropriate interpretive statement may encourage the patient to talk and provide an opportunity to move him or her to an area in which the anger and frustration can be vented in privacy. For example, if an angry patient shouts, "You had better not touch me!" it is probably best to respond by saying to the patient, "All right, John, I won't touch you if it bothers you. Can you tell me what bothers you about being touched?" rather than saying to the patient, "I don't intend to touch you" or "I will touch you if I have to" or "Don't be so afraid of being touched." The first suggested response leaves room for the patient to talk about the reasons for his not wanting to be touched and to allow the staff member an opportunity to enter into a discussion with him. Of course, the patient may or may not have enough insight to understand his or her discomfort in being touched. Observing the patient's wishes whenever possible, avoiding a power struggle, and being willing to talk with the patient might later lead to the establishment of a relationship in which the patient might learn to trust the staff member.

Because a basic and pervasive sense of worthlessness and inadequacy is thought to underlie much of the paranoid patient's behavior, it is usually not helpful to use flowery language, flattery, or overabundance of praise to try to improve the patient's poor self-concept or self-image. It is difficult to "convince" most patients of their worth, but it is particularly difficult to persuade a suspicious patient of increased worth. A staff member also runs the risk of having paranoid patients reject such verbalizations outright, thus breaking off the potential for therapeutic relationships. In grandiose patients, such staff behavior may reinforce the patients' feelings of grandiosity and may, at best, be inappropriate therapy for them.

Staff members and patients alike are frequently intimidated or made to feel extremely uncomfortable when the suspicious patient appears to be visually locked in on them. The "paranoid stare" occurs when patients stare intently, trying to observe and understand everything that is taking place in their environment. Such patients miss very little. For example, when staff members or others look away from staring patients, those patients sometimes feel that others are afraid of them or that others cannot tolerate the scrutiny of such a righteous person. If a staff member is in a visual confrontation with a paranoid patient, it is best to not avoid the stare but to observe the patient closely for a brief period. The patient may then decide that the staff member is not afraid and is willing to pay close attention to what the patient has to say. A long, staring duel may be avoided if staff members move quickly to distract the patient by suggesting some diversional activity or directing the patient's attention to a picture in a magazine or on the wall. Alternatively, a staff member might confront the staring patient by interpreting the stare as a bid for attention and say, "You seem to be trying to get my attention, John. Is there some way I can be of help?"

Paranoid patients seem to have a great many religious delusions. A staff member might listen quietly as the patient talks about a delusion and then take the first opportunity to ask for help with some particular task or to engage him or her in a more reality-oriented conversation. Make as little reference as possible to the delusional concerns. Argument is inappropriate and useless because the patient will feel compelled to defend the delusion. If discussion about the content of the delusional perception cannot be avoided, it is often appropriate to state something like the following: "John, I know you believe the FBI is after you but it doesn't seem that way to me. I'm not going to convince you they aren't after you and you aren't going to convince me they are, so why don't we take a walk and you can tell me about things you like to do when you aren't worried about the FBI." This approach is straightforward, acknowledges the patient's position, is not argumentative, does not demean the patient, and permits a graceful way to move on to other topics.

The suspicious or paranoid patient typically has a strong fear of developing a close relationship with another person. This is related to the fear of being rejected, and the patient can feel rejection only if close relationships are established. These patients are most likely to establish a relationship with a staff member who is honest and forthright. If Mr. Jones believes that you are going to hurt him, simply reassuring him that you are not going to hurt him will not allay his suspicions. However, if a staff member recognizes Mr. Jones' suspiciousness by saying, "I know you don't trust me and that's all right. I just want to talk," Mr. Jones may be able to understand that he is not going to be rejected because he is distrustful.

Another way of managing patients who present outlandish demands or who, as mentioned, demand acceptance of obviously delusional ideas is to say to the patient, "I know you believe you have a lightbulb burning inside your head but I can't see it." To say anything more might lead to an argument the staff member could not win and might escalate the patient's anger. If pushed, you might say, "I know you believe it's true, but you wouldn't ask me to believe something I don't know to be true, would you?" That last statement runs the risk of asking for a rational response from an irrational person, but all rationality is not always lost, even in people with irrational thoughts and beliefs. If you don't believe that, just look at some of our politicians!

A reason for not agreeing with a patient's delusions is that patients frequently retain some contact with reality and will be quite mistrustful if they seem able to convince a staff member that a delusion is true. Patients often do not want the delusion to be true but cannot bring themselves to alter their belief. If Mr. Jones has convinced the staff member of the truthfulness of his delusion, he may have enough rationality to know that the staff member may not be as mentally healthy as he is, or it may increase his fearfulness that his delusional material is indeed verifiably true.

In many cases, patients' stories are close enough to rationality that it is difficult to know whether a patient is being truthful. For example, one of the authors once treated a patient who was convinced a family member was trying to steal money and property left to her by her father. She was so convincing that the author had to recommend that an attorney be brought in to evaluate the situation. In fact, she was right. Just because a patient is irrational about one thing does not mean he or she cannot be rational about other things. Always try to verify things that are not obviously absurd. For example, it might be difficult to verify a delusion such as, "I'm on a special mission to prepare the way for aliens from Mars. I'm a martian princess and I own half the land on the planet." Not only would that statement be difficult to verify but, until we hear something new from UFO headquarters, we are probably safe in assuming that the patient is delusional.

To sum up these last few comments, a rule of thumb may be appropriate: *Do not participate in a patient's mental games, because you do not know the rules and therefore cannot hope to win.*

Finally, it is important to realize that a patient's suspiciousness of and attentiveness to surrounding activities frequently make the patient a source of anxiety and provocation for staff members. A paranoid patient may make offensive, yet accurate, criticisms of staff members, unit policies, and unit procedures. It is of absolute importance that staff members not respond to these criticisms by becoming anxious or by rejecting the patient. That is a difficult lesson. The paranoid patient is likely to be kind at times and vicious at others. This inconsistency in behavior makes the paranoid patient difficult to manage successfully. It is the staff's responsibility to provide such patients with firm, consistent, supportive care.

▼ KEY POINTS ▼

Managing Suspicious Behaviors

1. In addition to fearful and distrustful behavior, the suspicious or paranoid patient tends to be quarrelsome and aloof.

2. Paranoid patients feel ill at ease in interpersonal relationships and tend to interpret minor oversights as significant personal rejections, often finding slights or injustices where none exist.

3. Projection is the major defense mechanism used by paranoid patients. They project their own hostility and aggressive impulses onto other people and perceive hostility and rejection from others.

4. Suspicious patients frequently show good ego strength, appear to be capable people, feel they do not need to rely on anyone else, and react with hostility when their opinions are challenged.

continued on page 298

Key Points continued

5. It is not in the best interest of the patient or the staff member to argue. Paranoid patients may perceive that they must defend their position and will feel quite self-righteous about venting their hostility.

6. Paranoid patients sometimes try very hard to win staff members to their side because they see staff members as authority figures.

7. Such patients usually have an extreme commitment to their position; reasoning, by definition, is lost on the irrational patient.

8. It is probable that making an appropriate interpretive statement such as, "You seem quite angry" may encourage the patient to talk and will afford the patient an opportunity to privately vent anger and frustration.

9. Because a basic sense of worthlessness and inadequacy underlies much of the paranoid patient's behavior, it is usually not helpful to use an overabundance of praise to try to improve the patient's self-concept. The patient may think you are being kind in order to take advantage of him or her.

10. The "paranoid stare," characteristic of the suspicious patient, occurs when patients stare intently, trying to observe and understand everything that is taking place in their environment.

11. If a staff member is in a visual confrontation with a paranoid patient, it is best to not avoid the stare but to observe the patient closely for a brief period and then try to distract the patient.

12. Paranoid patients often have religious delusions. A staff member should listen quietly and take the first opportunity to engage them in a more reality-oriented conversation.

13. The suspicious or paranoid patient has a strong fear of developing a close relationship with another person and most likely will establish a relationship with a staff member who is honest and forthright but not overly friendly.

14. One way of managing patients who present outlandish demands or who demand acceptance of obviously delusional ideas is to say, "I know you believe it's true, but you wouldn't ask me to believe something I don't know to be true, would you?"

15. Patients frequently retain some contact with reality and may be quite mistrustful if able to apparently convince a staff member that a delusion is true.

Key Points continued

16. Just because a patient is irrational about one thing does not mean he or she cannot be rational about other things. Always try to verify statements that are not obviously absurd.

17. A good rule of thumb may be: Do not participate in a patient's mental games because you do not know the rules and, therefore, cannot hope to win ("winning" means helping the patient).

18. The paranoid patient is likely to be kind at times and vicious at others. This inconsistency in behavior makes the paranoid patient difficult to manage successfully.

Annotated Bibliography

Blise, M. L.: Everything I learned, I learned from patients: Radical positive reframing. *Journal of Psychosocial Nursing and Mental Health Services,* 1995, 33(12):18–25.

Explains how a process of reframing can help patients with paranoid delusions to develop less-threatening explanations and choices in their perception and management of their delusions.

Davidhizar, R.: A manager's dilemma: Paranoid thinking. *Nursing Management,* 1992, 23(9):66–68.

Discusses the prevention and control of paranoid thoughts with employees. The roles of self-concept, employer, and employees in dealing with paranoid thought are explored.

Epstein, L. J.: Paranoid illness in the elderly. *Consultant,* 1980, 20(9):95–102.

Relates range of etiologic factors contributing to paranoid behavior in the elderly. Author states opinions on the goals of treatment.

Grossberg, G. T., and Manapalli, J.: The older patient with psychotic symptoms. *Psychiatric Services,* 1995, 46(1):55–59.

Reviews the last 10 years of literature of general medical causes of psychotic symptoms in persons over age 65. Specifically discusses the role of drug and other toxicities as causes of paranoia in the elderly.

Hales, D., and Hales, R. E.: *Caring For The Mind: The Comprehensive Guide To Mental Health Nursing.* New York: Bantam Books, 1995, pp. 548–556.

Discusses the personality traits and lifestyle patterns of the paranoid and suspicious patient, including the frequency of occurrence of paranoia in the United States and the numerous options available for treating paranoid and suspicious behaviors.

Hawes, M. J., and Bible, H. H.: The paranoid patient: Surgeon beware! *Ophthalmic Plastic and Reconstructive Surgery,* 1990, 6(3):225–227.

Provides a case example of a plastic surgeon's work with a patient with a paranoid disorder. Includes suggestions for detecting and managing such patients.

Lehman, L., and Kelley, J. H.: Nursing interventions for anxiety, depression and suspiciousness in the home care setting. *Home Healthcare Nurse,* 1993, 11(3):35–40.

Reviews general concepts of the patient experiencing anxiety, depression, and suspiciousness. The authors give specific illustrations of the nursing care involved in this patient population.

Mizsur, G. L.: Depression and paranoia: Is your patient at risk? *Nursing,* 1995, 25(2):66–67.

Discusses methods of determining the level of risk associated with depressed patients with paranoid thoughts.

The Quality Assurance Project: Treatment outlines for paranoid, schizotypal and schizoid personality disorders. *Australian and New Zealand Journal of Psychiatry,* 1990, 24:339–350.

Presents treatment outlines for paranoid, schizotypal, and schizoid personality disorders, using advice from expert committees, review of the literature, and opinions of practicing psychiatrists.

Williams, D.: Nursing care of the paranoid patient. *Advanced Clinical Nurse,* 1990, 5(6):12–15.

Gives the nurse a well-developed nursing care plan to deal with the paranoid patient in the medical-surgical setting.

Post-Test

True or False. Circle your choice.

T   F   1. Usually a patient's delusions have some basis in reality.

T   F   2. It is therapeutic for a patient to discuss his or her delusion at length.

T   F   3. The paranoid patient is likely to be warm and kind one moment and then become very anxious the next moment.

T   F   4. The major defense mechanism used by the paranoid patient is projection.

T   F   5. Suspicious patients often interpret minor oversights as personal rejection.

T   F   6. Because a basic sense of worthlessness and inadequacy underlies much of the paranoid patient's behavior, it is helpful to use flattery and a great deal of praise to improve the patient's self-image.

T   F   7. Paranoid patients may have a great many religious delusions.

Multiple Choice. Circle the letter you think represents the best answer.

Situation. Mr. White is a 49-year-old man who has spent much of his life drifting from place to place. He was admitted to the hospital because of extreme suspiciousness of others and visual hallucinations. The next four questions apply to Mr. White's situation.

1. Which approach by the staff would be the most threatening to Mr. White?
   a. Forthright and honest.
   b. Friendly and emotionally detached.
   c. Warm and nurturing.
   d. Permissive and reserved.

Post-Test

(continued)

2. Mr. White is sitting quietly next to a staff member in the dayroom. He seems to be mumbling to himself. Which comment would best serve to get the patient's attention?
   a. "Tell me what you are thinking, Mr. White."
   b. "Why are you mumbling, Mr. White?"
   c. "I understand you are angry, Mr. White."
   d. "Let's look at this magazine, Mr. White."

3. You are talking with Mr. White and suddenly he says, "What are you asking me all this for? I've already told this to my doctor. I suppose you're trying to find out if my answers will be the same." Which of the following responses would be best?
   a. "Why do you think I would do that?"
   b. "I'm only trying to help you."
   c. "It seems to you I've been prying."
   d. "I'm sorry you feel that way. Let's talk about something else."

4. The chief mental mechanism Mr. White is using is:
   a. Rationalization.
   b. Reaction formation.
   c. Projection.
   d. Introjection.
   e. Conversion reaction.

Situation. Mr. Green has voluntarily admitted himself to the state hospital upon the urging of his physician. Mr. Green has lived alone most of his life and has no known friends. Recently, he has been phoning his neighbors, accusing them of "bugging" his house and plotting to kill him. The next two questions apply to this situation.

5. During the admission procedure, Mr. Green refuses to take off his clothes and get into bed. Which approach by the staff member would be most helpful at this point?
   a. Get another staff member to assist in removing the patient's clothes.
   b. Leave the room and send an orderly to undress the patient.
   c. Find out why the patient does not want to undress.
   d. Let the patient wear his street clothes.

Post-Test

(continued)

6. Mr. Green is angrily telling you people's actions against him. Your best response is:
   a. To say nothing.
   b. "I don't blame you for being angry. That's a terrible thing for them to do."
   c. "Why are you angry at me? I haven't done anything to you."
   d. "It doesn't really make any sense, does it, that your neighbors would be doing this?"
   e. "It must be difficult to feel all alone and threatened like that."

Care for Depressed Patients

OBJECTIVES: Student will be able to:

1. Identify symptoms of depression.
2. List techniques for managing depressed behaviors in patients.
3. Identify a "beginner's trap" when dealing with suicidally depressed patients.
4. Help a depressed patient increase self-esteem.
5. State the one thing depressed patients should almost never be told not to do.
6. Cite several specific statements appropriate for the depressed patient who is crying.
7. Respond appropriately when a depressed patient becomes overly attached to a staff member.
8. Identify different modes of treatment for depression.

The depressed patient is the patient who usually gets the most sympathy from a therapeutic staff. However, if a patient's depression does not lift as treatment progresses, he or she may experience a great deal of rejection and hostility from staff members.

Depressed patients have such a multiplicity of symptoms and problems that effective management is difficult. These patients frequently have decreased appetite, significant weight gain or weight loss, loss of interest in activities of daily living, difficulty sleeping, and many other physical problems. Usually, their self-esteem is poor and, when depression is severe, personal hygiene is neglected. Depressed patients are likely to be tearful, upset, and apathetic. Because their activity level is low, they have a predisposition to certain physical problems. Bedsores, skin rashes, boils, scalp infections, constipation, and nutritional deficiencies may occur. These problems may be reduced or prevented by attentive staff, although extra effort is required.

The treatment of depressed patients requires a great deal of careful observation and supportive therapy. Frequently patients' lives are at stake because of suicidal feelings. These patients often have exaggerated feelings of guilt and believe that their lives are not worth living. Sometimes their feelings of uselessness and worthlessness are so strong that they feel they do not deserve to live and would rather die. During this time, it is important to prevent these patients from destroying themselves while trying to help them understand that times and circumstances change as does the availability of love objects and that they may hope for a better situation at some time in the future. Most depressed patients, however, are strongly oriented to the present and have very little wish to consider a future for themselves. They lose sight of the fact that circumstances do change, and they seem to believe that their situation will always be as painful and hurtful as it is at present.

Inexperienced staff members sometimes allow themselves to become trapped by agreeing not to disclose a patient's suicidal thoughts. Staff members should never agree to keep anything concerning a patient's welfare from other staff members or from the patient's physician. If, in reality, the patient did not want the information known, it is unlikely he or she would share it with anyone.

It is important to recognize that depressed patients frequently deny their need for human companionship and for the support of persons in their environment. Although depressed patients may indicate that they do not want to talk and do not want company, they are usually comforted by someone's paying attention to them and by knowing that someone is willing to talk to them. This subtly bolsters their self-esteem and helps them to feel that they are worthwhile individuals. Even if patients do not appear to notice that a staff member is present, it is quite likely that they take comfort in the knowledge that someone cares enough to sit with them in their misery. If at all possible, patients should be encouraged to talk about their feelings and problems. Patients' verbalizations should be responded to in an understanding and nonjudgmental way. Patients should be supported in their efforts to talk about their problems and should be permitted to express their discomfort and hurt feelings by crying if they feel the need to cry. Patients should almost never be told not to cry.

Sometimes a crying or weeping patient causes discomfort among staff members. A crying patient, however, usually responds to a calm, soothing voice and an arm around the shoulders. Comments such as "Everything will be all right" and "the sun will shine tomorrow" are not comforting to the patient because they are not consistent with the patient's feelings. Instead, depressed patients should be encouraged to talk about what makes them feel like crying. Comments such as "Would you like to talk about what is making you cry?" or "something must be hurting you very much" may encourage the patient to talk. The idea is to focus on the patient's feelings and not so much on the content of the patient's words or the solution to his or her problems.

Depressed patients also suffer from sleep disturbances. They may require medication for sleep and may need to talk or sit with someone before they can calm their fears and become sleepy. In other cases, depressed patients may sleep 12 to 14 hours a day to escape feelings of guilt and depression.

Because depressed patients have low activity levels, it is often necessary to encourage them to participate in a wide range of activities so that they may begin to re-establish social relations that have been neglected. Involvement in as many activities as possible should be encouraged. This is particularly true of activities that permit the establishment of social relationships that increase the patient's confidence and improve self-esteem. Depressed patients usually need to establish relationships on a one-to-one basis. As their condition improves, they can be encouraged to become involved in group interactions. Sometimes when depressed patients do not believe they can help themselves, they willingly take steps to help others. Such interactions may prove to be quite therapeutic.

Depressed patients should be encouraged to get out of bed, go to breakfast, go to all their meals, make up their beds, and attend to matters of personal hygiene.

Staff members can help depressed patients regain pride in their personal appearance by making sure that they are provided with clean, attractive clothing and that they are neatly dressed and well groomed. Family members should be encouraged to bring favorite articles of clothing or perhaps a new shirt or a new dress. Barbers and beauticians may be needed to help with improving patients' physical appearance. Staff members, however, should be careful not to overwhelm depressed patients with too many extravagances because the patients may respond by withdrawing further, believing they are not worthy of all the attention.

Small meals, selected from favorite foods and presented attractively, help to restore lost appetites and improve nutrition. It may be helpful to sit with such patients and offer verbal encouragement. Sometimes staff members must feed severely withdrawn patients.

It is important to not be critical of the level of involvement that a patient might show in an activity. Proficiency will improve with regular exposure and a developing interest in the activity. In the beginning, praise and reinforcement for simply showing up at a particular activity are important, and any effort made toward involvement should also be supported with encouragement. Frequently, efforts to involve a patient in activities require a number of attempts. Staff members need not become discouraged or irritated if the patient does not respond immediately to their efforts. Persistence and kind, gentle persuasion often result in the desired involvement. Force is not helpful. It instead produces resentment or guilt feelings and more withdrawal. New patients, especially, need time to adjust to the clinic or ward routine and to learn what is expected of them.

On occasion, a crying, whiny patient will become attached to a particular staff member and may make the staff member's life difficult. In such cases, it is helpful if other staff members approach that patient with suggestions for activities and with requests for assistance at some minor task. This encourages interaction with other staff members. Encouragement to become involved in activities that require spending time doing something independently or with another patient is desirable.

It is likely that a few patients will remain withdrawn despite intensive efforts by the staff to draw them out and get them involved in activities. In such cases, visits at regular intervals by particular staff members enable these patients to look forward to company. These visits should take place even if they result in no conversation or interaction with the staff members. During such visits, the staff member might perform small tasks for the patient to let the patient know of the staff's care and concern. If the patient is in bed, a staff member might smooth the bedcovers, quickly brush the patient's hair, suggest makeup, a change of bedclothes, or some other aspect of personal care. Without appearing overly cheerful, a staff member's positive outlook on life and a discussion of activities that might interest the patient are helpful. Patients should be encouraged to attend activities of interest and even to attend some activities that may not be of particular interest but could simply help pass the time.

In talking with the depressed patient, a staff member might try a broad range of topics. Usually even severely depressed patients are interested in something. The trick is to discover that "something" and then to use it to further the patient's interest in other activities.

It is critically important to remember that, although depressed patients may not show it, they want and are much in need of a relationship with another person. They are often afraid that they will not be able to fulfill their part of a relationship and thus are reluctant to become involved. Once involved, however, much therapeutic good can be accomplished. Because depressed patients almost always have poor self-esteem, they may respond well to assisting staff members with minor tasks. This allows patients to feel somewhat special and important, thus improving their self-esteem. A patient may have a particular talent or characteristic that can be pointed to with respect and admiration by a staff member and by other patients. Ancillary therapy activities such as art, occupational, recreational, adventure, and music therapies frequently offer an opportunity for patients to accomplish something that can be recognized and appreciated by staff members and patients.

Two other modes of treatment for depressed patients are electroconvulsive shock therapy (ECT) and medication (psychopharmacology). Because both of these treatment modes have been discussed in detail previously (Chapters 10 and 11), they are not repeated here. It is sufficient to say that they require special attention and must be taken into consideration in planning treatment for a given patient. It may be helpful to review those procedures when beginning to care for depressed patients.

▼ KEY POINTS ▼

Managing Depressed Patients

1. The depressed patient often has a multiplicity of symptoms and problems that make effective management difficult.

2. Because depressed patients' activity level is low, they have a predisposition to physical problems such as skin rashes, malnutrition, and constipation. These problems may be reduced or prevented by attentive staff.

3. Treatment of the depressed patient requires careful observation and supportive therapy; the patient's life is often at stake because of suicidal feelings.

4. Most depressed patients are strongly oriented to the present and give little consideration to the future. An aim of therapy is to shift their focus to appropriate considerations for the future.

5. Do not agree to hold in confidence a patient's suicidal thoughts. A staff member should never agree to keep anything concerning a patient's welfare from other staff members or from the patient's physician.

6. Depressed patients frequently deny their need for human companionship and for the support of persons in their environment. Although they may not show it, depressed patients want and need relationships with other persons. It is often necessary to encourage them to participate in activities in order to re-establish social relations.

continued on page 310

Key Points continued

7. Patients should be encouraged to talk about their feelings and problems. Patients' verbalizations are better responded to in an understanding and nonjudgmental way.

8. A crying patient usually responds to a calm, soothing voice and an appropriate therapeutic touch. The idea is to focus on feelings and not so much on the patient's words.

9. Depressed patients suffer from sleep disturbances and may require medication, need to talk, or sit with someone before they can calm their fears and become sleepy.

10. Patients who are depressed may sleep 12 to 14 hours a day to escape feelings of guilt and depression. They should be encouraged to get out of bed for meals, to make up their beds, and to attend to matters of personal hygiene. Making sure that depressed patients are neatly dressed and well groomed helps them regain pride in their personal appearance.

11. When depressed patients do not believe they can help themselves, they sometimes willingly take steps to help others.

12. Small meals, selected from favorite foods and presented attractively, help to restore lost appetites and improve nutrition.

13. Do not be critical of a patient's level of involvement in a particular activity. Proficiency improves with regular exposure and a developing interest in the activity.

14. If a crying, whiny patient becomes attached to a staff member, it is helpful if other staff members approach the patient with suggestions for activities and requests for assistance at some minor task.

15. It is likely that a few patients will remain withdrawn despite intensive efforts by the staff. However, even severely depressed patients are interested in something, and discovering that something may further the patient's interest in other activities.

16. Because depressed patients almost always have poor self-esteem, they may respond well to assisting staff members with minor tasks.

17. A patient may have a talent or characteristic that can be pointed to with respect and admiration by others.

18. Two other modes of treatment for depressed patients are medication and electroconvulsive shock therapy (ECT). It may be helpful to review those procedures when beginning to care for depressed patients.

Annotated Bibliography

American Psychological Association: *Prevalence of Depression and the Effectiveness of Psychotherapy in Ameliorating Depressive Symptoms.* Washington, D.C.: American Psychological Association, 1991.

Examines through research study the prevalence, cost to employers, and effectiveness of treatment of persons suffering from depression.

Andrews, B., and Brown, G.: Self-esteem and vulnerability to depression: The concurrent validity of interview and questionnaire measures. *Journal of Abnormal Psychology,* 1993, 102(4):565–572.

Examines various measures of self-report questionnaires on depression.

Bell, I. R., and Gelenberg, A. J.: Mood disorders. In: Conn, H. F., and Others (eds.): *Conn's Current Therapy.* Philadelphia: W. B. Saunders, 1993, pp. 1113–1122.

Examines the types of depression, medical and organic causes, and use of a decision tree to facilitate a proper diagnosis and treatment plan.

Copenhaver, M.: Better late than never: Of reminiscence and resolution. 1995, *Journal of Psychosocial Nursing,* 33(7):17–22.

Discusses assessment techniques for depression in the elderly.

Hewitt, P. L., and Flett, G. L.: Dimensions of perfectionism in unipolar depression. *Journal of Abnormal Psychology,* 1991, 100(1):98–101.

Examines through research study the hypothesis that self-oriented perfectionism, other-oriented perfectionism, and socially prescribed perfectionism are related differentially to unipolar depression.

Joseph, S. G.: Facing the darkness. *Insight,* 1991, 12(2):25–31.

Discusses the combination of biologic, psychological, and social factors contributing to depression in women.

Swanson, B., Cronin-Stubbs, D., and Colletti, M.: Dementia and depression in persons with AIDS: Causes and care. *Journal of Psychosocial Nursing and Mental Health Services,* 1990, 28(10):33–39.

Discusses the importance of distinguishing depression from AIDS dementia complex and presents treatment plans for both disorders to promote the quality of life.

Ugarriza, D. N.: Postpartum affective disorders: Incidence and treatment. *Journal of Psychosocial Nursing,* 1992, 30(5):29–36.

Divides postpartum depression into three distinct syndromes: postpartum "blues," postpartum psychosis, and postpartum depression. Provides treatment issues surrounding each postpartum affective disorder.

Winokur, G., Coryell, W., Endicott, J., and Akiskal, H.: Further distinctions between manic-depressive illness (bipolar disorder) and primary depressive disorder (unipolar depression). *American Journal of Psychiatry,* 1993, 150(8):1176–1181.

Examines differences of bipolar and unipolar depression and takes into account family background, medical history, and childhood traits for diagnosis.

Zerhusen, J. D., Boyle, K., and Wilson, W.: Out of the darkness: Group cognitive therapy for depressed elderly. *Journal of Psychosocial Nursing and Mental Health Services,* 1991, 29(9):16–21.

Examines through research study the benefits of nurses' facilitating cognitive group therapy with nursing home residents suffering from depression.

Post-Test

True or False. Circle your choice.

T   F   1. The depressed patient usually has poor self-esteem.

T   F   2. Often depressed people feel so worthless that they feel they do not deserve to live.

T   F   3. Depressed patients often convey a strong need for companionship.

T   F   4. Upon approaching a tearful, depressed patient, it is helpful to remind him or her that things will be better tomorrow.

T   F   5. Depressed patients frequently suffer from sleep disturbances.

T   F   6. A high activity level is often seen in the depressed person.

T   F   7. A staff member caring for a depressed patient should have a friendly, cheerful outlook to encourage the patient to feel the same.

T   F   8. Two important modes of treatment of the depressed patient are medication and electroconvulsive therapy (ECT).

T   F   9. Depressed patients should be encouraged to talk about their feelings and problems.

T   F   10. Depressed patients should not be encouraged to participate in activities but should be left alone to participate at their own pace.

Multiple Choice. Circle the letter or number you think represents the best answer.

1. While planning activities for the depressed patient, the staff member should understand that the patient needs:
   a. Variety and challenge to lift him or her out of depression.
   b. Competitive activities with the group.
   c. Activities that require exertion of energy.
   d. Simple and structured activities at first.

Post-Test

(continued)

2. Which of the following are characteristic of depression:
   a. Early morning wakening.
   b. Good appetite.
   c. Lack of guilt feelings.
   d. Worse in the late afternoon.
   e. Enjoys life.
      (1) a and d.
      (2) a, b, and e.
      (3) c and e.
      (4) c, d, and e.
      (5) None of the above.

Situation. Mrs. Brown, a 35-year-old mother of three, part-time bookkeeper and part-time cosmetics salesperson, was brought to the hospital by her husband. Mrs. Brown had become progressively unable to sleep, eat, talk, or perform housework. She sat for long periods, smoking one cigarette after another, seemingly unaware of people or things around her. The next two questions apply to this situation.

3. Mrs. Brown's depression is probably the result of:
   a. Paralyzing fear.
   b. Conflicting responsibilities.
   c. Physical exhaustion.
   d. Internalized aggression.

4. The feeling Mrs. Brown is most likely to demonstrate during her depression is:
   a. Suspicion.
   b. Fear.
   c. Loneliness.
   d. Worthlessness.

5. An attempt to commit suicide is most likely to occur during which of the following phases of hospitalization?
   a. Immediately following hospital admission.
   b. At the point of deepest depression.
   c. When depression begins to lift.
   d. Shortly before hospital discharge.

Post-Test

(continued)

6. Mrs. Adams expresses to a staff member that she is feeling depressed about the recent death of her father. Which of the following responses by the staff member communicate understanding and acceptance?
   a. "I know just how you feel."
   b. "Everyone gets depressed when a loved one dies."
   c. "This must be very difficult for you."
   d. "Try to think positively. He was ill only a short time and didn't have to suffer long."

CHAPTER
17

Care for Suicidal Patients

OBJECTIVES: Student will be able to:

1. Identify the number one suicide site in the world.
2. State the reason men are often more successful in suicide attempts than are women.
3. Relate the role of genetics in suicidal behavior.
4. Identify suicide attempts that should be taken seriously.
5. Describe different treatment modes for dealing with the suicidal patient.
6. State the most common reason for suicide.
7. Name the most common stimulus for suicide.
8. List at least five behavioral clues to possible suicidal intention.
9. List steps to create a safe environment for the suicidal patient.
10. List therapeutic approaches to the suicidal patient in each category of the Suicidal Intention Rating Scale.

In the United States, suicide is the 10th leading cause of adult deaths and the 3rd leading cause of death in college students. Suicidal deaths persist despite the advent of psychotropic drugs, open door hospitals, community mental health centers, suicide prevention centers and hotlines, and a significant increase in the number of professionals available to treat patients.

It has been estimated that more than 27,000 Americans die each year by their own hand. Alec Roy (1989), a suicide expert and researcher, reports that the Golden Gate Bridge in San Francisco is the number one suicide site in the world. He further reports that about 75 people kill themselves every day in the United States, and many experts believe this figure is far below the actual number of suicides. These experts reason that many suicides are made to look like accidents or are recorded as such to protect the feelings of surviving family members. It is also difficult, and sometimes impossible, to collect life insurance when the insured commits suicide.

For each completed suicide, estimates suggest 10 to 20 unsuccessful attempts. Statistics further show that men are more likely than women to succeed in committing suicide. The difference is that men and women choose different types of suicide weapons. By using firearms, knives, poisons, ropes (hanging), or automobiles, men end their lives in painful, violent ways that are extremely lethal. Women prefer drugs, often those that have been prescribed by a physician. Because it takes time for drugs to be absorbed from the stomach into the circulatory system, overdoses are often discovered and medical treatment provided before death occurs. This method also provides the opportunity for a change of mind by telling someone of the attempt.

The possibility of suicide is higher for certain groups of people than it is for the general population and some evidence suggests that genetic factors may predispose people to suicide. In addition to those in genetically vulnerable groups, these groups include persons who have previously attempted suicide, the terminally ill, the elderly, the alcoholic, the severely emotionally ill, persons in families with successful suicides among members, and people associated socially with persons who have made suicide attempts. Highly stressful situations and the availability of lethal weapons also increase the likelihood of a suicide attempt.

TREATMENT

All suicidal attempts should be taken seriously. Health team members sometimes find this difficult, especially if a person has made several superficial suicide attempts. Someone may say, "Oh, they're just trying to get attention." This statement may be true to some extent, but it is therapeutically significant that a person can be so starved for human attention that he or she resorts to such drastic measures.

The human desire to be loved and feel worthwhile is universal. Suicidal patients desperately wish to communicate and relieve their feelings of worthlessness, abandonment, rejection, helplessness, and hopelessness. Their inability to do so may result in a sense of rage or anger directed toward themselves. Something as temporary as losing a job may create such momentary feelings of worthlessness that a person commits suicide. The suicidal person's anger is often the result of a world perceived as nonsupportive, uncaring, and demanding, and the person feels so incapable of changing those circumstances that the only way to address that anger and resolve the feelings of frustration is to take his or her life. Thus, the rage against an uncaring world that does not meet the suicidal person's needs is turned inward and the person removes himself or herself from that uncaring, nonsupportive world.

Shneidman (1986) reports the most common reason for suicide is to seek a solution; the most common goal, cessation of consciousness; the most common stimulus, intolerable psychological pain; the most common stressor, frustrated psychological needs; and the most common emotions, hopelessness and helplessness. Other motivational factors in suicide include identification with someone who has killed himself or herself, revenge, sacrifice, religious fantasies about joining a lost loved one, punishment of a jilting lover, punishment for any number of acts against the suicidal person, and cult ideologies such as those adhered to by the followers of Jim Jones at Jonestown. In adolescents, family turmoil, loss of love objects, and physical and psychological illness are leading causes of suicides. Data indicate that an adolescent dies of suicide in the United States every 90 minutes.

Unfortunately, many suicidal patients do not realize that they are unhappy, depressed, or anxious. They may not be aware of the cause of their suicidal impulses or the fact that they need help. Frequently, an overinvolvement in work, career, or love objects is found in the preattempt history of the suicidal patient. For example, a young wife who merges her identity with that of her husband, thus losing her own sense of capability, may attempt suicide if something happens to break up that relationship. Such overidentification frequently masks underlying feelings of worthlessness, insecurity, and inadequacy. To feel worthless is to feel unloved, unlovable, and unwanted. Self-esteem is significantly reduced.

A suicide attempt should be viewed as an effort by the individual to communicate emotional pain and a need for help. It should also be taken as a signal that something is drastically wrong in the individual's life and that change and improvement are necessary if the person is to survive.

Research indicates that a vast majority of patients who commit suicide have openly expressed their intention to kill themselves well in advance of the act. Many of these people have discussed their plight with friends and relatives. They may have been told that they should not have such thoughts or have been completely ignored and thus rejected. In fact, Shneidman (1986) says the most common interpersonal act in suicide is communication of the intent to commit suicide. Any time someone reacts to a suicidal patient in a rejecting manner, the patient's desire to commit suicide may be increased because his or her feelings of worthlessness have once again been reinforced.

Suicidal persons need someone with whom they can talk, someone willing to listen, and someone sincerely interested in their problems. Anyone with emotional or physical problems may be suicidal. This is especially true if the individual has suffered a recent loss, such as the death of a loved one, loss of a body part, divorce, loss of positive feelings of self-worth due to divorce, business losses, or loss of a job. As mentioned earlier, terminally ill patients are likely candidates to attempt suicide. This is especially true if they believe that their impending death is likely to be painful.

Recognizing Behavioral Clues

Depressed patients constitute a large group of potential suicides. Because these patients tend to stress physical complaints rather than suicidal ideas, the staff may overlook their suicidal potential. Thus, to help prevent suicides among such patients, health team members must pay particular attention to the patients' emotional state. For example, when patients who have been agitated and upset suddenly become calm, outgoing, and happy for no apparent reason, they may be "telling" that they have decided to commit suicide. Patients seem to actually feel relieved and happier after deciding that the solution to their problems is to end their lives.

The following are other behavioral clues that may indicate a suicide attempt. Patients exhibiting such behaviors deserve your close attention:

1. Patients who have extreme difficulty sleeping and especially those who also experience early morning (3 to 6 A.M.) awakenings.
2. Patients who continually talk about committing suicide and, particularly, those who have made a previous attempt.
3. Patients who express feelings of hopelessness and helplessness.
4. Patients who are very tearful and dwell on sad thoughts.
5. Patients who show the vegetative signs of depression (loss of sleep, appetite, and interest in their appearance and usual activities).
6. Patients who show unusual interest in getting their affairs in order and who may even try to give away their belongings.
7. Patients who are hallucinating (hearing voices, seeing things, and so forth) or who feel persecuted or both. Patients who are hallucinating may commit suicide if the voices tell them to do so, if

they attempt to get away from those voices, or if they are trying to escape from the frightening creatures they see.

Creating a Safe Environment

The creativity shown by patients in finding weapons with which to harm themselves is truly amazing. If you consider the fact that many suicide attempts seem to occur as a result of a momentary uncontrollable impulse (common in personality disorders and alcoholics), the necessity for making sure that weapons are not available becomes obvious. Patients have broken mirrors, lightbulbs, and lamps and then used the glass to cut themselves. They have been known to wet themselves completely and then try to electrocute themselves by sticking something metal in an electrical outlet. They may try to stab themselves with pens, pencils, nail files, or dull dinner knives; to hang themselves with belts, simple household string, or knotted bed sheets; to poison themselves by eating abrasive cleansers or drinking shaving lotion, mouthwash, or lighter fluid; or to drown by submerging themselves in the bathtub. They may also try to drown themselves by holding their head underwater in the sink, pouring gargling solution down their nose or sticking their head in a mop bucket full of water. Others may jump out of windows, step in front of cars, or set themselves on fire. Depressed patients may simply refuse to eat in an attempt to starve. There are many other suicide methods not already listed, and it is a real challenge to stay one step ahead of patients in keeping the patients' environment as safe as possible.

Suicidal patients often need to remain under constant supervision, and alertness is the staff's best defense. If the staff maintains a warm, friendly, supportive attitude while carrying out assigned responsibilities, patients may reap a special benefit. Not only will they be prevented from ending their lives before treatment has had a chance to work, but also they may feel that all the attention they are receiving means that they are truly important and that people care about what happens to them. Perhaps they may even begin to feel that life really is worth living.

Techniques for Effective Interaction

To relate effectively to suicidal patients, health team members should realize that these patients may feel particularly discouraged and hopeless if they do not perceive a steady improvement in their condition.

Such feelings are increased if these patients are led to believe that their lack of improvement is due to poor motivation or lack of will power.

Some specialists in suicide believe that, instead of placing the responsibility for improvement on the skills of the staff or on the patient's willpower, the responsibility should be assigned to the medication the patient is receiving. This tends to neutralize the patient's sense of guilt and thus reduces symptoms. Realizing that it takes days to weeks for some of the antidepressants to reach an optimal therapeutic level in the bloodstream, the staff can approach the patient in an optimistic and hopeful way. Such knowledge may also make it easier for the patient to understand and tolerate a slower than expected rate of recovery. Because suicide is permanent, the necessity of communicating a sense of hope to these patients is of utmost importance. Life circumstances and personal aspirations vary and change. If, therefore, a patient is prevented from committing suicide and is able to internalize a sense of hope, there is a significant possibility for a good recovery. The authors are constantly impressed with the fact that intensely suicidal patients shake their heads in wonder after their suicidal crisis has passed and seem to not understand their own behavior. Many realize they would have killed themselves but for the work of the staff—and most are truly grateful.

In working with suicidal patients, mental health workers may expect that a great deal of time will be spent with a few patients who generate crisis after crisis by making repeated suicide attempts. Dealing with such patients is often exasperating and anxiety provoking. Perhaps one of the reasons for this anxiety is that staff members perceive the anger the patient is experiencing but are unsure of the way to deal with it. Unfortunately, the most common way of reacting to anger is to respond with anger. If the staff reacts in this manner, the patient feels more rejected and the anger is increased. Staff members must realize that the ability to react appropriately is essential. They must be interested in, and understanding toward, the patient, but they must not assume the patient's emotional burdens and attitudes. When they do so, they become ineffective in helping the patient deal with suicidal feelings.

It is important to remember that patients expect staff members to be calm and controlled even in the face of a patient's hostility and anger. Patients depend on the staff to recognize destructive elements in their behavior that they cannot see and to provide a safe, structured environment in which they can regain a sense of hope. Suicidal crises can best be handled with genuine human concern and understanding. An honest attempt on the part of staff to reach out and help will eventually be accepted by most suicidal patients.

Suicidal Intention Rating Scale

Because treatment plans vary with the intensity of a patient's suicidal impulses, a Suicidal Intention Rating Scale (SIRS) that has been developed and found useful by the authors is presented. It provides a systematic procedural guide that can be used in the day-to-day management of hospitalized suicidal patients. It is the responsibility of the patient's doctor or the RN in charge of the unit to rate the patient and then notify the rest of the staff of the preventive measures to be instituted. Even though all hospitals do not use such a tool, it is included to suggest some practical approaches to the care of the suicidal patient. A recent survey of public and private psychiatric hospitals indicates that most hospitals follow a procedure similar to the one presented here when caring for the suicidal patient.

The SIRS values and suggested therapeutic approaches are as follows:

0. A SIRS value of zero (0) is assigned to a patient when there is no evidence that the patient has (or has had in the past) suicidal ideas that have been brought to the attention of another person.

Nursing Approach: A patient with a SIRS value of 0 follows usual admission procedures and hospital routines.

1+. A SIRS value of 1+ is assigned to a patient when there is some evidence of suicidal ideas but no actual attempts. This patient does not have a history of repeatedly threatening to commit suicide.

Nursing Approach: A patient with a SIRS value of 1+ follows usual admission procedures and hospital routines. However, the patient should be quietly and unobtrusively observed and evaluated for evidence of recurrence of suicidal thoughts.

2+. A SIRS value of 2+ is assigned to a patient when (*a*) there is evidence that the patient has attempted suicide in the past but is not now actively thinking about suicide or (*b*) when the patient is having suicidal ideas but is not threatening suicide. For example, the patient may say, "I have thought about suicide but I don't believe it is the way out."

Nursing Approach: A patient with a SIRS value of 2+ follows usual admission procedures and hospital routines. The patient is allowed to use the following items but must return them to be locked up after use:

    a. Shaving kit (including razor, blade, aftershave, cologne, shaving cream).
    b. Mouthwash in glass bottles.
    c. Belts.
    d. Fingernail files and fingernail clippers.
    e. Knives of any description, including penknives. These may be used under supervision only.
    f. Hair picks and hair lifts.
    g. Any cosmetics in glass containers.
    h. Hairspray.
    i. Plastic clothes coverings.

3+. A SIRS value of 3+ is assigned to a patient who has been making serious suicidal threats. For example, the patient may have said, "If they don't stop bothering me, I'm going to kill myself."

Nursing Approach: Upon admission a patient with a SIRS value of 3+ must be searched to determine if there are instruments on his person, in his clothes, or in his room that may possibly be used for self-destruction. This procedure should be performed in a professional manner, with the staff taking extreme care to protect the patient's dignity. The patient will then be allowed to use the following items only under direct supervision:
    a. Shaving kit (including razor, blade, aftershave, cologne, shaving cream).
    b. Mouthwash in glass bottles.
    c. Belts.
    d. Fingernail files and fingernail clippers.
    e. Knives of any description, including penknives.
    f. Hair lifts or hair picks.
    g. Any cosmetics in glass containers.
    h. Hairspray.
    i. Plastic clothes coverings.
    j. Medications brought in on admission.
    k. Coat hangers.
    l. Lamps or any breakable item from the patient's room.
    m. Eyeglasses (*Note:* These should be removed only when a patient is extremely suicidal and may use the glasses as a weapon. It must be kept in mind, however, that the removal of eyeglasses may add to confusion and depression.)

Such a patient should be observed at least every 30 minutes or more often, if at all possible. Eating meals in the dining room is permissible, but a staff member should be present at the table during the meal.

Unless otherwise ordered by the physician, the patient is not permitted to leave the unit for recreational or occupational therapy activities and visitors are restricted to immediate family.

> *Note:* It is wise to encourage patients with a SIRS rating of 3+ or below to stay out of their rooms and in the company of other patients and staff. They can thus be watched more closely. Usually other patients on the unit know when a patient is suicidal. They often take it upon themselves to help watch the patient and notify staff members of behavioral changes.

4+. A SIRS value of 4+ is assigned to a patient who has been brought to the hospital because of an active suicide attempt or as a precaution against such an attempt.

Nursing Approach:

a. The patient is admitted to a seclusion room. This is for protection, not punishment. Staff members should take care to explain the need for this procedure. It is much easier to observe and limit behavior in a smaller area, but the staff should spend as much time as possible with the patient, interacting on a one-to-one basis. With the permission of the attending physician, a family member or members acceptable to the patient should stay around the clock while the patient is in seclusion.

b. The nurse in charge will search the patient's clothing and body, taking care to conduct the search in a professional manner, with concern for the patient's dignity. A very thorough search should be carried out. Sometimes it is necessary to carefully check the patient's hair, ears, between toes and fingers, and other parts of the body where harmful objects might be concealed. In females, the admitting physician may consider it necessary to examine the vaginal area to be sure that nothing has been concealed there. This may seem to be an extreme precaution; however, a loaded .22-caliber pistol has been found in a vagina. There are numerous cases of drugs' being concealed in this manner by females, as well as rectally by both males and females.

c. The patient will be clothed in a hospital gown.

d. Any clothing, supplies, or other items that are brought to the hospital, and which may be needed when suicidal precautions are removed, will then be placed in the patient's locker outside the seclusion room. All unnecessary items brought to the hospital will be sent home.

e. All items brought to the hospital by the family will be thoroughly inspected by the nurse on duty and anything that might be used in a suicide attempt will not be given to the patient.

f. The door to the seclusion room should be locked at all times when the patient is alone.

g. Meals will be served in the seclusion room and only paper dishes used if a staff member is unavailable to supervise a meal. If at all possible, a staff member should spend time with the patient during meals.

h. It may be necessary to remove all linen from the bed, and a staff member must stay with any patient trying to commit suicide by banging his head on the walls or door of the seclusion room.

i. Anytime the patient is allowed out of the security room, a member of the hospital staff must be in attendance.

j. Under no circumstances will the patient be allowed to leave the psychiatric unit without a direct order from the attending physician. In cases in which the patient has permission of the attending physician, the patient should be accompanied by an attendant at all times (for example, to x-ray department, laboratory, and so forth).

k. Visitors will be restricted altogether. The only persons allowed to visit will be those with specific permission from the attending physician.

Ideally, all patients assigned a 2+, 3+, or 4+ suicidal rating would be closely or continuously observed on a one-to-one basis (one staff member to one suicidal patient). In most hospitals such a staffing ratio is impossible, and many hospitals now use closed-circuit TV monitoring to provide constant supervision for one or more patients simultaneously. Drastic intervention procedures such as placing the suicidal patient in a seclusion room or searching the patient for potential weapons may become necessary. These protective measures are used to prevent suicides until treatment measures such as medication and psychotherapy begin to take effect. The items taken from the patient or the fact that a patient is placed in seclusion is not as important as the manner in which these procedures are performed.

All suicidal patients should be watched closely at shift change and in the early morning hours. Patients who have been unable to sleep all night often decide that they are not going to face another such night and make a suicide attempt. Others who are waiting for an unobserved chance to commit suicide often find one during the confusion of increased activity occurring at shift change.

After visiting hours or activity periods, it may be necessary to closely check the environment, and possibly the patient, for objects (potential weapons) that may have been given to the patient or unintentionally left by a visitor. When workers must make repairs, staff members must be sure that patients do not take tools and that the workers do not leave supplies on the unit.

If you find a patient who has attempted suicide or who is about to do so, do not leave the patient. If alone, call out for help. Then, while waiting, speak to the patient in a calm, reassuring manner. If the patient wants to talk about his or her feelings, allow him or her to do so. If not, try to distract the patient from the suicidal intention by whatever means available.

If you find a patient who is already unconscious, call for help and then start appropriate first aid measures.

▼ KEY POINTS ▼

The Suicidal Patient

1. Suicide is the 10th leading cause of adult deaths and the 3rd leading cause of death among college students in the United States.

2. It has been estimated that more than 27,000 Americans die each year by their own hand.

3. Many suicides are made to look like accidents or are recorded as such to protect the feelings of surviving family members.

4. For each completed suicide, estimates suggest 10 to 20 unsuccessful attempts. Further, men are more likely to succeed than are women, primarily because of their choice of weapons.

5. The possibility of suicide is higher for certain groups of people than for the general population, and evidence suggests that genetic factors may predispose people to commit suicide.

6. Highly stressful situations and the availability of lethal weapons increase the likelihood of a suicide attempt.

7. Be careful at shift changes, mealtimes, and other times when staff attention may be divided. These times are often chosen by patients to carry out a suicidal attempt.

Recognizing Behavioral Cues of a Suicidal Patient

8. Depressed patients constitute a large group of potential suicides. Because these patients tend to stress physical complaints rather than suicidal ideas, the staff may overlook their suicidal potential.

continued on page 328

Key Points continued

9. Behavioral cues that may indicate the possibility of a suicide attempt include:

   - Extreme difficulty sleeping.
   - Continuous talk about committing suicide.
   - Feelings of hopelessness and helplessness.
   - Dwelling on sad thoughts and being tearful.
   - Vegetative signs of depression.
   - Unusual interest in getting personal affairs in order.
   - Suddenly appearing calm, at peace, and happy. This may indicate the patient has found the "solution," i.e., suicide.
   - Visual or auditory hallucinations or both.

Creating a Safe Environment for the Suicidal Patient

10. Many suicide attempts seem to result from a momentary uncontrollable impulse. The necessity for ensuring that weapons are not available becomes obvious.

11. Suicidal patients often need to remain under constant supervision. Alertness is the staff's best defense.

12. A warm, friendly, supportive attitude will help patients feel that they are important and that people care about what happens to them.

Treatment of Suicidal Patients

13. **All suicide attempts should be taken seriously.** It is therapeutically significant that someone can be so distressed that he or she resorts to such drastic measures.

14. Suicidal patients desperately wish to communicate and relieve their feelings of worthlessness, abandonment, rejection, helplessness, and hopelessness.

15. The suicidal patient's anger is often directed toward a perceived nonsupportive and uncaring world that the patient wishes unconsciously to destroy; the only way to destroy that world may be to remove one's self from it.

16. The most common reason for suicide is to seek a solution; the most common goal, cessation of consciousness; the most common stimulus, intolerable psychological pain; the most common stressor, frustrated psychological needs; and the most common emotions, hopelessness and helplessness.

Key Points continued

17. Family turmoil, loss of love objects, and physical and psychological illness are the most common factors leading to adolescent suicide.

18. Many suicidal patients may not be aware of the cause of their suicidal impulses or the fact that they need help.

19. Frequently, one finds in the preattempt history of the suicidal patient an overinvolvement in work, career, or love objects.

20. Suicide attempts should be viewed as an effort to communicate emotional pain and need for help.

21. Research indicates that a vast majority of patients who commit suicide have openly expressed their intention to kill themselves well in advance of the act.

22. Shneidman (1986) says the most common interpersonal act in suicide is communication of the intent to commit suicide. Anytime someone reacts to a suicidal patient in a rejecting manner, the desire to commit suicide may be increased.

23. Suicidal persons need someone with whom they can talk, someone willing to listen, and someone sincerely interested in their problems. This is especially true if the individual has suffered a recent loss.

Techniques for Effective Interaction with the Suicidal Patient

24. Depressed or suicidal patients may feel particularly discouraged and hopeless if they do not perceive a steady improvement in their condition.

25. Some specialists in suicide believe that responsibility for improvement should be assigned to the medication the patient is receiving. It may take days to weeks for some antidepressants to reach an optimal therapeutic level in the bloodstream, allowing the staff to approach the patient with hope.

26. Intensely suicidal patients often cannot believe their behavior after their suicidal crisis has passed. Many realize they would have killed themselves, and most are grateful for the staff's intervention.

27. In working with suicidal patients, health team members may expect that a great deal of time will be spent with a few patients who generate crisis after crisis by making repeated suicide attempts.

continued on page 330

Key Points continued

28. Staff members must realize that the ability to react appropriately is essential. Do not empathize to the point of assuming the patient's emotional burdens and attitudes.

29. It is important to remember that patients expect staff members to be calm and controlled even in the face of the patient's hostility and anger.

30. Use a Suicidal Intention Rating Scale (SIRS) to gauge the intensity of a patient's suicidal impulses, thereby allowing more effective management of the patient.

31. All patients assigned a 2+, 3+, or 4+ suicidal rating using the SIRS should be closely or continuously observed on a one-to-one basis.

32. Drastic intervention procedures such as placing the suicidal patient in a seclusion room or searching the patient for potential weapons may become necessary.

33. All suicidal patients should be watched closely at shift change and in the early morning hours. Patients who have been unable to sleep all night may refuse to face another night or may be waiting for an opportunity to attempt suicide during a shift change when they are unobserved.

34. After visiting hours or activity periods, it may be necessary to closely check the environment, and possibly the patient, for potential weapons.

35. If you find a patient who has attempted suicide or who is about to do so, do not leave the patient. If alone, call out for help and then start any appropriate first aid measures. Distract the patient from the suicidal intention by whatever means available.

Annotated Bibliography

Cooper, C.: Patient suicide and assault: Their impact on psychiatric hospital staff. *Journal of Psychosocial Nursing,* 1995, 33(6):26–29.

Discusses the aftermath of patient suicide and patient assault on staff and how it can be disruptive both on and off the job.

Davis, A. T., and Schrueder, C.: The prediction of suicide. *The Medical Journal of Australia,* 1990, 153:552–554.

Reviews the literature addressing suicide prediction, role of the clinician in evaluating the risk of suicide, and directions for future research.

Kaplan, M. L., Asnis, G. M., Lipschitz, D. S., and Chorney, P.: Suicidal behavior and abuse in psychiatric outpatients. *Comprehensive Psychiatry,* 1995, 36(3):229–235.

Examines the relationship between suicidal behaviors and histories of abuse in psychiatric outpatients.

King, M. K., Schmalin, K. B., Cowley, D. S., and Dunner, D. L.: Suicide attempt history in depressed patients with and without a history of panic attacks. *Comprehensive Psychiatry,* 1995, 36(1):25–30.

Examines the differences in the frequency of suicide attempts in individuals with or without panic attacks.

Linehan, M. M., Tutek, D. A., Heard, H. L., and Armstrong, H. E.: Interpersonal outcome of cognitive behavioral treatment for chronically suicidal borderline patients. *American Journal of Psychiatry,* 1994, 151(12):1771–1776.

Discusses the positive effect of behavior therapy techniques on patient behavior.

Peterson, L. G., and Bongarm, B.: Repetitive suicidal crises: Characteristics of repeating versus nonrepeating suicidal visitors to a psychiatric emergency service. *Psychopathology,* 1990, 23:136–145.

Discusses the characteristics of patients seen in the hospital setting multiple times in a 1-year period for suicide attempts.

Rickelman, B. L., and Houfek, J. K.: Toward an interactional model of suicidal behaviors: Cognitive rigidity, attributional style, stress, hopelessness, and depression. *Archives of Psychiatric Nursing,* 1995, 9(3):158–168.

Explores major theoretical models and research findings regarding the interaction of selected cognitive factors and discusses the implications for nursing research.

Schotte, D. E., Cools, J., and Payvar, S.: Problem-solving deficits in suicidal patients: Trait vulnerability or state phenomenon? *Journal of Consulting and Clinical Psychology,* 1990, 58(5):562–564.

Research study examining the stability of interpersonal problem-solving skills in suicidal patients.

Valente, S. M.: Deliberate self-injury: Management in a psychiatric setting. *Journal of Psychosocial Nursing,* 1991, 29(12):19–25.

Discusses self-injury, the potential dangers, and how to manage these behaviors in a psychiatric setting.

References

Roy, A.: Suicide. ed. 5. In: Kaplan, H. I., and Sadock, B. J. (eds.): *Comprehensive Textbook of Psychiatry, Vol. 2,* Baltimore: Williams & Wilkins, 1989, p. 1414.

Shneidman, E.: Some essentials of suicide and some implications for response. In: Roy, A. (ed.): *Suicide.* Baltimore: Williams & Wilkins, 1986.

Post-Test

Judgment Exercises. Although a doctor or an RN usually rates the patient's suicidal potential, try to rate the following patients according to the SIRS scale given in this chapter. Knowledge of this scale and the signs and symptoms that patients exhibit in each category will make you a better observer of the behavior of suicidal patients. You often will be the one that reports to other team members any behavior that indicates the need for a change in suicidal precautions. Rate the following patients according to the type of SIRS rating they should be given.

1. Mrs. Brown, a 30-year-old divorced mother of three, has been hospitalized on the psychiatric unit for 2 weeks because of severe depression. She has spent most of this time alone in her room, crying and pacing the floor. She has been your patient during her entire hospitalization, and on several occasions she has verbalized to you her belief that the only solution to her problems is to end her life. She has also expressed such feelings to other staff members. You come on duty one morning and, much to your surprise, Mrs. Brown is in the dayroom and cheerfully says, "Good morning" as you approach her. She then immediately states the following: "You can stop worrying about me now. I know everything's going to be all right."

2. Mrs. Green is admitted to the hospital because of severe depression that began 3 weeks after the death of her husband. She says that she guesses she has thought about suicide but that she has never seriously considered taking her life.

3. Mrs. Farmer, a 23-year-old female, is admitted to the unit. She immediately begins to order people around and to be generally uncooperative. She says that she wants to kill herself because nobody likes her.

4. A private detective, Mr. Jones, is admitted to the unit following a self-inflicted gunshot wound to the head. He says that he is tired of the world and that he no longer wishes to live. He says that as soon as he gets out of the hospital he will kill himself.

Post-Test

(continued)

According to your hospital's routine, what approach would be used with each of these patients? (Be specific.)

1. Mrs. Brown:

2. Mrs. Green:

3. Mrs. Farmer:

4. Mr. Jones:

Short Answer. Answer as briefly and specifically as possible.

1. For each successful suicide attempt, records indicate approximately how many unsuccessful attempts?

_____

_____

_____

2. What specific groups in the general population are more likely to attempt suicide?

_____

_____

_____

3. What is an individual who has made a suicidal attempt trying to communicate?

_____

_____

_____

4. For a mental health worker in a hospital setting, what is one of the best defenses in the prevention of suicide?

_____

_____

_____

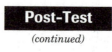

(continued)

5. List three behavioral clues that indicate the possibility of a suicide attempt.

a. _____

b. _____

c. _____

True or False. Circle your choice.

T   F   1. In the United States, suicide is the 10th leading cause of adult deaths.

T   F   2. Women are more likely to be successful in their suicide attempts than are men.

T   F   3. When individuals have made several superficial suicide attempts, it is not necessary to take them seriously because they are trying only to get attention.

T   F   4. Research indicates that a majority of individuals who have successfully committed suicide have expressed their intention in some form before doing so.

T   F   5. Patients often appear quite happy or relieved once they have decided that suicide is the answer to their problems.

T   F   6. All suicidal attempts should be taken seriously.

T   F   7. Patients who are hallucinating (e.g., hearing voices, seeing things) may commit suicide because the voices they hear tell them to do so.

T   F   8. A SIRS value of 1+ is assigned to a patient when there is evidence that the patient has attempted suicide in the past but is not now actively thinking about suicide.

T   F   9. A patient admitted with a SIRS of 4+ is admitted to a seclusion room for punishment.

T   F   10. A suicide note is a bid for attention and should not be taken seriously.

Post-Test

(continued)

T   F   11. It is usually harmful for a patient to talk about suicidal thoughts and his or her attention should be diverted from such topics.

T   F   12. A suicidal patient whose spirits seem to suddenly improve should be observed closely, for it is likely he or she has decided on a suicidal plan and intends to carry it through.

T   F   13. Professionals in the field of medicine usually respond in a positive manner toward patients who have attempted suicide.

T   F   14. The more violent or painful the suicide method chosen, the more serious the intent of suicide.

T   F   15. Persons who abuse alcohol or drugs are prone to suicidal behavior.

Matching. Match the letter(s) of the appropriate SIRS value(s) in column B with the statements in column A (more than one answer may be used).

Column A	*Column B*
1. Allowed shaving kit with razor and blade.	a. SIRS 0
	b. SIRS 1+
2. No evidence that the patient is actively thinking about suicide but evidence shows a previous attempted suicide.	c. SIRS 2+
	d. SIRS 3+
	e. SIRS 4+
3. "If I don't get some relief, I'm going to kill myself."	
4. Admitted and remains in seclusion room for patient's own protection.	
5. No history or evidence of suicidal ideas.	
6. Admitted to hospital because of an active suicidal attempt.	

Post-Test

(continued)

Multiple Choice. Circle the letter or number you think represents the best answer.

1. Among adults, suicide is the _____ cause of death in the United States.
   a. 1st.
   b. 5th.
   c. 10th.
   d. 15th.

2. Which of the following losses might be significant enough to motivate a person to attempt suicide?
   a. Death of a loved one.
   b. Loss of health due to a chronic illness.
   c. Loss of a job.
   d. Loss of a loved one via divorce.
   e. Loss of beauty.
       (1) a only.
       (2) a, b, and e.
       (3) b, c, and d.
       (4) All of the above.

3. A person attempting suicide is likely to have recently experienced which of the following feelings?
   a. Guilt and a wish for punishment.
   b. Hopelessness.
   c. Anxiety.
   d. Worthlessness.
   e. Exuberance.
       (1) b only.
       (2) a and d.
       (3) a, b, c, and d.
       (4) All of the above.

4. Establishing a therapeutic relationship with the suicidal patient contributes to which of the following:
   a. The patient's feelings of self-worth.
   b. The patient's desire to live.
   c. A feeling of being overprotected and dependent.
   d. The patient's belief that others want him or her to live.

Post-Test

(continued)

(1) a only.
(2) b and c.
(3) a, b, and d.
(4) All of the above.

5. Which of the following behaviors might be clues preceding a suicidal act?
   a. Sudden changes in behavior from depression to cheerfulness.
   b. Talking directly or indirectly about suicide.
   c. A history of a previous suicidal attempt.
   d. Giving away items of great sentimental or monetary value.
      (1) a and c.
      (2) a, b, and c.
      (3) a, c, and d.
      (4) All of the above.

Care for Patients Who Have Lost Contact with Reality

OBJECTIVES: Student will be able to:

1. Identify behaviors associated with a patient who has lost contact with reality.
2. Cite a reason bizarre behaviors sometimes become reinforced.
3. State an appropriate response to socially inappropriate behavior from a patient who is out of touch with reality.
4. Identify a reason hallucinating patients should not be left to spend time alone.
5. Define and give an example of a *delusion,* an *illusion,* and a *hallucination.*
6. State an appropriate response when a hallucinating patient asks if you can hear the voice he or she is hearing.
7. Identify statements a student or staff member should *never* tell a hallucinating patient.

Patients who hallucinate or exhibit other bizarre behavior are usually suffering from one of the psychotic disorders (schizophrenia, senile dementia, manic-depressive psychosis, among others). Such behaviors, however, may occur with organic brain disease, traumatic injury to the brain, high fever, or ingestion of certain drugs such as LSD or other hallucinogens. Regardless of the cause, these patients pose unique problems for staff members and can be quite upsetting to other patients.

If the symptoms are recognized soon enough, quiet attention and support from staff members can often keep patients who are hallucinating or delusional from losing control. Therefore, staff members must constantly be alert and attuned to behavioral cues that indicate impending problems. For example, a manic patient may first exhibit loud talk, rapid pacing, and grandiose ideas before becoming agitated and destroying the dayroom.

On the other hand, staff members must be careful not to reinforce bizarre behavior. This happens when the behaviors exhibited by patients get them what they want. For example, if a female patient begins dancing up and down the hall with her dress tucked in her panties to get attention, the staff should kindly, but firmly, instruct the patient to go to her room. She should be escorted, if necessary. When the patient has no audience, the behavior will likely cease. If the staff or patients stop to watch, clap, or giggle, the patient's inappropriate behavior will be rewarded and will most likely be repeated.

Patients who show bizarre behavior often need help in understanding the reason their behavior is inappropriate and the effect it has on others. They may benefit from appropriate confrontation with the fact that their behavior is not socially acceptable. Such confrontations should be made only by a staff member who is well trained and experienced in psychotherapeutic techniques.

Patients who are hallucinating or showing other bizarre behaviors do not respond well to demands or orders. They do, however, usually respond to kind but firm structuring (instructions in appropriate behavior).

Patients who are totally out of contact with reality exhibit behavior that is also bizarre but that is far more disturbing. Staff and patients are often at least tolerant of vulgar language, unusual makeup, or other inappropriate behavior but may be frightened by people who hear voices, see visions, and act in unusual ways because of their hallucinations. Three types of reality distortions indicate that a patient may have lost contact with reality. They are delusions, illusions, and hallucinations.

A *delusion* is a false belief that cannot be corrected by reason. For example, a delusional patient may believe that someone is trying to poison him or her by putting something in the food, and, therefore, the patient may refuse to eat.

An *illusion* is a falsehood or misinterpretation of a real sensory impression or image. For example, Mrs. Jones thinks she sees a man in her room when it is only the shadow of her bathrobe hanging on the door, or Mr. Brown thinks he hears a gunshot when he actually heard a car backfire as it passed his window. Illusions become a problem only when the patient will not reconsider his or her perceptions when given factual information about the stimulus causing the misperception.

A *hallucination* is an idea or perception that does not exist in reality. Patients who hear voices telling them to do things when no one is talking or patients who see things that no one else sees are said to be hallucinating. The most common hallucinations are visual and auditory, but patients occasionally smell things (olfactory), taste things (gustatory), or feel things (tactile) that are not real.

These patients should be shown a great deal of kindness and concern, because their hallucinations, delusions, or illusions are often quite frightening. Voices may say scary things to them, tell them to do dangerous or evil things, or tell them to kill themselves or someone else (command hallucinations). They may see snakes slithering on their beds or feel lice or worms crawling all over their bodies. Although none of this is really happening, it is very real to hallucinating patients, and they are often panic-stricken. It is helpful to stay with these patients until their prn medication can begin to calm them. Sometimes they will become quieter and more in contact with reality if they are simply removed from the environment (often busy, rushed, and overstimulating) in which they started to lose touch. Talking to the patient in a quiet, soothing manner is also helpful, especially if the nurse tries to steer the conversation back to reality. For example, Mrs. Smith states that she has just heard God telling her how to save the world. Instead of asking the patient to explain further, which would focus on the hallucination, the staff member might try to draw the patient's attention back to reality by commenting on the needlework the patient has been doing and asking to be shown how to do a particular stitch.

Patients who tend to lose contact with reality should not be allowed to spend a great deal of time alone because this situation encourages their bizarre behavior. Some authorities believe that hallucinations begin because a person is lonely and anxious and has no "real" person to talk with. Patients then "create" someone in their mind with whom they can have an interpersonal relationship. In the beginning, the imagined people or voices tell the patient what the patient wants to hear and provide relief from anxiety. Thus, the patient begins to allow more time for the imagined relationship and less time for real people. Such a patient needs to be around other people and, if possible, to sit and talk quietly with someone. A staff member who cares can help a great deal if the caring attitude and feeling are communicated to the patient. Staff members must begin to replace the imaginary people with real relationships. Certainly, there are other theories about the reasons patients hallucinate, most recognizing the role of biochemical and bioelectrical processes in the brain. We know, for example, that prolonged sleep deprivation produces hallucinations in persons without mental illness and that drug or alcohol withdrawal also produces hallucinations.

When a patient experiences a hallucination or delusion, he or she should be told that the staff member knows that the patient is upset and knows that the patient hears the voices or sees the snakes, but that the staff member cannot hear or see them. The staff member must serve as a healthy role model and someone with whom the patient can test the real and the unreal. For this reason, it is extremely important for staff members never to tell a patient they, too, can hear the voices or see the snakes.

Some authorities suggest that, after a staff member has established a working relationship with a patient, the staff member should tell the patient to dismiss the voices any time the patient is hallucinating. For example, the staff member might say, "Mrs. White, tell those 'voices' to go away. I'm real; they are not." Once again, focus the patient's attention on something else—something real. This action is sometimes called *grounding*—that is, grounding the person in reality by stating or reviewing certain facts.

Finally, it is important that staff members not argue with patients who are hallucinating. Arguing forces patients to defend their false perceptions and may cause them to become violent. Avoid making statements that might be misinterpreted by patients and always try to be supportive of patients' feelings about their perceptions without supporting the misperceptions themselves. For example, the patient who says he is being chased by FBI agents would not benefit from a staff member's saying, "Mr. Jones, it's ridiculous for you to believe FBI agents are after you. That's nonsense. Just stop believing that and you'll be all right." Neither would it be helpful to respond by saying, "Gee, that really sounds interesting, Mr. Jones. Please tell me more about it." It would be better to respond by saying, "Mr. Jones, I know you believe the FBI is after you, but it doesn't seem that way to me. It is a very pretty day. Why don't we take a walk?" Then try to interest Mr. Jones in things that are reality-oriented.

▼ KEY POINTS ▼

Patients Who Have Lost Contact with Reality
1. Patients who hallucinate or exhibit other bizarre behaviors are usually suffering from one of the psychotic disorders.

2. Other conditions that may produce this type of behavior include organic brain disease, traumatic injury to the brain, high fever, sleep deprivation, alcohol withdrawal, or ingestion of hallucinogenic drugs.

Key Points continued

3. If recognized soon enough, quiet attention and support from staff members can often keep hallucinating or delusional patients from losing control.

4. Be alert and attuned to behavioral cues that indicate impending problems, and be careful to not reinforce the bizarre behavior.

5. Patients who show bizarre behavior often need help in understanding the reason their behavior is inappropriate and the effect it has on others.

6. Patients who are hallucinating or showing other bizarre behavior do not respond well to demands or orders but instead require instructions on appropriate behavior.

7. Three types of reality distortions indicate that a patient may have lost contact with reality: delusions, illusions, and hallucinations.

8. A *delusion* is a false belief that cannot be corrected by reason.

9. An *illusion* is a falsehood or misinterpretation of a real sensory impression or image.

10. A *hallucination* is an idea or perception that does not exist in reality.

11. Hallucinations, delusions, and illusions are very real to patients and often create panic. It is helpful to stay with these patients until their prn medication can begin to calm them or to remove them from the environment in which they started to lose touch.

12. Patients who tend to lose contact with reality should not be allowed to spend a great deal of time alone because this encourages withdrawn or bizarre behavior.

13. Some authorities believe that hallucinations begin because a person is lonely and anxious and has no "real" person to talk with. The person then "creates" someone in his or her mind with whom the person can have an interpersonal relationship. There are other theories as well.

14. These patients need to be around other people and to sit and talk quietly. A staff member can be very helpful by communicating a caring attitude to the patient.

15. When a patient experiences a hallucination or delusion, the patient should be told the staff member understands that the patient

continued on page 344

Key Points continued

hears or sees something but that the staff member cannot hear or see it. It is extremely important that staff members never tell a patient they, too, can hear the voices or see the images.

16. After a staff member has established a working relationship with the patient, the staff member may tell the patient to dismiss the voices any time the patient is hallucinating; the staff member may also use other grounding techniques.

17. It is important that staff members not argue with a patient who is hallucinating. Staff members should always try to be supportive of a patient's feelings without supporting the misperceptions themselves.

Annotated Bibliography

Blair, D. T., and Hildreth, N. A.: PTSD and the Vietnam veteran: The battle for treatment. *Journal of Psychosocial Nursing and Mental Health Services,* 1991, 29(10):15–20.

Focuses on the professional bias, personal issues, countertransference, and pathological staff dynamics encountered by many patients treated for post-traumatic stress disorder (PTSD). Also presents characteristics of PTSD and the complications of diagnostic confusion in treatment.

Chapman, T.: The nurse's role in neuroleptic medications. *Journal of Psychosocial Nursing and Mental Health Services,* 1991, 29(6):6–8.

Discusses adverse side effects of neuroleptic medications for the treatment of schizophrenia. Patients were allowed to express their attitudes concerning the need for these medications.

Curl, A.: Agitation and the older adult. *Journal of Psychosocial Nursing and Mental Health Services,* 1989, 27(12):12–14.

Focuses on agitation in elderly patients that is caused by delirium, dementia, parkinsonism, and depression and on appropriate management of these behaviors by nursing staff.

Dauner, A., and Blair, D.: Akathisia: When treatment creates a problem. *Journal of Psychosocial Nursing and Mental Health Services,* 1990, 23(10):13–17.

Explains the symptoms and dangers of akathisia (a side effect of antipsychotic medications) and gives several case examples of patients suffering from these symptoms.

Deutsch, L. H., and Rovner, B. W.: Agitation and other noncognitive abnormalities in Alzheimer's disease. *Psychiatric Clinics of North America,* 1991, 14(2):341–349.

Presents the behavioral symptoms of Alzheimer's disease, such as agitation, wandering, passivity, psychosis, and sleep disturbances and discusses the importance of understanding the nature and treatment of these symptoms.

Dzurec, L. C.: How do they see themselves? Self-perceptions and functioning for people with chronic schizophrenia. *Journal of Psychosocial Nursing and Mental Health Services,* 1990, 28(8):10–14.

Describes through research study the relationship between the self-perceptions of schizophrenic patients and their level of daily functioning.

Ehmann, T. S., Higgs, E., Smith, G. N., Altman, T. S., Lloyd, D., and Honer, W. G.: Routine assessment of patient progress: A multiformat, change-sensitive nurses' instrument for assessing psychotic inpatients. *Comprehensive Psychiatry,* 1995, 36(4):289–295.

Discusses a new assessment tool for nurses that incorporates both interview and observational data into a comprehensive assessment of psychiatric patients.

McFarlane, A. C.: Individual psychotherapy for post-traumatic stress disorder. *Psychiatric Clinics of North America,* 1994, 17(2):393–408.

Discusses the competitive relationship among various schools of therapy and the need for a conceptual model. The authors also provide a model reflecting the differential role of traumatic experiences in determining which of several subsets of symptoms may occur in post-traumatic stress disorder.

Swanson, B., Cronin-Stubbs, D., and Colletti, M.: Dementia and depression in persons with AIDS: Causes and care. *Journal of Psychosocial Nursing and Mental Health Services,* 1990, 28(10):33–39.

Discusses the importance of distinguishing depression from AIDS dementia complex and presents treatment plans for both disorders to promote the quality of life.

Ugarriza, D. A.: A descriptive study of postpartum depression. *Perspectives in Psychiatric Care,* 1995, 31(3):25–32.

Reports on a study of postpartum depression, including the favorable response of postpartum psychoses to conventional treatment.

Post-Test

True or False. Circle your choice.

T   F   1. Patients who are hallucinating or exhibiting other bizarre behaviors respond best to direct demands.

T   F   2. A patient who hears voices telling him or her to do things when no one is talking is said to be experiencing an illusion.

T   F   3. The most common hallucinations are visual and auditory.

T   F   4. Patients who tend to lose contact with reality should be left alone a great deal of the time because it tends to decrease their bizarre behavior.

T   F   5. Some authorities believe that hallucinations begin because a person is lonely and anxious with no "real" person to talk with.

T   F   6. A delusion is a false belief that cannot be corrected by reason.

Multiple Choice. Circle the letter or number you think represents the best answer.

1. Which of the following is not appropriate when responding to disoriented, confused, or incoherent patients?
   a. Giving the patient necessary information and assistance as needed.
   b. Assisting the patient to hurry through activities so he or she gets exposure to all areas of the ward routine.
   c. Be kind and firm, yet help the patient when appropriate.
   d. Provide reality-oriented conversation topics.

2. When working with a person who has a distorted perception of reality, the mental health worker will generally be most effective if he or she:
   a. Encourages the patient to discuss the voices he or she hears.

Post-Test

(continued)

   b. Continually tries to draw the patient's attention to the here and now.
   c. Avoids all unnecessary physical contact.

3. In working with a patient who is hallucinating, appropriate approaches include:
   a. Carefully watching what one communicates nonverbally.
   b. Providing a structured environment.
   c. Conveying to the patient that you believe the "voices" are real.
   d. Asking concrete, reality-oriented questions.
   e. Increasing social interaction rapidly.
   (1) a, b, and c.
   (2) a, b, and d.
   (3) b, d, and e.
   (4) c, d, and e.
   (5) All of these.

Short Answer. Answer the following as briefly and specifically as possible.

1. List two psychiatric disorders mentioned in this chapter that are likely to have hallucinations as one of their major symptoms.

   a. _____

   b. _____

2. What behavioral clues are indicative of a patient that is about to lose control?

   _____

   _____

   _____

3. List the three types of reality distortions that indicate that a patient has lost contact with reality.

   a. _____

   b. _____

   c. _____

Post-Test

(continued)

4. Define an *illusion*:

_____

_____

_____

5. Define *hallucination*:

_____

_____

_____

Care for Patients Who Have Neurological Deficits

OBJECTIVES: Student will be able to:

1. Define the terms *JOCAM* and *affect.*

2. Define and give an example of *confabulation.*

3. State the reasons change should be held to a minimum in patients with neurological deficits.

4. Describe the role and importance of *structure* in caring for neurologically impaired patients.

5. State a proper response when a neurologically impaired patient is affectively inappropriate in a given situation.

6. Give three examples of behavior that would be most effective with a patient with organic brain syndrome.

Mental health professionals have coined the acronym *JOCAM* to describe the group of symptoms often shown by patients who suffer from neurological deficits. Of course, patients with other psychiatric illnesses may exhibit these same behaviors and the approach to them may be the same. When used in reference to a patient, the acronym *JOCAM* means that the patient has difficulty in the following areas:

J = Judgment
O = Orientation
C = Confabulation
A = Affect
M = Memory

When working with patients who exhibit behaviors indicating problems in those areas, staff members must maintain a warm, accepting attitude. Because these patients often show poor judgment, they must be supervised closely to prevent them from bringing physical harm to themselves (e.g., wandering off or getting lost, falling, drinking or eating inappropriate things, taking baths that are too hot, not paying adequate attention to environmental hazards). Often these patients know they are confused and become quite frustrated and agitated because they cannot correct the problem. Measures such as supportive understanding from the staff, a supervised warm bath, a well-lighted room that eliminates shadows that may be misinterpreted, soft music, or mild tranquilizers may be used to help these patients relax.

Some patients with neurological deficits have excellent memories for past events but forget new information and experiences rather quickly. The staff may need to repeat information several times. The staff should use a kind, quiet tone of voice and give simple, short explanations and answers, especially when patients' attention spans may be short. Loud voices and long explanations tend to bewilder these patients and may not be remembered at all.

Because it is embarrassing to not be able to remember, patients who are forgetful often make up information to fill in information gaps and cover up the things they have forgotten. This is called *confabulation*. It is important, therefore, to listen carefully to a patient's words. If the information is made up or incorrect, the patient should be corrected in a gentle, nonpunitive manner. A staff member might say, "I know you're having trouble remembering where you lived last year but your family says it was with your son, not in a home for the aging" or "I know you miss your mother but she died a long, long time ago." If such explanations bother the patient or worsen his or her depression, you might try distracting the patient from the thoughts and say, "I know you miss your mother. Would you like to help me with this game? I think it goes like this," and engage the patient in the game.

Calendars with large print and clocks with large numbers and hands help keep patients with neurological deficits oriented to date and time. These items should be placed around the unit in the areas in which patients spend most of their time. Ideally, a large clock and calendar should be in every patient's room.

It may also be helpful to label certain areas, such as the nurse's station and the bathrooms, and even to put the patient's name in big letters on his or her bedroom door. Staff members should wear easy-to-read, large-print name tags at all times, and it is helpful if the tag also states the person's position (e.g. RN, aide, dietitian, social worker).

When patients with neurological deficits are admitted to the hospital unit or come to a community mental health center for treatment, they should be carefully oriented to their new environment. These patients are extremely sensitive to change and may become confused in new surroundings. They like to follow a stable routine, and changes make them feel anxious and insecure. These patients should not be hurried and should be assisted whenever they need help. Because they may not always ask for assistance when they really need it, the staff must observe them carefully and give assistance when the situation warrants it. Mr. Green may be able to dress himself but may put his shoes on the wrong feet or may forget how to tie his shoelaces. Mr. Jones may remember the general location of the bathroom but may forget which is for the men and which is for the women. He may, therefore, use the wrong one. Patients with these problems should never be scolded or embarrassed in front of other patients or staff members. Instead, staff members should help them correct the inappropriate behavior or learn the necessary task. These problems occur because older patients with neurological impairments often have trouble generalizing their learning experiences. For example, an older man who learns to walk with the aid of a walker in physical therapy may be unable to remember how to use it when he returns home or to his room on the unit. Therefore, elderly patients must be taught in a setting similar to the one in which they will use whatever skill is being learned, or they should have supervised practice in that area.

When neurologically deficient patients talk in a manner that seems nonsensical or confused, they might be told that the staff member does not understand what they are saying and the subject might be changed back to a reality-oriented topic.

Confusion can be kept to a minimum by allowing patients to bring familiar objects from home such as a favorite chair, nightstand, or pictures of their families. Also, it is helpful to place their personal items (clothing, toilet articles, etc.) in an area to which the patient has easy access. If Mrs. Jones is found wandering around nude, she should be taken back to her room and helped to dress. The reason Mrs. Jones was wandering around nude may be that she was tired of wearing the same dirty dress and couldn't find her clean ones, which were unintentionally "hidden away" in her suitcase on the top shelf of the closet, out of reach and out of mind.

Another way to help decrease confusion and forgetfulness is to teach patients to use lists or appointment books or both. If Mrs. Green has trouble remembering her daily schedule, help her write it down in a small notebook so that she can renew it as needed. If she forgets and asks a staff member about a scheduled event, she can be referred to her notebook. A list taped next to the mirror in his bathroom may help Mr. Green remember to shave, comb his hair, and brush his teeth each day. Lists and appointment books are a socially acceptable means of keeping someone from forgetting important matters and may even improve the patient's self-esteem.

Sometimes normal unit activities such as a simple birthday party for another patient can confuse a patient with a neurological deficit. If this happens, the patient should be removed to a quieter area. A staff member should stay with the patient while he or she eats his cake in peace and quiet so that the patient does not feel that he or she is being rejected or punished.

Affect refers to the feeling tone experienced with an emotion. The usual descriptive terms for affective states are flat (showing no feeling tone, masklike face, monotone voice), dysphoric (showing no joy, sad), constricted or bland (showing limited affect), euphoric (showing too much affect), appropriate (showing appropriate feeling tone for the emotion being expressed), and inappropriate (showing feeling tone not matched to the emotion being expressed). Patients with problems of JOCAM are often described as having flat affects. They seem to be neither happy nor sad and show little, if any, emotion about anything; they simply exist. Sometimes, however, their affect may be quite inappropriate. Patients may cry uncontrollably because they cannot open a letter, or they may laugh when they hear that a friend has died. When such patients have reason to be upset, they need to express their feelings, even when an inappropriate emotion is used. The appropriate emotion can sometimes be obtained by simply telling the patient, "I know you are upset. You might feel better if you cried." The suggestion is tailored to the situation. This technique structures the situation for the patient and gives information about the type of behavior expected. Another technique the staff can use in handling excessive emotional outbursts is distraction. Mrs. Brown, a patient who is crying uncontrollably, may be stopped by calling her attention to an interesting activity occurring across the room or by involving her in that activity.

The language of patients with neurological deficits may also be inappropriate. If Mr. Jones swears and screams obscenities at a staff member who has moved his eyeglasses from their usual resting place, the staff member might respond in the following manner: "Mr. Jones, you're right. I should have put your glasses back where you keep them. I'm sorry, but screaming and swearing will only make people angry. Next time, try not to get so upset. Just ask for what you want and we will help you." If this is too long an interaction for the patient's neurological condition, shorten it by saying, "You're right. Just ask if you need anything else." This acknowledges the patient's frustration and provides structure without involving a long interaction.

When a patient's behavior must be corrected, the correction should occur immediately after the inappropriate behavior takes place and it should be done privately. Otherwise, the patient may not remember what he or she said or did that should be changed and may become embarrassed or angry. When a patient acts in an appropriate way or learns a new task, be sure to give immediate feedback in the form of praise and approval.

It is the responsibility of staff members to recognize that neurologically impaired patients depend on routine and structure to help them stay oriented. Anything that disturbs their "world" is likely to upset them. In the previous situation, it was, in fact, the staff member who caused the situation leading to Mr. Jones' inappropriate behavior.

Patients with neurological deficits are not always hopeless. Drugs are now available to help clear the patient's thinking by increasing the brain's metabolism and use of oxygen. Further, great strides in helping such patients cope with their environment and illness can be made by a kind, understanding staff that rewards appropriate behavior and re-channels inappropriate behavior.

Staff members must remember that other physical problems such as infection, kidney dysfunction, high fever, or adverse drug reaction may cause or exacerbate the behaviors described in this chapter. Staff members must be constantly alert for the possibility of such factors when JOCAM difficulties are discovered.

▼ KEY POINTS ▼

Patients with Neurological Deficits

1. Mental health professionals have coined the acronym *JOCAM* to describe the group of symptoms often shown by patients suffering from neurological deficits.

2. *JOCAM* means that the patient has difficulty in the following areas:

> J = Judgment
> O = Orientation
> C = Confabulation
> A = Affect
> M = Memory

continued on page 354

Key Points continued

3. These patients must be supervised closely to prevent them from bringing physical harm to themselves.

4. Patients know they are confused and become quite frustrated and agitated because they cannot correct the problem.

5. Patients with neurological deficits have excellent memories for past events but forget new information and experiences rather quickly.

6. The staff should use a kind, quiet tone of voice and give simple, short explanations and answers.

7. Patients who are forgetful often make up information (*confabulation*) to fill in information gaps and cover up the things they have forgotten.

8. Calendars with large print and clocks with large numbers help keep patients with neurological deficits oriented to date and time.

9. It may be helpful to label the nurse's station, the bathrooms, and the patient's bedroom door.

10. Patients with neurological deficits should be carefully oriented to their new environment. They are extremely sensitive to change and may become confused in new surroundings.

11. Patients should be assisted whenever they need help. Keeping in mind that these patients may not always ask for assistance, the staff must observe them carefully.

12. When neurologically deficient patients talk in a nonsensical manner, they should be told that the staff member does not understand what they are saying and the subject should be changed back to a reality-oriented topic.

13. Confusion can be kept to a minimum by allowing patients to bring familiar objects from home such as a favorite chair, nightstand, or pictures of their families.

14. To help decrease patients' confusion and forgetfulness, teach them to use lists or appointment books or both.

15. Normal unit activities such as a simple birthday party for another patient can confuse a patient with a neurological deficit.

16. *Affect* means the feelings experienced with an emotion. Patients with problems of JOCAM are often described as having flat affects.

Key Points continued

17. Sometimes, the affect may be quite inappropriate in that patients may cry uncontrollably while performing the simplest of tasks. On the other hand, they may laugh when they hear that a friend has died.

18. The patient's situation must be structured and the patient given information about the type of behavior expected.

19. Another effective technique in handling excessive emotional outbursts is distraction.

20. The language of patients with neurological deficits may also be inappropriate. The staff member should acknowledge the patient's frustration and provide structure.

21. When a patient is being corrected, the correction should occur immediately after the inappropriate behavior takes place and it should be done privately.

22. Patients with brain impairments depend on routine and structure to help them stay oriented.

23. Drugs are now available to help clear the patient's thinking by increasing the brain's metabolism and use of oxygen.

24. Infection, kidney dysfunction, high fever, or adverse drug reaction may cause or exacerbate the behaviors described. Be alert for the possibility of such factors when JOCAM problems are discovered.

Annotated Bibliography

Abraham, I. L., Holroyd, S., Snustad, D. G., Manning, C. A., Brasher, H. R., Diamond, P. T., and Heisterman, A. A.: Multidisciplinary assessment of patients with Alzheimer's disease. *Nursing Clinics of North America,* 1994, 29(1):113–128.

Discusses psychological and biologic manifestations of Alzheimer's disease and provides a protocol for nursing assessment.

Beck, C., Heacock, P., Mercer, S., and Walton, C. G.: Dressing for success: Promoting independence among cognitively impaired elderly. *Journal of Psychosocial Nursing and Mental Health Services,* 1991, 29(7):30–35.

Presents ideas on fostering independence in the cognitively impaired population to discourage excess disability.

Curl, A.: Agitation and the older adult. *Journal of Psychosocial Nursing and Mental Health Services,* 1989, 27(12):12–14.

Focuses on agitation caused by delirium, dementia, parkinsonism, and depression and the appropriate management of these behaviors by nursing staff.

Deutsch, L. H., and Rovner, B. W.: Agitation and other noncognitive abnormalities in Alzheimer's disease. *Psychiatric Clinics of North America,* 1991, 14(2):341–349.

Presents the behavioral symptoms of Alzheimer's disease, such as agitation, wandering, passivity, psychosis, and sleep disturbances and discusses the importance of understanding the nature and treatment of these symptoms.

Fallon, B. A., and Nields, J. A.: Lyme disease: A neuropsychiatric illness. *American Journal of Psychiatry,* 1994, 151(11):1571–1583.

Discusses this multisystemic illness that may affect the central nervous system, causing neurological and psychiatric symptoms.

Hoover, S. D.: Impaired personal boundaries: A proposed nursing diagnosis. *Perspectives in Psychiatric Care,* 1995, 31(3):9–13.

Describes and discusses the physical, emotional, intellectual, and spiritual dimensions of personal boundaries and their significant role in neurosis.

Lohr, J. B.: Oxygen radicals and neuropsychiatric illness: Some speculations. *Archives of General Psychiatry,* 1991, 48:1097–1106.

Explores the relationship between free radicals and neuropsychiatric conditions marked by the gradual development of psychopathological symptoms and movement disorder. Radical-induced damage may be important in Parkinson's disease, tardive dyskinesia, metal intoxication syndromes, Down syndrome, schizophrenia, Huntington chorea, and Alzheimer's disease.

Masters, J. C., and O'Grady, M.: Normal pressure hydrocephalus: A potentially reversible form of dementia. *Journal of Psychosocial Nursing and Mental Health Services,* 1992, 30(6):25–28.

Discusses the symptoms, diagnosis, etiology, treatment, and nursing care for normal pressure hydrocephalus (NPH), a form of dementia that has proven to be reversible.

Richter, J. M., Roberto, K. A., and Bottenberg, D. J.: Communicating with persons with Alzheimer's disease: Experiences of family and formal caregivers. *Archives of Psychiatric Nursing,* 1995, 9(5):279–285.

Discusses the decreased cognitive functioning of Alzheimer's patients and examines the communication processes used by family members and formal caregivers.

Samuel, W. A., Henderson, V. W., and Miller, C. A.: Severity of dementia in Alzheimer disease and neurofibrillary tangles in multiple brain regions. *Alzheimer Disease and Associated Disorders,* 1991, 5(1):1–11.

Examines through research study the relationship of numbers of neurofibrillary tangles (NFTs) in selected cortical and subcortical sites to the duration of clinical disease and the severity of dementia.

Scott, A. L., and Dumas, R. E.: Personal space boundaries: Clinical applications in psychiatric mental health nursing. *Perspectives in Psychiatric Care,* 1995, 31(3):14–19.

Discusses a nursing intervention used with neurotic patients with personal space boundary issues. The intervention incorporates the interactive effects of cognition, affect, and behavior.

Post-Test

Multiple Choice. Circle the number or letter you think represents the best answer.

1. Organic brain disorders are caused by:
   a. Interpersonal traumas.
   b. Anatomic damage.
   c. Physiological damage.
   d. Trauma to the psyche.
   e. A too-strong superego.
      (1) a, d, and e.
      (2) b, c, and d.
      (3) d and e.
      (4) a, b, and c.
      (5) b and c.

2. Choose the items that can be features of organic brain disorders:
   a. Impairment of memory for past events.
   b. Impairment of judgment.
   c. Good control of emotions.
   d. Personality changes.
   e. Hallucinations.
      (1) All of the above.
      (2) b, d, and e.
      (3) a, b, and c.
      (4) a, c, and e.
      (5) None of the above.

3. Confabulation is:
   a. A type of hallucination.
   b. An effective medication.
   c. Fragmented thinking.
   d. Echolalia.
   e. Filling in memory gaps.

4. In treating a patient with organic brain disorder caused by cerebral arteriosclerosis, the mental health worker should:
   a. Understand the patient's personality before illness.
   b. Give individualized care.

(continued)

  c. Know that memory for recent events is better than memory for past events.
  d. Provide a disordered environment.
  e. Be optimistic, emphatic, and clear.
    (1) All of the above.
    (2) None of the above.
    (3) a, b, c, and d.
    (4) a, c, and d.
    (5) a, b, and e.

5. The relatively permanent impairment of cerebral function occurring in chronic organic impairments produces defects in:
  a. Memory.
  b. Orientation.
  c. Judgment.
  d. Comprehension.
  e. Affect.
    (1) a, b, c, and e.
    (2) a, b, and c.
    (3) a, b, c, and d.
    (4) All of the above.

6. The premorbid personality of a patient with organic brain disorders:
  a. Usually has little to do with the type of illness he or she develops.
  b. Usually determines the behavior he or she shows.
  c. Is usually impossible to determine.
  d. Usually is the opposite of that shown.

7. A senile patient is withdrawn and negativistic. The best approach to the patient might be:
  a. "Would you like to go to your room where you can be alone?"
  b. "I need a partner to play checkers with me."
  c. "Your family will be terribly disappointed if you don't go to occupational therapy."
  d. "Your doctor wants you to participate in activities."

Post-Test

(continued)

8. Which of the following is not appropriate when responding to disoriented, confused, or incoherent patients?
   a. Giving patients necessary information and assistance as needed.
   b. Assisting patients to hurry through activities so they are exposed to all areas of ward routine.
   c. Be kind and firm, yet help patients when appropriate.
   d. Provide reality-oriented conversation topics.

True or False. Circle your choice.

T   F   1. Organic brain disorders (chronic type) can be reversible.

T   F   2. Good psychological adjustment to life prior to the onset of cerebral arteriosclerosis is a determining factor in the prognosis of the disease.

T   F   3. Patients with organic impairments often have short memory spans.

T   F   4. It is frequently helpful to "make an example" for other patients by choosing a particular neurologically impaired patient to keep correcting until he or she does almost everything in the desired manner.

T   F   5. Patients should not be allowed to bring personal items from home because it only makes them cry and want to go home.

Short Answer. Answer the following as briefly and specifically as possible.

1. Fill in the term that corresponds to the letter given:
   J =
   O =
   C =
   A =
   M =

Post-Test

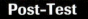

(continued)

2. The best way to explain something to an organically impaired person is:

_____

_____

_____

3. Neurologically impaired patients often have difficulty in maintaining a good orientation to a new environment. List five things a mental health worker can do to reduce disorientation.

   a. _____
   b. _____
   c. _____
   d. _____
   e. _____

4. When it is necessary to correct a patient, why should it be done immediately following the inappropriate behavior?

_____

_____

_____

5. The two most important factors in helping neurologically impaired patients to stay oriented are:

_____

_____

_____

The Journey

What is this affliction that causes the pain,
　　that produces feelings of inferiority and shame?
What is this force that drives me to be,
　　something I hide and fear others might see?
How do I handle the turmoil within,
　　and how long do I wait for my soul to mend?
How do I handle the despair that I feel,
　　when I don't know fantasy—and I don't know real?

I must lay down my guilt and give up my lies,
　　and I'll view the world through different eyes.
Say goodbye to the past, anticipate the new,
　　reach out to others, giving them a chance too.
I must know that I'm worthy and know that I'm strong,
　　with my new inner peace, I will not go wrong.
What was this affliction that caused the pain?
　　And what will I do with the insight I've gained?
I will live out my life one day at a time
　　knowing whatever the outcome, the decision is mine.
Feelings still surface every now and then,
　　But none that would take me to where I have been.

—*Diane Quinn*

Care for Patients with Eating Disorders

DIANE QUINN, RN, MSN

OBJECTIVES: Student will be able to:

1. Define anorexia nervosa, bulimia nervosa, and compulsive overeating.

2. Explain the potential importance in anorexia of a casual remark from a significant other about a girl's figure or weight.

3. Identify several psychological and behavioral characteristics associated with anorexia nervosa.

4. Explain why satisfaction of hunger plays a minimal role in bulimia.

5. Tell how looking at a patient's hand may allow one to identify a bulimic, even if he or she denies it.

6. Discuss the central role of control in bulimic dynamics.

7. State why compulsive overeaters might benefit more from addiction treatment than from diets.

8. Plan appropriate nursing interventions for patients with eating disorders.

Although there are no absolute standards of beauty, we learn at an early age what is attractive and acceptable and what is not. Because our society often equates beauty with thinness, many adolescents and young adults are obsessed with their physical appearance. In their quest for the ideal, they practice extreme and bizarre eating behaviors.

Some risk their lives by denying their need for food; others with unmet needs turn to food for consolation.

Eating is one of the earliest forms of nurturance and is the process by which attachment between infant and mother begins. Eating represents parental love for many people, but for others eating is symbolic of quite a different parental relationship. Throughout life, attitudes toward food continue to impact on human interaction. When the bond between certain individuals and food becomes more than a life-sustaining activity, then quality of life is compromised. In addition, current emphasis on personal control and cultural pressures for thinness have created a preoccupation with physical appearance and produced a major healthcare concern in the United States.

Anorexia nervosa, bulimia nervosa, and compulsive overeating are the three major eating disorders discussed in this chapter. Unfortunately, their etiology is unclear, the physiological and psychological complications are debilitating, and the cure is uncertain. Effective treatment is complex and involves skilled interventions based on knowledge and understanding of the disorder. Patients with eating disorders offer a challenge to every health professional involved in their care, and the nurse's role is often critical.

ANOREXIA NERVOSA

Anorexia nervosa is a severe form of self-starvation that may lead to death. Essential characteristics of the disorder include extreme weight loss (usually of more than 25 percent of beginning body weight), intense fear of fatness, disturbed body image, bizarre attitude toward food, and amenorrhea in females. Anorexia nervosa occurs predominantly in adolescent females with above-average intelligence and the disorder's incidence increases with socioeconomic status. The onset of anorexia nervosa is associated with stressful life situations with which the individual is unable to cope. It is not unusual, however, for one event to mark the beginning of a rigid program of food avoidance. Case histories are often complex but certain patterns emerge. Consider the following:

> Carla is a shy, soft-spoken girl who was considered a loner by her friends and a "model" daughter by her parents. Carla described herself as very active and ambitious but admitted that no accomplishment had ever resulted in her feeling satisfied with herself.
>
> At 16, Carla applied for a part-time modeling job at a local department store. When she did not get the job, the 5'6", 130-pound Carla was con-

vinced it was because she was too fat. She decided to diet. Carla only nibbled in her family's presence, and when they questioned her eating behavior, she minimized their questions regarding her well-being.

Carla spent many hours vigorously exercising. She weighed herself several times a day. If she didn't like what the scales showed, she exercised more.

Carla masked her thinness with loose-fitting clothes. One evening Carla's mother walked into Carla's room and was frightened by her daughter's emaciated body. The next day Carla visited the family physician, who encouraged Carla to eat more and prescribed vitamins. To Carla's mother, the physician's advice was, "Don't worry, it's just a phase she is going through."

On Carla's 17th birthday, her parents threw her a surprise party, complete with cake and ice cream. Carla reacted by screaming accusations at her parents: "You are trying to make me fat! I don't want to gain any weight! Take it away, take it all away!"

Carla was admitted to the psychiatric unit of the local hospital. Her admission weight was a mere 92 pounds. Carla's parents were unaware of their daughter's condition.

The Process of Treating Eating Disorders

History

Obtaining accurate data from the patient with anorexia nervosa may be difficult. The anorectic may be unable or unwilling to provide the necessary information. The family, however, is usually able to describe the patient's behavior in great detail. Typically, the anorectic has been well-adjusted, highly conforming to aggressive parental expectations, perfectionistic, and achievement-oriented. These young adults are described as impeccably groomed and orderly. As the condition worsens, this compulsive neatness is sometimes replaced with a lackadaisical attitude toward hygiene and appearance. Other characteristics of anorectics include empathy and sensitivity toward the feelings of others, and an intense fear of criticism.

A history often reveals that an anorectic began dieting with a casual remark from a significant other about the individual's figure or weight. When body image plays such a critical part in one's self-esteem, misperceptions of self-worth are enough to initiate a pattern of self-destructive behaviors.

Anorectics may begin by skipping desserts and sweets and progress to skipping meals. As food restriction increases, exercise increases.

Many anorectics lose considerable weight and avoid weight gain by restricting intake and exercising. Unsure of the degree of control they do have, some resort to vomiting and abusing laxatives, enemas, and diuretics.

Signs and Symptoms

Because anorectics may appear healthy, considering the degree of emaciation, novice nurses may have difficulty assessing the condition's severity.

Anorexia nervosa patients perceive themselves as overweight, no matter how thin they may be. Despite severe wasting, patients may deny that anything is wrong and can always find some body part they believe is fat (Chitty, 1992). Anorectics may insist that everyone is unduly concerned.

Anorectics think endlessly about food and they are obsessed with controlling their own intake. Even though they deliberately refuse to eat, anorectics' appetites are not suppressed. They usually have a broad knowledge of the nutritional and caloric value of food. Although they rarely eat the food themselves, anorectics may collect cookbooks and recipes, prepare elaborate meals, and take great pleasure in watching others eat. This food refusal is exhilarating to these patients, therefore they withdraw from anyone who encourages them to eat.

Anorectics have an insatiable compulsion for vigorous exercise. They may engage in lengthy aerobics sessions or jog for miles every day. Terrified of gaining even a pound and losing control, anorectics push themselves to greater endurance levels until they experience a sense of triumph. Anorectics may maintain academic excellence by increasing hours of study, continue to be active in sports and other extracurricular activities, hold several part-time jobs, and sleep as few as 2 to 3 hours a night.

Anorectics frequently deny having a weight problem and insist they feel fine. They plead with their parents to cease nagging about eating behaviors and body weight. They are proud of their self-denial and their low weight and just want to be left alone. Anorectics admit feelings of loneliness and isolation, but have difficulty forming healthy relationships.

The anorectic patient appears emaciated and skeletal: The cheek bones are prominent, the eyes are sunken, and the upper torso appears particularly thin with the ribs and clavicles highly visible. When the disorder is in the advanced stages, fine downy hair (lanugo) may be-present on the face, trunk, and extremities, the hands and feet may be cold and mottled, and other symptoms include bradycardia, hypotension, anemia, and high serum calcium levels (indicating osteoporosis).

Nursing Interventions

Once the patient's life is out of danger, treatment focuses on restoring normal nutrition and eating habits and dealing with psychological issues associated with the eating problem (Lucas, 1991).

Ineffective coping, misperceptions of body image, and poor self-esteem are subjective emotional experiences of the anorectic. Nursing interventions to promote improvement in these areas are included in the following discussion.

Trust is the foundation of the therapeutic relationship. In therapeutic relationships, there are certain expectations of both the nurse and patient. The nurse is responsible for maintaining the therapeutic relationship and guiding it toward the achievement of goals. The attitudes and skills of the nurse are of crucial importance to successful treatment. Chitty (1992) emphasizes that anorectics are extremely resistant to change. Progress may be slow, and, at best, recovery may be defined as a lessening of the symptoms.

Promoting Improved Nutrition. If the patient is medically unstable, intravenous (IV) therapy or tube feedings may be necessary. Nurses must evaluate their own strengths and have an honest awareness of their feelings toward patients if treatments are to be carried out in a nonjudgmental manner. Daily weights and accurate intake and output measurement (I&Os) are effective interventions for monitoring progress.

Nurses must avoid discussing food and eating behaviors with patients. Such self-centered issues reinforce maladaptive behaviors by allowing patients to avoid dealing with the hidden causes of the disorder. Refer patients for dietary consultation and assist with the development of realistic dietary goals.

Provide for a stress-free mealtime environment. Because large meals overwhelm anorectic patients, small frequent ones are more manageable and will be better accepted by them. Anorectics are masterminds of manipulation and procrastination; therefore, it is helpful to set time limits for meals. Acknowledge efforts of patients who meet the established goals, but remember that due to their mistrust of others, anorectics will not accept excessive praise.

Behavioral interventions such as rewards for new adaptive behavior may be incorporated into the management plan for the anorectic.

Privileges need to be linked to caloric intake, however, and not to weight gain. Consistency in the treatment approach must be maintained throughout hospitalization to prevent manipulation of the staff by the patient.

Promoting Effective Coping. Nurses must be sincere in their approach to anorectic patients. Using empathy and active listening shows concern for the patients. At first, patients may be in a dependent patient role, but as their conditions improve, nurses should encourage patients to assume more responsibility for their behavior and feelings. Having patients participate in their treatment planning fosters independence and maturity and facilitates the development of healthy coping mechanisms.

The nurse must demonstrate a belief in the patient's ability to improve maladaptive behaviors and must provide encouragement for accomplishments. The patient should be allowed some flexibility in daily routines, but the treatment team must set and maintain limits. Limit-setting not only provides the structure necessary to ensure the safety of the patient but reflects a sense of caring.

Patients need to be encouraged to explore their fears and feelings about gaining weight. Help them understand and accept these fears. Gaining insight into their relationships with others can help the patients deal with their disorder. As patients risk self-disclosure, their anxiety may intensify. The nurse must have advanced preparation and the skills necessary to prevent a new crisis. For the inexperienced nurse, spending time with the patient, observing the behavior and documenting it accordingly, is a valuable contribution to the success of the treatment.

Promoting Improved Perception of Body Image. Body image reflects a person's attitude and reveals something about the individual's self-concept. Body image constantly changes in response to a person's life experiences and perceptions. During adolescence, when the fear of rejection is great, perceptions of body size and weight play a major role in self-concept.

Anorectics have extreme misperceptions of their body size. No matter how thin they are, what they see in the mirror is someone who needs to lose weight. Staff members must encourage anorectic patients to express these feelings, be accepting of the patients' mental mistakes, and help the patients to accept both their strengths and weaknesses.

Promoting the Patient's Feelings of Self-Worth. Anorectics refuse to accept reinforcement for anything less than perfection. Help patients identify and focus on their positive attributes, and encourage patients to ventilate their feelings in whatever ways they are comfortable.

Nurses must offer unconditional acceptance of both the negative and positive feelings expressed by patients. Discounting patients' feelings will only increase their humiliation. Acceptance helps patients to realize that negative feelings are normal, that mistakes are tolerated, and that perfection and acceptance are not synonymous. For anorectics, the ability to compromise indicates progress and a greater level of personal awareness.

Prognosis and Outcome

The effect of interventions in the treatment of anorexia nervosa is not well understood and the outcome is uncertain. Some anorectics recover whereas others become permanently incapacitated or die. Resolution of the underlying psychological problem, as well as nutritional counseling, is crucial to recovery. Comerci, Kilbourne, and Harrison (1989) point out that early motivation for change is believed to be a good prognostic sign.

BULIMIA NERVOSA

Bulimia nervosa, more commonly known as binge eating, is the frequent compulsion to ingest large amounts of food in a short period of time (usually less than 2 hours). Bulimia nervosa is a disorder closely related to anorexia nervosa in that feelings of lack of control and distorted body image are present, but bulimia is a distinct eating disorder in itself. Bulimia is characterized by episodes of overeating and purging through self-induced vomiting, laxative and diuretic use, fasting, or vigorous exercise. These episodes are followed by post-binge guilt, self-deprecating thoughts, and depression. Bulimia occurs in anorectic, normal weight, and obese individuals. Most bulimics are white females of high school or college age, middle to upper middle class, well educated and intelligent.

Nicole, a 21-year-old part-time secretary and full-time nursing student, came to the Mental Health Department because of binge eating. She complained that she was concerned about her body image and weight, but she regularly went on eating binges that lasted 2 to 5 days. These episodes left her nauseated and weak. Nicole expressed feelings of guilt and shame over her lack of willpower. She admitted to abusing alcohol and drugs.

The initial interview with Nicole revealed a significant family and psychosocial history. Nicole lived with her mother, her alcoholic stepfather, and a sister who was viewed by the family as the "pretty one." Nicole related a history of sexual abuse by her grandfather between the ages of 10 and 13. She confided in her mother on several occasions regarding her grandfather's incestuous behavior but was told by her mother, "You will get over it." Nicole had never mentioned it again.

Psychotherapy with Nicole involved helping her to identify inner conflict and self-defeating behaviors. As she began to discuss her feelings openly and honestly, the need for indirect expression of her anger lessened and the binge eating subsided.

History

The nurse may be astonished by the bulimic's obsession to control eating and the inability to do so. The consumption of food is described more as an addiction, an escape from life's pressures, than a means of satisfying hunger. There is usually a failure at many "quick" weight loss endeavors, causing the patient to lose control and binge. Weight fluctuations are common with bulimics, as are night binges.

Family characteristics, as perceived by the bulimic, include a high level of conflict, low emphasis on independence, and little appreciation for the open expression of feelings (Laraia and Stuart, 1990).

Many bulimics are former anorectics, whereas others may become anorectic. The nurse must keep in mind that these two conditions, although different, often co-exist. Bulimics, like anorectics, are usually very secretive about their eating habits. Feeling ashamed, the bulimic will often withhold information about symptoms.

Signs and Symptoms

Patients with bulimia nervosa have feelings of low self-esteem, lack of control, worthlessness, and guilt. They are embarrassed and ashamed of their binges (eating three to four bags of chips, two to three pizzas, and several dozen cookies is not unusual). Bulimics live in a state of mental chaos. They want to give up on life and they want to keep their habit. Binging is their means of escaping life's pressures but it results in feelings of worthlessness.

Anxiety, limited impulse control, unsatisfactory interpersonal relationships, and chronic depression are characteristics of this disorder. Bulimics are preoccupied with food and cannot delay gratification, therefore gorging becomes a compulsive ritual. Unlike anorectics, bulimics recognize their bizarre eating behaviors, and may self-refer to an eating disorders program.

Bulimic patients usually are of average or slightly above-average weight. Their appearance may not offer any significant clues to the disorder. Bulimic patients are usually older and more outgoing than anorectics. They may engage in impulsive behaviors such as gambling, shoplifting, and alcohol or drug abuse. On the unit, bulimics may steal others' food.

Physical signs of bulimia nervosa include hoarseness and esophagitis, enlarged parotid glands, dental enamel erosion, muscle weakness, and lacerations of palate and calluses on knuckles (called Cooper's sign) due to self-induced vomiting. In the advanced stages, amenorrhea may be present. Bulimic patients may complain of weakness and fatigue. Laboratory tests may reveal electrolyte abnormalities; potentially fatal cardiac arrhythmias could occur.

Nursing Interventions

For the bulimic patient, the goal of nursing interventions is to promote effective coping skills—to help the patient recognize anxiety-producing events and to avoid binging and purging in response to anxiety (Chitty, 1992). To establish a therapeutic relationship with the bulimic, the nurse must be genuine and reassuring. Scheduled contact with the patient should be provided. The nurse should define in simple terms the role and responsibilities for both the patient and nurse. Once trust is established, help the patient identify the situations that produce anxiety. What were the coping behaviors prior to binging and purging? What are healthier ways of handling anxiety?

Patient contracts may be useful with bulimics. Contracts define the expectations of the patients as well as the reinforcement from the staff. The contracts should be a mutual endeavor between the patients and their nurses and must be renegotiated at intervals. Such a contract might look like the following (adapted from Steckel, 1982, p. 44.).

Patient Contract

I, _____ , will _____
         (patient)   (behavior)

in return for _____ .
                               (reinforcement)

Patient _____

_____ Nurse

_____ Date

(Room at the bottom of the contract page should be used to record information about items in the contract that may need further explanation or that need to be spelled out in greater detail. The space may also be used to record other information needed by either the patient or the therapist.)

Promoting Effective Coping. Help the patient to identify the triggers that cause binging. What emotions precipitate the binging? Fear? Boredom? Anger? Loneliness? Once these high-risk situations are identified, the nurse can help the patient identify alternate behaviors, that is, exercise, a hobby, or a warm bath. Encourage the patient to express feelings that have been suppressed because they were considered unacceptable. Help the patient to identify healthier ways to express those feelings.

The exaggerated sense of guilt and inferiority that bulimics feel is overwhelming. Role-playing with the nurse is an effective way for patients to deal with these feelings and experiment with new behaviors.

Involve the patients in their discharge planning. Compliance is improved when they have an active part in goal-setting. Discharge plans for bulimics should include the productive use of time, appropriate expression of feelings, and nutritional counseling. Goals should be realistic. One small win can reinforce another and build confidence.

Intrafamilial conflicts reinforce maladaptive eating behaviors; therefore, the patient's family must be included in the plan of care for the patient. Listen to the family's concerns and fears about the patient's bulimia. Encourage family members to identify their own strengths and weaknesses and to explore together their own coping mechanisms. Encourage the family to share their feelings with one another. Help the family understand the needs of the patient. Social support is an important determinant in one's ability to make stressful decisions. Make appropriate referrals to community resources.

Prognosis and Outcome

Generally, the prognosis for bulimia is less favorable than for uncomplicated anorexia nervosa. Polivy and Thomsen (1988) point out that the abnormal cycle of binging and purging is difficult to break because, to bulimics, it means control over the body as well as control in other areas of personal functioning. Serious complications, including death, may occur as a result of electrolyte imbalances. Comerci, Kilbourne, and Harrison (1989) note that because depression is so prevalent in bulimics, the risk of suicide is also greater.

COMPULSIVE OVEREATING

Compulsive overeating has not long been recognized as an addiction. Treatment has historically focused on obesity, a symptom of compulsive overeating, rather than the addiction itself.

Obesity is generally defined as body weight exceeding the recommended weight by 20 percent. Obesity is found among the affluent as well as in lower socioeconomic groups and is common among both women and men. Obesity is most prevalent between the ages of 20 and 50 years.

Emotional factors have always been linked with obesity. In times past, emotional disturbances were viewed as causes of obesity, but it is now believed that these disturbances are the result of obesity.

The nurse cannot assume that all obese individuals are emotionally disturbed, because many appear to be well adjusted. The focus of the following discussion will be on the obese patient who is psychologically impaired.

> Phillip is 44 years old, 6'1", and weighs 300 pounds. He has been on many diets over the past several years. The last attempt at weight loss consisted of grapefruits and eggs, lasted 2 weeks, and netted a total weight loss of 3 pounds.
>
> Phillip went to a private psychiatrist with complaints of depression. He reported that his problems began 8 years ago when his wife left him. Unable to find a satisfying relationship with another woman, Phillip turned to food for comfort. His weight had escalated from a previous 200 pounds.

Phillip was so discouraged every time he looked into the mirror that he would consume huge quantities of food just to feel better. His sense of satisfaction was short-lived, however, and soon after binging he would feel guilty. He stated that he felt he was under constant scrutiny by others and perceived himself as a total failure.

Psychotherapy with Phillip involved helping him to explore his feelings about the meaning of obesity and body image. With encouragement and support from his therapist, Phillip began to explore feelings about his relationships with others. Soon he began assuming responsibility for himself. With the help of his therapist, Phillip was able to set realistic weight-loss goals, initiate an exercise program, and identify healthier coping strategies.

History

Most obese patients report a lifetime of noncompliance with various weight-loss methods. Between-meal snacking and late-night eating are common to the obese. Because genetics and family traditions or beliefs contribute to obesity, obtaining family histories is useful. People with eating disorders are likely to have a history of chemical dependence. Any pre-existing medical conditions, as well as any medications, should be ruled out as causes of weight gain. Many obese people live sedentary lifestyles and engage in few recreational activities.

Signs and Symptoms

Not only do obese individuals suffer from the stigma of obesity, but they are blamed for being fat. Fat is not valued in our society as thinness is, thus overweight people are stereotyped. Such societal labels as "lazy," "weak," and "self-indulgent" add to patients' poor self-esteem. These individuals are not weak. They are, in fact, usually very determined overachievers, searching for acceptance from others, and grateful for any crumb of human kindness. Patients who compulsively overeat may feel hopeless over their failure to lose weight. It is important to recognize that obesity is a complex problem and the relationship people have with food is influenced by many biopsychosocial factors.

Many obese patients live out their fantasies through food. Roth (1985) believes that, "Many compulsive overeaters eat because they don't know that they are allowed to express the anger they carry inside" (p. 64). Emotions were meant to be expressed; if they are not, they can all be displaced onto food. Because food asks nothing in return, it is perceived as safer and more predictable than interpersonal relationships for those who fear rejection.

Obese people tend to be less active than normal-weight individuals, but the total energy expenditure is no different than it is in the non-obese. The reason for this is that it requires increased energy to move the excess body fat.

The pain that the compulsive overeater experiences comes not from the weight gain or from the negative comments about their body. The pain comes from within as these messages are translated into a measure of self-worth. To some, in a culture where the social pressures for body thinness are so powerful, being fat is the ultimate failure.

Obesity may result in feelings of depression, anxiety, low self-esteem, and social isolation. These negative mood states may produce the need to turn to something that never fails us—food.

Nursing Interventions

The nurse must approach the obese patient in a supportive, nonjudgmental manner and accept the patient as a person. The ultimate goal of treatment for the compulsive overeater is to help the patient achieve a balance between caloric intake and energy expenditure. Nursing interventions should focus on teaching the patient good nutrition, improving the patient's current nutritional status, and promoting social interaction and a sense of well-being.

Teaching Good Nutrition. Some obese patients demonstrate a basic knowledge of good nutrition, although many others have a nutritional knowledge deficit. The nurse must recognize that patients' negative self-concepts potentiate the need for emotional nurturing, that is, food. Because of their impulsiveness and inability to delay gratification, many compulsive overeaters cannot distinguish emotional hunger from biologic hunger.

The nurse can discuss the basic food groups with patients and encourage them to select favorites from each group. Emphasize to patients the importance of examining food labels. Written nutritional materials are also helpful.

Improving Nutritional Status. Help the patients establish realistic goals for improving their nutritional status. Help the patients explore ways to change eating habits. Establishing programs of exercise helps patients to achieve a more acceptable energy balance.

Keeping a food journal helps the patient identify patterns of eating as well as the relationship between emotions and eating. Review the journal with the patient weekly and help the patient identify techniques for dealing with the urge to eat. Stress to the patient that relapse may be prevented by using delay and distraction strategies in high-risk situations.

Give positive feedback when patients achieve any small weight loss. Slips in progress can provoke a variety of responses, generally assumed negative. Help patients to avoid overreacting to these experiences and use them constructively. Teach patients how to make healthy selections when dining out.

Promoting Social Interaction. For the socially isolated patient, the nurse can offer companionship while making no demands. Frequent, brief visits indicate interest and acceptance of the patient. Engage the patient in a noncompetitive one-to-one activity, progressing to group activities. Allow the patient the freedom to leave the group if anxiety becomes a problem. Recognize any time spent socializing as positive, and reinforce that behavior in the patient.

Promoting a Sense of Well-Being. Many compulsive overeaters experience feelings of hopelessness and social isolation but feel powerless to change. The nurse can promote hopefulness in obese patients by spending time with them. Encourage the obese patients to express both negative and positive feelings. Listen with an empathetic ear and accepting attitude.

Parent and Whall (1984) found that there was a positive relationship between physical activity and self-esteem. Encourage daily exercise for obese patients. Promote good grooming and hygiene because this heightens self-esteem.

Encourage patients to make eating the primary focus at mealtime. Teach the patients to eat slowly and put utensils down between bites. This can slow the eating process and demonstrate that change is possible.

Teach patients about obesity and its physiological and psychological implications. Involve them in the decision-making regarding their care. Reaching an understanding of their condition promotes hope. Encourage the patients to share experiences with other eating-disordered patients. Self-esteem increases with the ability to help others. Reinforce any expression of hopefulness.

Prognosis and Outcome

The key to successful weight loss is motivation. Compulsive overeaters must admit a personal need for help and commit to change. Without this, no amount of intervention from others will be effective. They must realize that losing the weight is only part of permanent weight control.

Maintenance of a normal weight is the ultimate goal. Patients must gain insight into their relationships with others as well as their relationship with food. In giving up the security of food and smothering relationships, self-doubt vanishes and a new freedom is found.

SUMMARY

Whatever the cause of eating disorders, all affected individuals demonstrate pathological coping skills. These maladaptive behaviors are manifested in the eating-disordered through physiological and psychological alterations, self-esteem disturbances, and body image distortions.

Recovery from eating disorders is a long journey filled with uncertainty. The eating-disordered must recognize the importance of small wins and cast their goals accordingly. They must come to realize and appreciate that balance is the way to physical and mental health. They must let down their psychological defenses, face their denial, and give up the struggle to be someone else. Colvin and Olson (1985) believe that these individuals must stop blaming others and go from self-delusion to self-honesty.

Patients may sometimes fail to respond to the best efforts and the nurse may feel defeated. The satisfaction that comes, however, with knowing that you have made a difference in these individuals' lives more than compensates for the frustrations along the way.

▼ KEY POINTS ▼

1. The society in which we live often equates beauty with thinness and many adolescents and young adults are obsessed with their physical appearance.

2. Eating is one of the earliest forms of nurturance, and is the process by which attachment between infant and mother begins.

3. Throughout life, attitudes toward food continue to impact on human interaction.

4. Anorexia nervosa, bulimia nervosa, and compulsive overeating are the three major eating disorders.

5. Effective treatment is complex and involves skilled interventions based on knowledge and understanding of the disorder.

---

continued on page 378

Key Points continued

Anorexia Nervosa

6. *Anorexia nervosa* is a severe form of self-starvation that may lead to death.

7. The disorder is characterized by extreme weight loss, intense fear of fatness, disturbed body image, bizarre attitude toward food, and, in females, amenorrhea.

8. Anorexia nervosa occurs predominantly in adolescent females with above-average intelligence and the disorder's incidence increases with socioeconomic status.

9. Onset is usually associated with stressful life situations with which the individual is unable to cope.

10. The anorectic may be unable or unwilling to provide necessary information to obtain a good history.

11. Typically, the anorectic has been well-adjusted, highly conforming to parental expectations, perfectionistic, and achievement-oriented.

12. The anorectic has a lackadaisical attitude toward hygiene and appearance, is empathetic and sensitive toward others, and has an intense fear of criticism.

13. Misperceptions of self-worth are often enough to initiate a pattern of self-destructive behaviors.

14. The anorectic may begin by skipping desserts and sweets and progress to skipping meals. Some resort to vomiting, and abusing laxatives, enemas, and diuretics.

15. Patients with anorexia nervosa perceive themselves as overweight, no matter how thin they may be.

16. Anorectics think endlessly about food and at the same time are obsessed with controlling their own intake.

17. They usually have a broad knowledge of the nutritional and caloric value of food, collect cookbooks and recipes, prepare elaborate meals, and take great pleasure in watching others eat.

18. Anorectics have an insatiable compulsion for vigorous exercise.

19. They frequently deny that they have a weight problem and insist they feel fine, when in fact, they are proud of their self-denial and their low weight and just want to be left alone.

20. The anorectic patient is emaciated and skeletal in appearance.

Key Points continued

21. Treatment should be aimed at restoring normal nutrition and eating habits while dealing with psychological issues.

22. Ineffective coping, misperceptions of body image, and poor self-esteem are subjective emotional experiences of the anorectic.

23. Chitty (1992) emphasizes that anorectics are extremely resistant to change.

24. If the patient is medically unstable, IV therapy or tube feedings may be necessary.

25. The nurse must avoid discussing food and eating behaviors with the patient. Instead, explore the patient's fears and anxieties about gaining weight.

26. Provide for a stress-free mealtime environment, keeping in mind that large meals overwhelm anorectic patients.

27. Acknowledge efforts of patients who meet the established goals but remember that anorectics will not accept excessive praise.

28. Behavioral interventions such as rewards for new adaptive behavior may be incorporated into the management plan for the anorectic. Rewards need to be tied to caloric intake—not to gaining weight.

29. The nurse must use empathy and active listening to show concern for the patient and should encourage patients to assume more responsibility for their behavior and feelings.

30. Demonstrate a belief in patients' ability to improve maladaptive behaviors and allow some flexibility in daily routines while continuing to maintain limits.

31. Patients need to be encouraged to explore their fears and feelings about gaining weight.

32. As patients risk self-disclosure, their anxiety may intensify. For inexperienced nurses, spending time with the patients to observe and document behaviors is a valuable contribution to the success of their treatments.

33. During adolescence, perceptions of body size and weight play a major role in self-concept.

34. Anorectics refuse to accept reinforcement for anything less than perfection. Help patients identify and focus on their positive

continued on page 380

Key Points continued

attributes and help them know that perfection and acceptance are not synonymous.

35. The effect of interventions in the treatment of anorexia nervosa is not well understood and the outcome is uncertain. Resolution of the underlying problem, as well as nutritional counseling, is crucial to recovery.

Bulimia Nervosa

36. *Bulimia nervosa* is the frequent compulsion to ingest large amounts of food in a short period of time.

37. Bulimia is characterized by episodes of overeating and purging through self-induced vomiting, laxative and/or diuretic use, fasting, or vigorous exercise.

38. Bulimia occurs in anorectic, normal-weight, and obese individuals, primarily white females of high school or college age, middle to upper middle class, well educated and intelligent.

39. The bulimic's consumption of food is an addiction, an escape from life's pressures rather than a means of satisfying hunger.

40. Bulimics often perceive their family life as one of conflict, low emphasis on independence, and little appreciation for the open expression of feelings.

41. Bulimia and anorexia nervosa often co-exist.

42. Feeling ashamed, the bulimic will often withhold information about symptoms.

43. Patients with bulimia nervosa have feelings of low self-esteem, lack of control, worthlessness, and guilt.

44. Anxiety, limited impulse control, unsatisfactory interpersonal relationships, and chronic depression are characteristics of this disorder.

45. Bulimics are able to recognize their bizarre eating behaviors and may self-refer to an eating disorders program.

46. The bulimic patient usually is of average or slightly above-average weight, is usually older than the anorectic, and may engage in impulsive behaviors.

47. Physical signs of bulimia nervosa include hoarseness and esophagitis, enlarged parotid glands, dental enamel erosion,

Key Points continued

muscle weakness, lacerations to palate, and calluses on knuckles.

48. The goal of nursing interventions is to promote effective coping skills in patients, helping them to recognize anxiety-producing events and to avoid binging and purging in response to anxiety.

49. Patient contracts, defining the expectations of the patient, and reinforcement from the staff may be useful with bulimics.

50. Help the patient to identify the triggers that cause binging (fear, boredom, loneliness, etc.).

51. The exaggerated sense of guilt and inferiority that bulimics feel is overwhelming. Role-playing is an effective way for patients to deal with these feelings and experiment with new behaviors.

52. Goals should be realistic. One small win can reinforce another and build confidence.

53. Intrafamilial conflicts reinforce maladaptive eating behaviors; therefore, the patient's family must be included in the plan of care for the patient.

54. The prognosis for bulimia is less favorable than for uncomplicated anorexia nervosa, perhaps because binging and purging represents control over body and other personal areas.

55. Comerci, Kilbourne, and Harrison (1989) note that because depression is so prevalent in bulimics, the risk of suicide is also greater.

Compulsive Overeating

56. Compulsive overeating has not long been recognized as an addiction. Historically, obesity has been the focus of treatment.

57. *Obesity* is generally defined as body weight exceeding the recommended weight by 20 percent.

58. It is found among all socioeconomic groups and is common for both women and men.

59. Although emotional factors have always been linked with obesity, one cannot assume that all obese individuals are emotionally disturbed.

continued on page 382

Key Points continued

60. Most obese patients report a lifetime of noncompliance with various weight-loss methods.

61. Genetics and family traditions or beliefs contribute to obesity; therefore, obtaining a family history is useful.

62. Patients with eating disorders are likely to have a history of chemical dependence. Any pre-existing medical conditions or medications should be ruled out as causes of weight gain.

63. Obese individuals suffer from the stigma of obesity and are blamed for being fat.

64. They are often very determined overachievers searching for acceptance from others.

65. Obesity is a complex problem and the relationship one has with food is influenced by many biopsychosocial factors.

66. Many obese patients live out their fantasies through food and some believe they eat because they think they are not allowed to express internal anger.

67. Obese people tend to be less active than normal-weight individuals.

68. The pain that the compulsive overeater experiences comes from within as negative comments about their body are translated into a measure of self-worth.

69. Obesity may result in feelings of depression, anxiety, low self-esteem, and social isolation.

70. The nurse can best approach the obese patient in a supportive, nonjudgmental manner and accept the patient as a person.

71. Nursing interventions should focus on teaching patients good nutrition, improving their current nutritional status, and promoting social interaction and lifestyle change.

72. Some obese patients demonstrate a basic knowledge of good nutrition, although others have a nutritional knowledge deficit.

73. Many compulsive overeaters cannot distinguish emotional hunger from biologic hunger.

74. Help the patients establish realistic goals for improving their nutritional status.

75. Keeping a food journal helps the patient identify patterns of eating and the relationship between emotions and eating.

Key Points continued

76. Give positive feedback when patients achieve any small weight loss.

77. For the socially isolated patient, the nurse can offer companionship while making no demands. This indicates interest and acceptance of the patient.

78. Many compulsive overeaters experience feelings of hopelessness and social isolation but feel powerless to change.

79. Parent and Whall (1984) found that there was a positive relationship between physical activity and self-esteem.

80. Encourage the patient to make eating the primary focus at mealtime.

81. Teach the patients about obesity and its physiological and psychological implications; involve them in the decision-making regarding their care.

82. Encourage the patient to share experiences with other eating-disordered patients. Self-esteem increases with the ability to help others.

83. The key to successful weight loss is motivation. The compulsive overeater must admit a personal need for help and commit to change.

84. When the security of food and smothering relationships are given up, self-doubt vanishes and a new freedom is found.

Annotated Bibliography

American Psychiatric Association: *Diagnostic and Statistical Manual of Mental Disorders,* ed. 4. Washington, D.C.: APA, 1994.

Chitty, K. K.: Eating disorders. In: Wilson, H. S., and Kneisl, C. R. (eds): *Psychiatric Nursing,* ed. 4. Redwood, Calif.: Addison-Wesley, 1992, pp. 469–486.

Chapter defines eating disorders and describes both historical and theoretical foundations of each. Major focus: nursing care plans and appropriate nursing interventions for both client and family.

Christie, C.: *Compulsive Eating, Anorexia, and Bulimia.* Berkeley, Calif.: Institute for Natural Resources, 1990.

Defines compulsive eating, bulimia, and anorexia. Profiles each to include etiology, symptoms, and treatment.

Colvin, R. H., and Olson, S. C.: In search of thinness: Secrets of people who have lost weight permanently. *New Woman,* November, 1985, pp. 77–83.

Authors identify four common phases that successful dieters experience during weight loss. Identifies strategies of once-obese, now permanently slim individuals.

Comerci, G. D., Kilbourne, K. A., and Harrison, G. G.: Eating disorders: Obesity, anorexia nervosa, and bulimia. In: Hofmann, A., and Greydanus, D. (eds): *Adolescent Medicine,* ed. 2. Norwalk, Conn.: Appleton & Lange, 1989, pp. 441–461.

Chapter reviews each eating disorder in detail including radiological and laboratory findings. Major focus on medical evaluation, assessment, and treatment.

deGroot, J. M., Rodin, G., and Olmsted, M. P.: Alexithymia, depression, and treatment outcome in bulimia nervosa. *Comprehensive Psychiatry,* 1995, 36(1):53–60.

Examines the relationship among women with bulimia nervosa and depression.

Deters, G. E.: Problems of nutrition. In: Lewis, S. M., and Collier, I. C. (eds): *Medical-Surgical Nursing: Assessment and Management of Clinical Problems,* ed. 2. New York: McGraw-Hill, 1987.

Chapter describes essential components of sound nutrition and medical and nursing management of bulimia and anorexia nervosa.

Gillberg, C., Rastam, M., and Gillberg, C.: Anorexia nervosa 6 years after onset: Part I. Personality disorders. *Comprehensive Psychiatry,* 1995, 36(1):61–69.

Examines the overrepresentation of certain personality traits in individuals who have previously been diagnosed with anorexia nervosa.

Laraia, M. T., and Stuart, G. W.: Bulimia: A review of nutritional and health behaviors. *Journal of Child and Adolescent Psychiatric Mental Health Nursing,* 1990, 3(3):91–97.

Epidemiology, physiology, and precipitating factors are reviewed. Treatment from a holistic approach is explored.

Lester, R., and Petrie, T. A.: Personality and physical correlates of bulimic symptomatology among Mexican American female college students. *Journal of Counseling Psychology,* 1995, 42(2):199–203.

Examines the physical correlates and personality of bulimic symptomatology in Mexican American female college students.

Lucas, A. R.: Eating disorders. In: Lewis, M. (ed): *Child and Adolescent Psychiatry.* Baltimore: Williams & Wilkins, 1991, pp. 573–583.

Chapter looks at adolescents and eating disorders from a developmental prospective. Biologic as well as psychological theories are discussed. Family and interpersonal dynamics as well as environmental and social influences are explored as causes of eating disorders.

Mallinckrody, B., McCreary, B. A., and Robertson, A. K.: Co-occurrence of eating disorders and incest: The role of attachment, family environment, and social competencies. *Journal of Counseling Psychology,* 1995, 42(2):178–186.

Examines the association between several psychosocial and psychosexual issues and eating disorders.

Owen, S. V., and Fullerton, M. L.: Would it make a difference? A discussion group in a behaviorally oriented inpatient eating disorder program. *Journal of Psychosocial Nursing,* 1995, 33(11):35–40.

Examines and evaluates a behaviorally oriented group for eating disorders in an inpatient program.

Parent, C., and Whall, A.: Are physical activity, self-esteem, and depression related? *Journal of Gerontological Nursing,* 1984, 10(9):8.

This study identifies the positive relationship between self-esteem and physical activity in the elderly.

Polivy, J., and Thomsen, L. Dieting and other eating disorders. In: *Handbook of Behavioral Medicine for Women.* (eds): New York: Pergamon Press, 1988, pp. 345–352.

Chapter focuses on eating disorders from compulsive eating to anorexia and bulimia and attempts to answer why the disorders are an issue in women's health.

Roth, G.: Feeling fat doesn't have to mean feeling you're a failure. *New Woman,* September, 1985, pp. 62–64.

Article examines perceptions of obese women in regard to self-worth and emphasizes positive self-talk.

Steckel, S. B.: *Patient Contracting.* Norwalk, Conn.: Appleton-Century-Crofts, 1982.

Sundermeyer, C. A.: *Emotional weight.* Ann Arbor: New Outlook, 1989.

Looks at the causes of obesity—both psychological and nutritional. Forces reader to identify true emotions and relationship with food.

Post-Test

Multiple Choice. Circle the best answer.

1. One predominant characteristic of anorectics is:
   a. Anxiety.
   b. Anemia.
   c. Depression.
   d. Preoccupation with food.

2. The percentage of total body weight lost in anorexia nervosa is often:
   a. 5%.
   b. 20%.
   c. 25% or more.
   d. 40% or more.

3. One of the diagnostic criteria for bulimia is:
   a. Weight loss of 15%.
   b. Refusal to maintain minimal body weight.
   c. Under 20 years of age.
   d. Awareness of abnormal eating patterns.

4. One of the many physical complications of binging and purging is:
   a. Hypotension.
   b. Pathological fractures.
   c. Decayed teeth.
   d. Throat cancer.

5. Characteristics of the compulsive overeater might include all of the following except:
   a. Knowledge deficit in regard to nutrition.
   b. Hopelessness.
   c. Social isolation.
   d. Laziness.

6. Treatment for the compulsive overeater should include all of the following except:
   a. Calorie restriction of 600 calories/day.
   b. Nutrition education.
   c. Keeping food records.
   d. Daily exercise.

Post-Test

(continued)

Short Answer. Answer the following questions as briefly and specifically as possible.

1. Describe the primary nursing interventions in the treatment of anorexia nervosa.

   _____

   _____

   _____

2. Describe the primary nursing interventions in the treatment of bulimia nervosa.

   _____

   _____

   _____

3. Describe the primary nursing interventions in the treatment of compulsive overeating.

   _____

   _____

   _____

True or False. Circle your choice.

T   F   1. The client with anorexia nervosa may have secret rituals about food.

T   F   2. Anorectics usually are not able to exercise because of their weakened condition.

T   F   3. The bulimic is usually very withdrawn.

T   F   4. The bulimic is very open and honest in regard to binging and purging.

T   F   5. The compulsive overeater should eat three well-balanced meals a day.

T   F   6. The compulsive overeater should be discouraged from expressing negative feelings.

CHAPTER
21

Care for Chemically Dependent Patients

OBJECTIVES: Student will be able to:

1. Identify factors that influence the use and abuse of alcohol.
2. State how TV and other media affect our social views on alcoholism and other drug abuse.
3. Identify the three categories of drinkers in the *DSM-IV.*
4. State why the "skid-row bum" idea of an alcoholic is misleading and inappropriate.
5. Tell why alcoholism as a lifestyle has so much appeal to alcoholics.
6. Differentiate between physiological and psychological dependence and state which usually comes first.
7. Identify the most prevalent defense alcoholics use to avoid accepting their disorder.
8. Identify Jellinek's four stages of alcoholism.
9. List symptoms associated with delirium tremens.
10. Define the term *cross tolerance.*
11. Identify methods of treatment for alcoholism and other drug abuse.

The abuse of alcohol and other drugs represents a significant problem for health authorities in the United States. In fact, alcohol abuse alone has been said to be the third-largest health problem in America. When abusers of other drugs are added to the ranks of those who abuse alcohol, the problem becomes even more devastating. Although many people believe that only members of the lower socioeconomic groups abuse alcohol and other drugs, statistics indicate that abusers are found in all socioeconomic groups.

Although athletes who die from cardiac arrhythmias associated with cocaine use frequently make the headlines, and large heroin and cocaine busts make sensational news stories, alcohol remains the most commonly abused drug in the United States. Alcohol is more readily available than other drugs, it is legal, and its use is socially accepted by our society. In fact, the drunk seems to occupy a special place in our society. If our friend, John Smith, gets drunk at a party, he is laughed at when he stumbles over a table, curses loudly, or makes a pass at a friend's wife. His behavior is often forgiven because he is not considered to be responsible because of his drunkenness. If Mr. Smith engaged in these behaviors under other circumstances, he would quickly become a social outcast or perhaps jailed for assault.

We are a nation of drug takers. The television daily presents the virtues of every conceivable form of pain relief, sleep inducer, muscle relaxer, and vitamin supplement. If creatures from outer space were to observe our television commercials and report back to their leaders, they probably would say that we are a nation of people who never sleep, who suffer constant low back pain, nasal congestion, bronchial spasms, gastric indigestion, tension headaches, aching feet, bloodshot eyes, and premenstrual pain and tension. They might also say that the life-sustaining substances on earth are so poor that they must be supplemented daily with many different kinds and colors of special vitamin tablets, and that indeed things are so bad that humans even have to have special foods for their animals that include the same kinds of supplements. Television commercials market all these various pills, along with alcoholic beverages, as a sure means of making life more tolerable, less boring, more exciting, and thus more pleasurable. Most drug abusers (remember that alcohol is a drug) drink or take pills in an attempt to withdraw or sedate themselves to escape from the realities, or as many say, the boredom, of the world in which they live.

Unfortunately, the most significant impact created by media advertising of alcohol and pills lies in the promotion of an attitude rather than promotion of the products themselves. For the most part, the products are not harmful. On the other hand, the attitudes created by the media indicate that it is okay for people to seek happiness, escape, excitement, or pleasure from a pill or a bottle with seemingly little regard for the possible psychological or physical addiction that may occur as a consequence of their drug-taking behavior.

The following sections present information related specifically to abusers of alcohol and other drugs. Although the two groups have similarities and differences (Table 21–1), they are presented separately to emphasize differences in treatment and management approaches.

Table 21–1. **Comparison of Alcoholics and Other Drug Abusers**

Similarities	Differences
1. Addicts in both groups come from all sociological and economic levels.	1. Men outnumber women 3:1 in drug abuse. The ratio of men to women for alcohol abuse is 1:1.
2. Basic personality structures for both include dependency, low self-esteem, inability to tolerate tension, immaturity, and difficulty in accepting responsibility for their own actions. Often blame their problems on someone else or on some event in their life.	2. Average age for alcoholic is substantially higher, being 30 to 55 years for the alcoholic and 16 to 25 years for other drug abusers.
3. Both cause psychological and physical dependence with psychological dependence occurring first.	3. Alcohol is much more socially acceptable than other drugs.
4. Often start habit for same reason—to feel accepted or gain a feeling of social well-being.	4. Usually takes longer to become addicted to alcohol than other drugs. Persons may become psychologically dependent on other drugs after first dose; not so with alcohol.
5. Both begin behavior leading to addiction because of psychological maladjustment and access to drugs and alcohol.	5. Alcohol withdrawal symptoms may appear from 1 to 8 days after last drink; drug withdrawal symptoms begin to occur 12 to 16 hours after last dose.
6. In advanced stages, both present poor general appearance and look extremely malnourished because they spend more on their habit rather than food.	6. Persons withdrawing from alcohol have tremors, increasing jitters, spasmodic gait, nausea and vomiting, loss of consciousness, convulsions, hallucinations, and death. Persons withdrawing from drugs other than alcohol often have teary eyes, persistent yawning, runny nose, increasing restlessness, hostility, and severe abdominal cramps.
7. Both cause severe economic problems for the addict and the addict's family due to cost of addiction.	

continued

Table 21–1. **Comparison of Alcoholics and Other Drug Abusers** *continued*

Similarities	Differences
8. Both have impaired judgment.	7. Alcoholic withdrawal is frequently a more acute medical problem.
9. Both types of addicts initiate treatment because of an acute medical problem or the concern of someone else for them—rarely of their own initiative; both use massive denial in treating, both need patience, understanding, consistency, a structured environment and empathy, not sympathy.	8. Alcohol is taken by mouth; other forms of drugs can be taken by mouth but are frequently taken intravenously or subcutaneously (skin popping) to increase and speed up the desired effect. Other drugs may also be sniffed or snorted.
10. Both need increasingly larger doses of their drug to produce the desired effect, with the end result being an increased intake not to feel good but to keep from feeling bad and to prevent withdrawal symptoms.	9. Unpredictable bad trips are often seen with drugs other than alcohol.
11. Both types of addiction cause severe medical complications.	10. Blood pressure, pulse, and respiration are depressed with overdose of drugs other than alcohol; in an alcohol overdose, pulse is often rapid (over 100), respiration is increased (often exceeding 30), but blood pressure is frequently normal.
12. It is often necessary in planning treatment to include family members.	11. Possession of drugs other than alcohol without a prescription is illegal, whereas alcohol is legally sold to anyone over 21 years of age.
13. Difficulty for people in medical field to accept drug abuse as an illness; therefore, they are reluctant to treat abusers and sometimes feel that they are wasting their time.	
14. Both addictions are curable but not arrestable.	
15. After initial addiction, both may become more of a physical problem than a mental one.	

ABUSE OF ALCOHOL

The *DSM-IV* divides alcohol abuse into two main subtypes, (1) alcohol-use disorders, and (2) alcohol-induced disorders. People who abuse alcohol are known by a variety of names ranging from problem drinkers to alcoholic, wino, lappster, derelict, or bum. The term *problem drinker* is usually applied to a person who does not have the obvious symptoms associated with clinically diagnosed alcohol dependence. *Alcohol dependent* is the term used by the *DSM-IV* to describe those persons with drinking characteristics generally called *alcoholism,* which along with the term *alcoholic* was coined in 1849 by Magnus Huss. Individuals are diagnosed as alcohol dependent when they have lost control of their drinking to the extent that interpersonal, family, and community relationships have become seriously threatened, disturbed, or significantly impaired. The term alcoholic will be used in this chapter as synonymous with the *DSM-IV* diagnosis of Alcohol Dependence.

Although alcoholics can be superficially witty, charming, and friendly, a great number of them are destructive and aggressive when they have been drinking. Long-term alcoholics tend to be pale, thin, and poorly nourished because they spend their money on alcohol rather than food and because they forget to eat when they are drinking. Long-term male alcoholics may have dilated blood vessels in their faces and a bulblike, fleshy nose, which is frequently referred to as a "whiskey nose." The alcoholic individual often has bloodshot eyes and a generally disheveled appearance. Poor personal and dental hygiene are likely as is a hoarse voice, hand tremors, and "the jitters." Alcoholics also tend to have a spasmodic work record or show decreased work proficiency. Of the approximately 5 to 10 million alcoholics in the United States today, only 5 percent are of the stereotyped Skid-Row-bum type. *Most do not fit the description just presented.* Instead, they are our neighbors, relatives, and friends. They go to work every day wearing neatly pressed clothes, they have families, go to church on Sunday, live in suburbia, and generally keep up a good front. With so much seemingly going for them, it is easy to wonder why such people become alcoholics.

Factors Influencing Alcoholism

Some authorities report that the alcoholic has ambivalent feelings about living and dying and that chronic alcoholism represents a slow form of suicide. Alcoholics often have a long-established pattern of self-medication using alcohol. They "medicate" themselves for promotions, weddings, new babies, job changes, and so forth, until finally they find themselves "medicating" in order to just make it through the day at the office. Many authorities see alcoholism as a lifestyle, a means of adjusting to a particular combination of circumstances and personality types. Health team workers frequently find in the history of an alcoholic a very poor mother-child relationship and significantly poor self-esteem. Many alcoholics have passive and dependent personality traits and thus have difficulty facing up to life's daily problems. They often lack the confidence to make choices and feel inadequate to face the basic tasks of life.

The alcoholic may be very angry about being so dependent and thus becomes frustrated and hostile. Because hostility often creates more hostility in relationships, alcoholics are likely to be rejected by others and may indeed begin to experience difficulty in meeting their basic needs because of such rejection. Alcoholics typically have difficulty tolerating tension and often appear to be either "wrapped up" in their own problems or in significant denial of their problems. Personality tests given to alcoholics frequently reflect a cyclic pattern in their personalities. Alcoholics feel tense and depressed and try to relieve these feelings by drinking. When they are rejected for becoming drunk, they become even more depressed and guilt-ridden. They then drink more to reduce their new feelings of guilt and depression, and a vicious cycle has begun.

Besides these psychological factors, a constitutional or genetic factor also appears to play a role in determining why some people who drink become alcoholic whereas others do not. Within the last few years a lot of effort has gone into demonstrating the presence of an alcohol "gene" that is passed on to the children of alcoholics. This gene is thought to make persons susceptible to becoming addicted more easily than the general population. Although there is still not a great deal of research data to substantiate this belief, and controversy continues about the gene theory, many people believe strongly that an inborn metabolic vulnerability causes people to become alcoholics. We do know that some individuals cannot tolerate alcohol and may become drunk after only one drink or may become pathologically intoxicated after using only a small amount of alcohol.

Social factors may also contribute to alcoholism. The ads for alcoholic beverages stress the "good life," and society in general is very accepting of the use of alcohol. An individual drinks with others and feels accepted. Cocktail parties abound and alcohol is served at practically every social function. Alcohol is generally considered to be a social facilitator and three out of four American adults drink to some extent.

Although many authorities believe that all drinkers begin to drink for the same reason, most do not believe that an individual chooses to become an alcoholic. That is, it is not an act of will. Rather, alcoholics begin to drink to sedate themselves so that they do not have to face the pain or boredom they perceive as inherent in living out their daily lives. The drinking temporarily makes it easier for them to face their problems, insecurities, shyness, disappointment, hurt, or perceived failure. As these individuals begin to drink more and more, their self-esteem problems are severely compounded. When they do go for treatment, they often speak of themselves as having a "drinking problem" and somehow divorce themselves as people from the "drinking problem". They often appear to be talking about someone other than themselves. Alcoholics often use massive denial as a defense mechanism and have much difficulty accepting personal responsibilities for their drinking problem. The process of being able to accept the fact that one is an alcoholic seems to be a major key in the treatment of alcoholism. Most treatment programs stress that once a person becomes addicted to alcohol, that person will always be addicted and can never regain the ability to tolerate alcohol. Alcoholics Anonymous (A.A.) and other such groups stress the fact that "recovered alcoholics" must never drink, and if they do drink again, they are considered to have relapsed.

Although many theories address the causes of alcoholism, there is very little disagreement over the fact that addiction to the drug is both psychological and physical. In fact, momentarily setting aside the gene theory, psychological dependence usually occurs before physical dependence. An individual drinks, feels relief, drinks more, feels more relief, and so on, and eventually becomes physically addicted. At that point, the alcoholism often becomes as much of a physical problem as a mental problem.

Physiological Effects

It is important to remember that alcohol is a poison and, therefore, is highly toxic to the body. It may sedate the drinker to the extent that the problems of daily life are more tolerable, but it irritates practically every organ system in the body. It inflames the gastrointestinal tract (including the pancreas and the liver), depresses the production of bone marrow and thus the production of red blood cells, and increases susceptibility to infection and bruises. Alcohol causes both brain-tissue changes and scar-tissue formation in the liver (cirrhosis) and may also cause significant damage to the heart. Alcohol decreases metabolic efficiency and reduces the ability to absorb vitamins. The liver may become increasingly enlarged, less functional, and, therefore, less able to rid the body of toxic substances. Because alcohol sedates the cerebral cortex, an individual who is drinking is less able to think discriminately, which results in impaired judgment and motor function. Therefore, when individuals are intoxicated, they are much more likely to fall and hurt themselves. Alcoholics who are seen in the emergency room setting should be carefully checked for subdural hematomas and other signs of trauma such as bruises, contusions, and fractures. Sexual impotence may also be a complication of alcoholism and further increases marital discord, which is prominent when one or both marriage partners are alcoholic.

Recognizing Alcoholic Tendencies

Because alcoholics tend to use denial as a defense against having to face their alcoholism, they are likely to go for a long time without treatment. Because alcoholics are not likely to identify themselves as such, it is helpful to treating professionals to be able to recognize a person who may be alcoholic. The following questions are provided as a means of assessing whether an individual may be an alcoholic. Of course, when asking these questions, it is important to keep in mind that the denial mechanism may cause the person being questioned to lie or to stretch the truth.

1. Have you ever lost work or been late for work because you were drinking?

2. Do you and your spouse ever argue about whether you drink too much?

3. Do your friends consider you to be a heavy drinker?

4. Are you quiet and withdrawn but become the "life of the party" after a few drinks?

5. Have you ever felt sorry about your drinking behavior?

6. Do you need a drink at certain times during the day, or do you usually drink throughout the day?

7. Do you often want a drink soon after waking in the morning?

8. Does drinking make it easier for you to get through the day?

9. Do you drink by yourself a good deal of the time?

10. Do you ever have difficulty recalling activities that occurred while you were drinking?

11. Do you feel better about yourself as a person when you are drinking?

A "yes" answer to any one of the preceding questions suggests the strong likelihood that an individual is alcoholic, and a "yes" answer to two or more questions increases the probability significantly.

The Alcoholic Process

The process of becoming an alcoholic has been broken down into four stages by Jellinek (1960):

1. *Prealcoholic Symptomatic Phase.* In this phase, alcohol is first used to avoid problems or bolster confidence during moments of stress or crisis. The drinking behavior takes the place of the development of adequate coping mechanisms, and as stress occurs more often, the individual's drinking becomes more frequent. The individual's ability to tolerate alcohol also increases.

2. *Prodromal Phase.* In this phase, the individual drinks heavily, which frequently leads to unconsciousness and memory blackouts. The individual cannot wait to get a few drinks but then feels guilty about drinking. There is usually no one to talk to about the problem.

3. *Crucial Phase.* During this phase, there is a loss of control; the individual is unable to abstain from drinking, often drinking continuously until nausea or unconsciousness results. The individual may exhibit grandiose or aggressive behavior while drinking along with remorse, self-pity, and resentment toward anyone who tries to prevent his or her drinking. Withdrawal symptoms will occur if the person stops drinking.

4. *Chronic Phase.* The behavior in this stage is marked by frequent "benders" and prolonged periods of intoxication. There is usually daily intake of alcohol in response to the physical "craving" that occurs as a result of metabolic changes. Nutritional deficiencies occur, as well as organ system difficulties and behavior problems. Individuals in this stage frequently lose their jobs because they are unable to work effectively. They are also likely to experience severe marital disruption and lose the family through divorce. If individuals in this stage are not treated, death may occur within a relatively short period as a result of malnutrition, infection, or acute problems that occur when they are unable to obtain alcohol. At this point, alcoholic hallucinosis (hallucinations after stopping drinking) and acute delirium tremens ("DTs") are likely.

Jellinek stresses the point that not all of the phases and symptoms are experienced by every alcoholic, and they do not always occur in the same sequence.

Treatment

Although we have already said that society tends to tolerate and even accept the individual who is drunk, patients who are diagnosed alcoholic are often rejected not only by family and friends but also by medical personnel who are assigned to care for them. Although medical personnel tend to view alcoholism as a disease and are usually able to view it more objectively than the alcoholic's family and friends, many are still ambivalent toward the alcoholic. The professional person may feel frustrated by alcoholics and unconsciously reject them. Some authorities believe that the longer one works with alcoholics, the more negative one becomes toward them. Alcoholics tend to relapse frequently and resume drinking; thus, it is often difficult for staff members to determine if alcoholics are making progress.

Medical personnel like to see their patients "get well" and do not like to see patients return. When alcoholic patients return time after time for detoxification, the treatment team has a tendency to become discouraged. The frequent return rate has been suggested as one of the main reasons alcoholics have difficulty finding acceptance among treatment team members. This is particularly true if patients do not appear to be trying to help themselves or if their willpower is so poor that the very afternoon they are discharged, they are returned to the unit unconscious from an alcohol overdose. One must remember, however, that alcoholism is a chronic illness and as in all chronic illnesses, the patient is subject to relapses.

Because alcoholics may not be well received by treatment teams, family members, and friends, it is no wonder that a great many people have difficulty admitting their alcoholism. Perhaps this is one reason individuals use the denial mechanism mentioned earlier as a defense against admitting their alcoholism. Alcoholics' massive use of denial is a major obstacle throughout the treatment process and often causes them to feel obligated to refuse treatment and detoxification, because to allow treatment would be to admit their alcoholic condition. The alcoholic's use of denial, abusive language, belligerence, and manipulative behavior are severely detrimental to good patient-staff relationships. At first it may be difficult to understand why alcoholics behave as they do, but examining the way they enter treatment makes it easier to see the reasons behind their behavior.

Ways of Entering Treatment. Alcoholics usually enter treatment in one of four ways. The most frequent way an alcoholic begins to receive treatment is through recognition of the alcoholic status by someone in the general hospital when the alcoholic has been admitted for some other reason. The patient may have sought medical attention for stomach ulcers, "nerves," urinary problems, liver disease, gastrointestinal problems or other physical complaints, or the patient may complain of depression or anxiety. Most often the physical illness is secondary to the primary problem of alcoholism. A second way alcoholics may enter treatment is that they are brought by the police after being picked up for public drunkenness. In the past, public drunks were thrown into jail to "dry out" and research indicates that many people died from DTs. Today, however, most states have legislation requiring that persons who are picked up for public drunkenness be taken to a hospital or a treatment center for alcoholics. The third way an alcoholic may begin treatment is when a family member, concerned friend, employer, or healthcare worker becomes aware of an individual's drinking problem and is able to convince the person to seek treatment. The fourth, and perhaps least likely, way for an alcoholic to begin treatment is through self-referral.

There is, however, one category of alcoholics who usually do seek treatment on their own initiative because they realize something is wrong and want help. This category is pathological intoxication, in which the individual becomes extremely intoxicated after only one or two drinks. Such individuals may be hostile, belligerent, and suicidal, or they may become severely depressed. For either type of reaction, symptoms usually last from a few hours to several hours, often with amnesia for the events. The cause of these idiosyncratic reactions is not known, but persons with a history of neurological trauma or neurological disease processes are more susceptible, as well as people who are fatigued or are in a weakened state from some other disease process.

Recognizing Signs and Symptoms

Because alcoholic patients are not likely to tell treatment team members that they are alcoholics, it is important for all team members to be aware of the signs and symptoms that indicate possible alcoholism. Of course, if the patient smells of alcohol when admitted, many people are immediately alerted to the problem. However, if there is no reason to suspect that a patient is drinking, one must become attuned to other symptoms. Alcoholics may not go into active DTs for a period of 1 to 8 days after their last drink. However, many other symptoms do appear 12 to 48 hours after the patient's last drink.

Anxiety and irritability are often the first symptoms to appear as the alcohol begins to be processed out of a patient's system. Patients may then develop shakiness or tremors, begin to make unreasonable demands, or have temper tantrums. They may become so nauseated that they vomit or show evidence of dehydration. Patients may be extremely restless, agitated, aggressive, or confused. Alcoholics can become disoriented and may sometimes begin to hallucinate. To keep environmental factors from increasing the hallucinating behavior of alcoholic patients, staff members need to maintain an attitude of caring concern and frequently reorient patients to reality and their environment. Explain to them who you are and restrict all visitors unless otherwise ordered. Place the patient in a quiet room with no shadows so that they will not be subjected to unnecessary stimulation from television, radio, other patients, or shadows on the wall (which are often misinterpreted as demons or people intending harm).

At any point during withdrawal, the alcoholic patient may begin to convulse and will die if not carefully managed. As a matter of fact, a significant number of patients in active DTs die if treatment is inadequate. Some patients continue to deny their alcoholism despite the presence of such significant and dangerous symptoms. One point of considerable interest to people working in general hospitals and outpatient clinics is the way to tell the difference between a drug overdose and an alcoholic withdrawal reaction. A general rule is that although both drug and alcohol withdrawals cause slowed motor responses, drowsiness, and confusion, in the toxic alcohol state, the patient's vital signs are usually elevated. The patient has rapid respiration, a rapid pulse (over 100), and normal blood pressure. In drug overdose, all vital signs are usually depressed. It is important to keep in mind, however, that alcoholics can become so acutely ill and have such poor circulation that they show a drastically lowered blood pressure. If this occurs, they must receive immediate emergency medical treatment to survive.

Methods of Treatment

Medical treatment of alcoholics in the prealcoholic and prodromal stages usually consists of some type of group therapy or, in some cases, individual psychotherapy. Treatment of alcoholics who are in the crucial or chronic phase not only requires group psychotherapy (there is no evidence that individual psychotherapy is beneficial) but often requires hospitalization or at least treatment in a special outpatient detoxification unit. Treatment of acute withdrawal from alcoholism is accomplished primarily through the use of medication. These patients are given intravenous fluids to combat dehydration and minor tranquilizers to help calm them and prevent seizures. Tranquilizers are also thought to help reduce anxiety and guilt.

Chlordiazepoxide (Librium) is the tranquilizer commonly used in the treatment of alcoholics, but other minor tranquilizers are also used. By the time alcoholics are in the crucial or chronic phase of alcoholism, they usually have decreased liver function due to cirrhosis or scarring of the liver, and Librium is not as difficult for the liver to metabolize as many of the other tranquilizers. Another reason physicians treat alcoholics with Librium is that although this drug is chemically similar to alcohol, it does not depress the brain centers.

Anticonvulsants may be needed to further reduce convulsive activity in these patients, and multivitamin therapy is essential to replace the vitamins lost due to poor nutrition. In particular, thiamine and B-vitamin deficiencies have been demonstrated to be associated with Wernicke-Korsakoff syndrome and peripheral neuropathy, respectively. Alcoholics must always be considered to have a malabsorption syndrome until proven otherwise. Antacids are given for gastric distress and antiemetics are given for severe nausea and vomiting. Again, it is important to realize that these patients are severely ill and may die without adequate care.

A great deal more than the appropriate use of medications is involved in the successful treatment of alcoholics. Most treatment programs make sure the alcoholic learns about the effects of alcohol on the body. Treatment teams try to provide alcoholics with psychological support while at the same time teaching them how to become more independent as they gradually learn to cope with the stress and problems involved in daily living. It is necessary to accept these patients without moralizing or blaming them for their behavior. On the other hand, it is necessary to help them begin to realize that they are responsible for their own behavior. Staff members need to be consistent and should not let alcoholic patients manipulate one staff member against another, as they often try to do. It is important to carefully evaluate physical complaints. If there are valid problems, they should be treated, but staff members should not let patients manipulate them into giving extra medications for nonexistent ills. At times, alcoholics going through detoxification become so desperate for alcohol that they will drink anything they think might have some alcohol content, including mouthwash and hair tonic.

It is important to point out realities to alcoholic patients and to try to keep them functioning in the "here and now." If they are expressing remorse about what has happened in their lives or are expressing unrealistic plans for their future, they may be doing so to avoid coping with current problems. Activities that increase the alcoholic patient's interaction with staff members and others help to build the patient's self-esteem. It is important to reward or reinforce appropriate behaviors exhibited by alcoholics and to be sure that they receive recognition for all accomplishments.

Insofar as outpatient or follow-up care is concerned, inpatient hospital staffs and outpatient clinic staffs are rather limited in their effectiveness. Maintenance of sobriety depends primarily on the alcoholic. Most treatment centers try to work with the families of alcoholics while the patient is in treatment. Their acceptance of the patient and willingness to help are vital links in the recovery process.

After their discharge, many alcoholics take a drug called Antabuse (disulfiram) to discourage them from drinking. If they take even one drink while on Antabuse, they may experience severe nausea and vomiting, redness of the face and trunk, headaches, heart palpitations, a drastic lowering of their blood pressure, and sometimes even death. Patients who have tried to drink while taking Antabuse indicate that the reaction is so severe that they will never drink alcohol again, at least not while they are on Antabuse. It should be noted that not all persons respond the same way to Antabuse; some patients can drink some amount of alcohol while on Antabuse whereas others will react strongly to very small amounts. Antabuse works by allowing an accumulation of acetaldehyde in the patient's system. Acetaldehyde is an extremely potent toxin that produces hypotension and nausea. The hypotension may produce shock, which can produce death. The drug is active for 3 to 5 days after its last ingestion.

One-to-one psychotherapy on an outpatient basis has not been shown to be successful in treating alcoholics. Group therapy programs such as those offered by Alcoholics Anonymous seem to be considerably more effective. Groups such as A.A. have a structured program with built-in rewards and reinforcements as well as built-in restrictions. A.A. gives alcoholics someone or something more powerful than themselves to lean on. Alcoholics know that if their resistance to taking a drink begins to slip, they can simply call their A.A. partner (called a sponsor) and they will receive help immediately. Perhaps A.A. groups are more successful in treating alcoholics because their members were once active alcoholics themselves. Not only do these people have greater empathy for the alcoholic, but they also have a personal understanding of the problems faced by the alcoholic. A.A. also sponsors a group called Al-Anon, which meets to help the families of alcoholics learn to deal effectively with their alcoholic family member. Regardless of the method, treating the alcoholic is a difficult task.

ABUSE OF OTHER DRUGS

Patients who abuse drugs other than alcohol also come from all socio-economic levels. Male addicts, however, outnumber female addicts 3:1. Most of these addicts show basic similarities in personality structure and can be described as rather unstable, immature, passive, dependent individuals. Their self-esteem is usually poor and they seem to lack a purpose in life. They tend not to become involved in social activities and have strong self-destructive tendencies. Many are self-centered and seem to relish playing the role of martyr. Such individuals have difficulty tolerating stress, anxiety, or pain and many have poor interpersonal relationships. Drug addicts have significant feelings of futility and have either real or imagined deprivations. Such psychological maladjustments, along with ready access to drugs and peer acceptance of taking them, very often sets the stage for such individuals to become addicts.

Before becoming addicted to a narcotic, an individual has usually experimented with other types of drugs. Sometimes the addicted patient was exposed to drugs accidentally. For example, when hospitalized, a patient may routinely receive medication for pain. Not only is the pain relieved but the medication causes the patient to feel good and forget or ignore many or most of his or her problems. After being released from the hospital, the individual may then start looking for some drug to take to feel as he or she did as a result of the pain medication in the hospital. An individual may become psychologically addicted after the very first dose. Physical addiction may occur after a short period of time if the drug is used on a regular basis. When drug abusers begin to have difficulty obtaining the high they once did, they will begin to experiment with new drugs and combinations of drugs. This is, of course related to the fact that after regular use of a drug, the body develops a tolerance for that drug, and it takes a larger and larger dose to produce the same "high." Many drug abusers say that the first high from a drug is the ultimate.

After a while the drug abuser begins to take the drug not to feel good but primarily to keep from feeling bad and to prevent withdrawal symptoms. At this stage, many drug abusers begin to feel sick a great deal of the time. They have headaches, gastrointestinal problems, and stomach cramps. The symptoms of these problems are similar to flu symptoms. In addition, addicts often have to stop working because they are either too high or too sick to function. As the addict's tolerance increases and larger and larger doses of the drug are required to get high, an overdose is likely to occur. This happens when individuals exceed their personal tolerance level or threshold for that particular drug.

Sometimes accidental overdoses occur because the strength of drugs such as heroin and cocaine is not carefully controlled from bag to bag. For example, most heroin in the past was only 5 percent pure, but now a random bag might be 80 percent pure, which could cause an overdose.

Individuals also get into difficulty because additives such as strychnine are sometimes used to dilute or "cut" the drug. Occasionally, suspected informers are intentionally overdosed by their suppliers.

When individuals develop a tolerance to a particular drug, they also develop a cross tolerance for other drugs in the same generic family. For example, an addict who has built up a tolerance for meperidine (Demerol) will not be able to obtain a high using heroin, and vice versa.

Because of the cost of many of these drugs, addicts are often forced to steal to support their habit. Female addicts frequently become prostitutes. One bag of heroin costs between $15 and $25, and because some addicts take as many as 10 to 15 bags a day, it is easy to see that they can easily develop a $200 to $400 per day habit. Persons addicted to cocaine have told the authors their habits run as much as $500 to $700 a day.

Although many people believe that it is the "doped-up" individual who commits crime, the truth of the matter is almost the reverse. An individual who has had a "fix" is highly unlikely to commit any crime. While under the influence of the drug, the addict's needs are at least temporarily satiated and he or she is usually not interested in anything, including food, sex, or more drugs. It is only when addicts are faced with the possibility of being without drugs that they turn to crime as a means of ensuring their supply. Because addicts frequently spend all their money, time, and effort supporting their addiction, they do not eat well and consequently usually develop significant malnutrition problems.

Adults may develop other serious problems due to side effects of taking drugs. For example, the heroin addict who takes his drug intravenously may develop infectious hepatitis from using contaminated needles, which also is one of the most certain ways of contracting the AIDS virus. Persons ingesting cocaine nasally may experience deterioration or necrosis of the tissues in the nasal area. Other possible complications include overdose, local infection, respiratory infection, severe constipation, and severe malnutrition, which generally weaken the body's defense system. The "rush" that the addict gets immediately after taking a drug has been compared with a sexual orgasm and for most addicts seems to erase any fear or consideration of possible side effects. After a fix, addicts may appear to be in a state somewhere between sleep and wakefulness where life has no problems. They are relaxed, content, and experiencing feelings of extreme well-being.

Although Demerol is the drug most abused by physicians and nurses, the general population also abuses many other types of drugs. Narcotics and analgesics are frequently abused, as are central nervous system stimulants such as the amphetamines, hallucinogenic drugs such as LSD, barbiturates (such as secobarbital [Seconal] and phenobarbital), and some of the minor tranquilizers such as Valium and Librium. Marijuana is one of the most commonly abused drugs after alcohol. The 1985 National Household Survey on Drug Abuse for the National Institute on Drug Abuse, reviewing nonmedical drug use, shows alcohol has been used at least once by 57 percent of people surveyed, cigarettes by 45 percent, marijuana by 24 percent, inhalants by 9 percent, stimulants by 6 percent, analgesics by 6 percent, cocaine by 5 percent, tranquilizers by 5 percent, sedatives by 4 percent, and hallucinogens by 3 percent. A review of several studies of the incidence of drug abuse, not including alcohol, suggests that between 5 and 7 percent of the population abuses drugs in such a way as to meet *DSM-IV* criteria for legitimate diagnosis of addiction or abuse.

When using alcohol, individuals have a pretty good idea of what to expect when they drink. Unfortunately, the same is not true for people who abuse other drugs. Individuals on amphetamines or hallucinogens are equally likely to have a good or bad trip. Even when they have a good trip, they may become quite depressed afterward, and many have strong suicidal impulses.

Treatment

Abusers of other drugs enter treatment in much the same manner as alcoholics. They may be seen by a physician because of an overdose or other medical complications or because they are brought to the treatment center by friends. Occasionally, addicts will seek help on their own. In general, the prognosis for any drug addict is not good, and the prognosis for heroin addicts is very poor. The cure rate for heroin addiction is said to be about 1 percent.

Recognizing Signs and Symptoms

Hospitalized patients who are suspected drug abusers should be observed carefully for the signs and symptoms of withdrawal. These may begin approximately 12 to 16 hours after the patient's last fix. These signs and symptoms include red or teary eyes, yawning, a runny nose, restlessness, and within about 48 hours, flulike symptoms that may include abdominal cramps. In some cases, the patient is quite hostile and paranoid and will refuse treatment if possible. Any time a treatment team member observes a large number of needle marks (tracks) on a patient's arms, hands, or legs, the possibility of drug abuse should be considered, especially if the patient has other characteristics associated with drug abuse.

Overdoses. In treating the drug addict who has overdosed, the so-called *ABCs* of an overdose should be observed. *A* is to establish an open airway, *B* is to breathe the patient, giving mouth-to-mouth resuscitation if other equipment is not available, and *C* is to provide cardiopulmonary resuscitation, often known as pumping. Some authorities add a "*D*," the administration of an antagonistic drug, which for narcotic overdoses is usually naloxone (Narcan). In cases of barbiturate overdoses, the doctor will administer an anticonvulsant drug.

After the immediate medical crisis has passed, the treatment of the drug-overdosed individual is very similar to that of the alcoholic. It is important to remember that the addict is usually a psychologically immature individual who is probably not accustomed to making decisions and is fairly dependent. Be candid with the addict but not judgmental. The addict needs patience and understanding but also structure and consistency. The addict can also be quite manipulative and may resort to trickery to get the medication he or she needs. An addict may prick a finger and place a drop of blood in a urine sample to fake a urinary tract infection. Because urinary tract infections are quite painful, that trick could be good for several analgesics. Both alcoholics and other drug addicts like to make others responsible for their behavior. It is necessary, therefore, to be sure that a staff member does not accept responsibility for the addict's behavior.

Methods of Treatment

Methadone maintenance programs, along with a variety of programs emphasizing individual, group, and family therapy, have been used to help heroin addicts. Methadone is a drug that is similar to heroin but does not produce euphoria. The addict does not stay high and is, therefore better able to function. Essentially, the methadone maintenance programs allow the addict to function by substituting one addictive agent for another with fewer incapacitating properties. Methadone is legal, and over a long period of time the physician may be able to decrease the dosage. Hopefully, the addict will eventually not need heroin or methadone. Methadone is fairly inexpensive and can also be used to entice patients into therapy groups if the physician insists that patients go to group therapy to obtain the methadone.

Whatever an individual's drug of choice, the goal of most therapy groups is to help people develop a different perspective of the world, become better educated about the ill effects of drugs on their physical and psychological well-being, appreciate that life is possible without drugs or alcohol, learn how to establish and maintain positive interpersonal relationships, develop more positive feelings of self-esteem, and engage in lifestyle changes that will support a drug-free existence. "Therapeutic communities" and "halfway houses" often provide an extended therapeutic opportunity to help addicts make the transition from drug dependency to being productive members of society.

Finally, do not forget that psychological problems are often associated with alcohol and drug abuse and dependencies. Anxiety, depression, and various psychosomatic complaints are often a part of the symptom picture. Those issues should be properly diagnosed and addressed if treatment is to be successful.

In summary, drug-dependent and alcohol-dependent individuals are generally difficult to treat. They often lack motivation and use a great deal of denial about the amount of drug or alcohol use. There are often psychological as well as physical complications. The etiology of drug and alcohol abuse is not always clear, and relatively little is known about exactly why people become addicted. Treatment activities often must be carried out against the patient's will and even if the patient "recovers," relapse is more the rule than the exception. Still, some addicts are rehabilitated; it is probably the success of those, and the hope of being able help more, that keep treatment teams involved in rehabilitation efforts.

▼ KEY POINTS ▼

Abuse of Alcohol

1. People who chronically abuse alcohol are known by a variety of names ranging from problem drinkers to alcoholic, wino, lappster, derelict, or bum.

2. The term *problem drinker* is applied to a person who has alcohol-related problems but does not have the obvious symptoms associated with clinically diagnosed alcoholics.

3. The *DSM-IV* does not use the term *alcoholic*. Instead it uses *Alcohol Dependence* as the diagnosis for describing the drinking characteristics and persons who have been called *alcoholics* since Magnus Huss coined the term in 1849.

---

continued on page 408

Key Points continued

4. Patients are diagnosed as alcoholics when they have lost control of their drinking to the extent that interpersonal, family, and community relationships have become seriously threatened or impaired.

5. Long-term alcohol-dependent persons tend to be pale, thin, and poorly nourished because they spend their money on alcohol and forget to eat when they are drinking.

6. Only 5 percent of alcoholics display the stereotypical characteristics of the Skid-Row-bum type.

7. The majority of alcoholics go to work every day wearing neatly pressed clothes; they have families, go to church on Sunday, live in suburbia, and generally keep up a good front.

8. Alcohol abuse alone has been said to be the third-largest health problem in America.

9. Statistics indicate that alcohol abusers are found in all socioeconomic groups.

10. Alcohol remains the most commonly abused drug in the United States, is more readily available than other drugs, and its use is socially accepted by our society.

11. We are a nation of drug takers; the television daily presents the virtues of every conceivable form of pain relief, sleep inducer, muscle relaxer, and vitamin supplement.

12. Television commercials market a large assortment of "pills" and alcoholic beverages as a sure means of making life more tolerable or pleasurable.

13. Many drug abusers drink or take pills in an attempt to withdraw or sedate themselves, or to escape from the realities or boredom of the world in which they live.

14. The most significant impact created by media advertising of alcohol and pills lies in the promotion of an attitude rather than promotion of the products themselves.

Factors Influencing Alcoholism

15. Some authorities report that the alcoholic has ambivalent feelings about living and dying and that chronic alcoholism represents a slow form of suicide.

16. Many see alcoholism as a lifestyle, a means of adjusting to a particular combination of circumstances and personality types.

Key Points continued

17. The history of an alcoholic often shows a very poor mother-child relationship and significantly poor self-esteem.

18. Many alcoholics have passive and dependent personality traits and have difficulty facing up to life's daily problems. However, no clinically validated "alcoholic" or "addictive" personality style exists.

19. Alcohol-dependent persons often lack the confidence to make choices, feel inadequate to face the basic tasks of life, and easily become frustrated and hostile.

20. Alcoholics are likely to be rejected by others and may begin to experience difficulty in meeting their basic needs.

21. They often appear to be either wrapped up in their own problems or in significant denial of their problems.

22. A constitutional or genetic factor has also been suggested as a possible reason for why some people who drink become alcoholics whereas others do not.

23. Social factors such as stress and social acceptance of drinking may also contribute to alcoholism.

24. Most authorities do not believe that an individual chooses to become an alcoholic; that is, it is not an act of will.

25. Drinking temporarily makes it easier for the alcohol dependent to face problems, insecurities, shyness, disappointment, hurt, or perceived failure.

26. The alcoholic's self-esteem problems often become severely compounded.

27. Alcoholics often use denial as a defense mechanism and have much difficulty accepting personal responsibility for their drinking problem.

28. Addiction to alcohol is both psychological and physical. Psychological dependence usually occurs before physical dependence.

Physiological Effects of Alcohol

29. It is important to remember that alcohol is a poison and is highly toxic to the body.

30. An individual who is drinking is less able to think discriminately, resulting in impaired judgment and motor function.

continued on page 410

31. Alcoholics in the emergency room setting should be carefully checked for subdural hematomas and other signs of trauma such as bruises, contusions, and fractures.

Recognizing Alcoholic Tendencies

32. Alcoholics tend to use denial as a defense against having to face their alcoholism, and they are likely to go for a long time without treatment.

33. The denial mechanisms associated with alcoholism may cause the person being questioned to lie or to stretch the truth.

Treatment of the Alcoholic

34. Patients who are diagnosed as alcoholics are often rejected not only by family and friends but also by the medical personnel who are assigned to care for them.

35. Alcoholics tend to relapse frequently, which sometimes makes it difficult for staff members to determine whether they are making progress.

36. Alcoholism is a chronic illness and as in all chronic illnesses, the patient is subject to relapses. However, the high relapse rate has been suggested as one of the main reasons alcoholics have difficulty finding acceptance among treatment team members.

37. The denial mechanism is brought into play by the individual as a defense against admitting alcoholism and is a major obstacle throughout the treatment process.

38. Alcoholics often enter treatment in one of four ways:
    a. through recognition of the alcoholic status by someone in the general hospital when the patient is admitted for some other reason.
    b. they are brought by the police after being picked up for public drunkenness.
    c. when a family member, concerned friend, employer, or health-care worker becomes aware of an individual's drinking problem.
    d. through self-referral.

39. One category of alcoholics who usually seek treatment on their own is those with pathological intoxication.

Key Points continued

Recognizing Signs and Symptoms

40. It is important for all team members to be aware of the signs and symptoms that indicate possible alcoholism. Active "DTs" may not occur for a period of 1 to 8 days after the last drink, but many symptoms appear within 12 to 48 hours. The symptoms include:
    a. experiencing shakiness or tremors.
    b. making unreasonable demands.
    c. throwing temper tantrums.
    d. becoming nauseated.
    e. showing evidence of dehydration.
    f. becoming extremely restless, agitated, aggressive, and confused.
    g. becoming disoriented and possibly experiencing hallucinations.

41. At any point during withdrawal the alcoholic may begin to convulse and may die if not carefully managed.

42. A general rule is that although both drug and alcohol withdrawals cause slowed motor responses, drowsiness, and confusion, in the toxic alcohol state the patient's vital signs are usually elevated.

43. In drug overdoses, all vital signs are usually depressed.

Methods of Treatment

44. Medical treatment of alcoholics usually consists of some type of group therapy or individual psychotherapy.

45. Alcoholics are sometimes hospitalized or at least treated in a special outpatient detoxification unit.

46. Treatment of acute withdrawal from alcohol is accomplished primarily through the use of medication.

47. Librium is the tranquilizer most commonly used in the treatment of alcoholics, but other minor tranquilizers are also used.

48. Anticonvulsants may be needed to further reduce convulsive activity in these patients, and multivitamin therapy is essential to replace the vitamin loss due to poor nutrition.

49. Alcoholics must always be considered to have a malabsorption syndrome until proven otherwise.

continued on page 412

Key Points continued

50. A great deal more than the appropriate use of medications is involved in the successful treatment of alcoholics; make sure alcoholics learn about the effects of alcohol on the body.

51. It is necessary to help alcoholics begin to realize that they are responsible for their own behavior.

52. At times, alcoholics going through detoxification become so desperate for alcohol that they will drink anything they think might have some alcohol content.

53. It is important to point out realities to alcoholic patients and to try to keep them functioning in the "here and now."

54. Reward or reinforce appropriate behaviors exhibited by alcoholics and be sure that they receive recognition for all accomplishments.

55. After discharge, many alcoholics take a drug called Antabuse (disulfiram) to discourage them from drinking. Taking even one drink while on Antabuse can result in serious illness.

56. One-to-one psychotherapy on an outpatient basis has not been shown to be successful in treating alcoholics. Group therapy seems to be substantially more effective because there is less opportunity to manipulate group members than an individual therapist.

Abuse of Other Drugs

57. Patients who abuse drugs other than alcohol also come from all socioeconomic levels; male addicts, however, outnumber female addicts 3:1.

58. Drug abusers' self-esteem is usually poor, and they seem to lack a purpose in life.

59. They tend not to become involved in social activities and have strong self-destructive tendencies.

60. Drug abusers have difficulty tolerating stress, anxiety, or pain and have poor interpersonal relationships.

61. Drug abusers have significant feelings of futility and have either real or imagined deprivations.

62. Before becoming addicted to a narcotic, an individual has usually experimented with other types of drugs or was exposed to drugs accidentally.

Key Points continued

63. Many drug abusers say that the first "high" is the ultimate, and the abuser begins to take the drug not to feel good but primarily to keep from feeling bad and to prevent withdrawal symptoms.

64. Sometimes accidental overdoses occur because the strength of drugs such as heroin and cocaine is not carefully controlled from bag to bag.

65. When an individual develops a tolerance to a particular drug, he or she also develops a cross tolerance for other drugs in the same generic family.

66. Because of the cost of many of these drugs, addicts are often forced to steal or commit other antisocial acts to support their habit.

67. An individual who has had a "fix" is highly unlikely to commit any type of crime. While under the influence of the drug, the addict's needs are at least temporarily satiated.

68. Adults may develop other serious problems due to the side effects that often occur as a result of taking drugs.

69. The "rush" the addict gets immediately after taking a drug has been compared with a sexual orgasm and seems to erase any fear of possible side effects.

70. Demerol is the drug most abused by physicians and nurses.

71. Narcotics and analgesics are frequently abused by the general population, as are central nervous system stimulants.

72. Studies of the incidence of drug abuse suggest that between 5 and 7 percent of the population abuses drugs in such a way as to meet *DSM-IV* criteria for legitimate diagnosis.

73. When using alcohol, individuals have a pretty good idea of what to expect when they drink. Unfortunately, the same is not true for people who abuse other drugs.

Recognizing Signs and Symptoms of Abusers of Other Drugs

74. Hospitalized patients who are suspected drug abusers should be observed carefully for the following signs and symptoms of withdrawal:
    a. red or teary eyes.
    b. yawning.

continued on page 414

Key Points continued

    c. runny nose.
    d. restlessness.
    e. flulike symptoms.

Treatment for Overdoses

75. In treating the drug addict who has overdosed, the ABCs of an overdose should be observed:
    A = establish an open airway
    B = breathe the patient
    C = provide cardiopulmonary resuscitation

76. The treatment of the drug-overdosed individual is very similar to that of the alcoholic.

77. The addict is usually a psychologically immature individual who is probably not accustomed to making decisions and is fairly dependent.

78. Both alcoholics and other drug addicts like to make others responsible for their behavior.

79. Methadone maintenance programs, along with a variety of programs emphasizing individual, group, and family therapy, have been used to help heroin addicts.

80. The goal of most therapy groups is:
    a. to help the person develop a different perspective of the world.
    b. to become better educated about the ill effects of drugs on their physical and psychological well-being.
    c. to help them appreciate that life is possible without drugs or alcohol.
    d. to help them learn how to establish and maintain positive interpersonal relationships.
    e. to develop more positive feelings of self-esteem.
    f. to engage in lifestyle changes that will support a drug-free existence.

81. Do not forget that psychological problems are often associated with alcohol and drug abuse and dependencies.

Annotated Bibliography

Allebeck, P., and Allgulander, C.: Suicide among young men: Psychiatric illness, deviant behavior and substance abuse. *Acta Psychiatrica Scandinavica,* 1990, 81:565–570.

A longitudinal study analyzing the role of psychiatric illness, as opposed to social and behavioral risk factors for suicide.

Bennett, J. B., and Jaquish, A.: The Winner's Group: A self-help group for homeless chemically dependent persons. *Journal of Psychosocial Nursing,* 1995, 33(4):14–19.

Discusses the success of a self-help group for the homeless and thus supports the value of providing such services.

Earley, P. H.: The changing face of addiction: Is everything I do an addiction? *Insight,* 1992, 12(3):2–7.

Explores the growth of the addiction movement, and provides information on what is and what isn't an addictive disease.

Foerster, D. W.: Turning back: The anatomy of relapse. *Insight,* 1992, 12(3):24–27.

Provides a definition and insight into the process of relapse from an addictive disease.

Goldenberg, I. M., Mueller, T., Fierman, E. J., et al: Specificity of substance use in anxiety-disordered subjects. *Comprehensive Psychiatry,* 1995, 36(5):319–328.

Examines the primary and secondary anxiety groups and onset of substance use disorder.

Haldeman, K.: Are elderly alcoholics discriminated against? *Journal of Psychosocial Nursing and Mental Health Services,* 1990, 28(5):6–11.

Discusses the prevalence of alcoholism in the elderly and the lack of programs designed to meet the need of this population.

Harvey, J. S.: Why does it happen? The latest research in addiction. *Insight,* 1992, 12(3):10–13.

Explores the cause of addiction and questions why some people become addicted whereas others do not.

Kokkevi, A., and Stefanis, C.: Drug abuse and psychiatric comorbidity. *Comprehensive Psychiatry,* 1995, 36(5):329–337.

Examines the relationship between substance abuse and Axis II diagnoses.

Kranzler, H. R., Kadden, R. M., Burleson, J. A., and others: Validity of psychiatric diagnoses in patients with substance use disorders: Is the interview more important than the interviewer? *Comprehensive Psychiatry,* 1995, 36(4):278–288.

Provides data on the concurrent, discriminant, and predictive validity of current substance use disorders and common comorbid diagnoses in a sample of 100 substance abuse patients.

Margolis, R.: Leaps of faith: A model for recovery. *Insight,* 1992, 12(3):18–23.

Discusses recovery of the addict with emphasis on the 12-step programs such as A.A.

Posig, M. T.: A conspiracy of silence: Women and recovery. *Insight,* 1992, 12(3):8–9.

Discusses the lack of equality in treatment for men and women in terms of recognition, treatment, and understanding.

Riley, J. A.: Dual diagnosis. *Nursing Clinics of North America,* 1994, 29(1):29–33.

Discusses the relevance of psychiatric-mental health nursing and dual diagnosis in regard to substance abuse and personality disorders.

Rubio-Stipec, M., Bird, H., Canino, G., Bravo, M., and Alegria, M.: Children of alcoholic parents in the community. *Journal of Studies on Alcohol,* 1991, 52(1):78–88.

Provides information on how alcoholism and adverse family conditions increase the risk of maladjustment in children.

Salloum, I. M., Mezzich, J. E., Cornelius, J., Day, N. L., Daley, D., and Kirisci, L.: Clinical profile of comorbid major depression and alcohol use disorders in an initial psychiatric evaluation. *Comprehensive Psychiatry,* 1995, 36(4):260–266.

Examines the coexistence of depression and alcoholism.

References

Jellinek, E. M.: *The Disease Concept of Alcoholism.* New Haven, Conn.: College and University Press, 1960.

National Institute for Drug Abuse: *National Household Survey on Drug Abuse.* Washington, D.C.: Alcohol, Drug Abuse, and Mental Health Administration, 1985–1986.

Post-Test

True or False. Circle your choice.

T F 1. Alcohol abuse has been said to be the third-largest health problem in the United States.

T F 2. Some authorities report that an alcoholic has ambivalent feelings about living and dying and that chronic alcoholism represents a slow form of suicide.

T F 3. Most alcoholics have aggressive and independent personality traits.

T F 4. Three out of four American adults drink to some extent.

T F 5. Alcoholics use the defense mechanism of denial most frequently and have difficulty accepting responsibilities for their drinking problem.

T F 6. In the prodromal phase of alcoholism there is a loss of control and the individual is unable to abstain from drinking.

T F 7. Alcoholics may go into active delirium tremens (DTs) any time from 1 to 8 days after their last drink.

T F 8. One-to-one psychotherapy is quite successful in treating alcoholism.

T F 9. Most authorities believe that all alcoholics begin to drink for the same reason.

T F 10. In the prealcoholic phase, drinking takes the place of the development of adequate copying mechanisms.

Short Answer. Answer as briefly and specifically as possible.

1. When are individuals diagnosed as being alcoholics?

_____

_____

Post-Test

(continued)

2. Describe the general physical appearance of a chronic alcoholic.

_____

_____

3. What appears to be the major key in the successful treatment of alcoholism?

_____

_____

_____

4. List three effects that alcohol has on the body.

a. _____

b. _____

c. _____

5. Describe the behaviors presented in the chronic phase of alcoholism as proposed by Jellinek.

_____

_____

_____

6. What is the most frequent way an alcoholic receives treatment?

_____

_____

_____

Multiple Choice. Circle the letter or number you think represents the best answer.

1. The best definition of an alcoholic is:
   a. A person who consumes alcohol every day.
   b. A person who regularly goes on "benders."
   c. A person who drinks to escape problems.
   d. A person who has developed a dependency on alcohol which causes him or her serious problems in living.

Post-Test

(continued)

2. The neurotic person uses alcohol:
   a. To build confidence.
   b. To escape responsibility.
   c. As a substitute for sex.
   d. To relieve anxiety.
   e. To consciously get mothering from others.
      (1) a, b, and d.
      (2) b and c.
      (3) a, b, c, and d.
      (4) c, d, and e.
      (5) All of the above.

3. The person with acute alcoholic hallucinosis most frequently experiences:
   a. Auditory hallucinations.
   b. Visual hallucinations.
   c. Tactile hallucinations.
   d. Olfactory hallucinations.

4. The defense mechanisms most commonly used by the alcoholic include all of the following except:
   a. Rationalization.
   b. Projection.
   c. Denial.
   d. Sublimation.

5. Alcohol is:
   a. A central nervous system stimulant.
   b. A central nervous system depressant.
   c. A fat oxidizer.
   d. A major tranquilizer.
   e. A volatile anesthetic agent.

6. When patients who are taking Antabuse consume alcohol in any quantity, they experience:
   a. Nausea, palpitations, and vomiting.
   b. Elation, grandiosity, and impotence.
   c. Headaches, dermatitis, and nocturnal sweats.
   d. Hepatitis and gastritis.

Post-Test

(continued)

7. The primary site for detoxification of alcohol is:
   a. The kidneys.
   b. The stomach.
   c. The intestines.
   d. The liver.
   e. The brain.

8. A patient is admitted with DTs. Possible observable symptoms are:
   a. Restlessness, tremors, and confusion.
   b. Depression, withdrawal, and tearfulness.
   c. Suspiciousness, depression, and unpredictability.
   d. Manipulation, stubbornness, and negativism.

9. The drug that is used specifically to help alcoholics refrain from drinking is:
   a. Morphine.
   b. Dilantin.
   c. Antabuse.
   d. Chlorpromazine.
   e. Librium.

10. Which of the following behavior patterns best describes the addicted individual?
    a. Ability to tolerate anxiety.
    b. Concern for the welfare of others.
    c. Inability to tolerate frustration.
    d. Inability to derive pleasure.

11. Care of a drug addict should involve observing the patient for immediate withdrawal symptoms, which include:
    a. Lacrimation, muscle twitching, rhinorrhea, and insomnia.
    b. Drowsiness, confusion, lability, and hallucinations.
    c. Tremors, euphoria, nausea, and palpitations.
    d. Inappropriate affect, restlessness, and impotence.

12. The most difficult problem in dealing with drug addicts is:
    a. Combating withdrawal symptoms.
    b. Keeping patients free of dependence on drugs.
    c. Obtaining family cooperation.
    d. Teaching them the danger of resorting to stronger drugs.

Care for Geriatric Patients

OBJECTIVES: Student will be able to:

1. Identify several factors involved in the elderly's loss of self-esteem.

2. Relate the effects of retirement and the assumption of the elderly role to self-perception.

3. Discuss the effect of lifelong adjustment patterns in the elderly.

4. Discuss the life task of reviewing successes and failures and how that may affect late-life satisfaction.

5. Cite the suicide rate among the elderly and reasons for it.

6. Identify major diseases occurring in the elderly.

7. Recognize the differential effect of medications on the elderly as compared to younger persons.

8. Cite a similarity between teenagers and the elderly.

9. Identify at least 10 basic principles of working with the elderly.

10. Identify several basic needs of the elderly.

Because aging begins at the moment of conception, it seems it should be considered a natural process of living. Unfortunately, that is not the case in our society. Americans, as well as most people in the Western world, have become so engrossed with the idea of youthfulness that to become old is often seen as a fate worse than death itself. Billions of dollars are spent each year on beauty aids, cosmetic surgery, and other "miracle" treatments by individuals seeking to prevent, or at least cover up, the telltale signs of aging.

This emphasis on youthfulness is not the only factor causing the elderly to feel they are no longer valued members of our society, but it seems to be the major culprit. The mere presence of the elderly seems to make younger generations uncomfortable, perhaps because their existence serves as a constant reminder that aging does indeed occur. Maybe this is part of the reason so many elderly are abandoned by their families and their society. One wonders what attitudes will prevail by the year 2000 when it is predicted that more than half of our country's population will be over age 55, with one-third being 65 years of age or older.

In addition to the normal day-to-day problems of living, the elderly must cope with special situations associated with old age and retirement. They tend to suffer a significant loss of self-esteem and often develop negative feelings about themselves. This loss of self-worth occurs for a variety of reasons, but retirement seems to be a major contributor. Our society values workers and often disregards nonproductive or unemployed individuals.

Retirement is viewed as the time in life when one is supposed to sit back, relax, and reap the benefits of years of hard work. Unfortunately, the mere act of reaching age 65 does not automatically change the work habits and attitudes an individual has developed over a lifetime. Many persons in Western cultures equate their worth as human beings with what they contribute to society as workers; therefore, to retire is to become worthless.

Retirement may also bring about a drastic reduction in income, which in turn contributes to the loss of self-esteem. Older individuals may no longer be able to afford to live independently of their children or may be forced to live in substandard housing. Inadequate nutrition may result from poor eating habits necessitated by a lack of money. Most often little, if any, money is left over for entertainment, recreational activities, or hobbies. Frequently, the older individual settles down into a life of drudgery and boredom and may become depressed.

Activities are further restricted by a loss of hearing, poor eyesight, and other physical ailments that occur with greater frequency as the individual grows older. Poor health, coupled with the loss of family and friends, forces the elderly to face the inevitability of death. Some older individuals have a greatly decreased ability to tolerate emotional stress and few resources or opportunities to compensate for their losses. In such cases, interest in living begins to diminish. Perhaps this loss of interest is a contributing factor to the results of a recent survey indicating that people live only an average of 60 months past retirement.

All people, regardless of age, need to love and be loved, have sufficient economic resources to meet basic physical needs, feel a sense of achievement, and receive recognition from others. Because elderly people begin to lose many of these satisfactions, a healthy adjustment to aging requires the ability to realistically appraise circumstances, making the most of the negative aspects and capitalizing on the positive. An elderly widow may not like the fact that she can no longer afford to live alone and must now live with a married daughter. On the other hand, she can make the most of the situation by offering to help with appropriate household chores and child care. By contributing in this manner, the grandmother may feel that she is a part of the family rather than a guest.

Emotional adjustment to old age is usually a continuation of life-long adjustment patterns. People often believe that they are going to change their ways when they get old. Instead of being "cantankerous," they say that they are going to become sweet and loving. There is little chance such a change will occur. Basic personality traits and ways of handling stress are formed early in life and if anything, the aging process exaggerates these traits and behaviors as the elderly person experiences the stress of losing authority, independence, and usefulness. The fact that people behave in ways that get them what they want is also not necessarily altered by age. The elderly may scream, yell, have temper tantrums, or become depressed or withdrawn in much the same way as they did early in life, if such behaviors helped to get what they wanted. On the other hand, they may be calm, quiet individuals who look at any new situation in an objective problem-solving manner, just as they did as well-adjusted young adults.

In mentally healthy individuals, the final years of life are years in which they have an opportunity to acknowledge their contributions to themselves, their families, and their society. They recognize that whatever they have done with their lives must now be accepted because they cannot live their lives over again. This is Erikson's eighth stage of development, Integrity versus Despair. For individuals who have been reasonably successful and who have developed healthy self-concepts, these tasks may be accomplished fairly easily. For individuals who have not been successful and thus do not feel reasonably fulfilled, aging is likely to bring a great deal of stress in the form of regret, guilt, and remorse, which form the psychological basis for despair. When elderly individuals cannot resolve such feelings, they often experience neurotic or psychotic disorders. Others may show significant behavioral disorganization as a result of their despair, which must be differentiated from the result of neurological impairment or disease processes.

Despite many potential problems, most elderly people in this country are alert, competent, and functioning with reasonable independence in their communities. As Caldwell (1975) says, "Advanced age is reached only by those who have proved themselves capable of survival." Available data suggests that only 5 percent of the elderly need custodial care and that only 1 percent are found in mental hospitals, taking up about 30 percent of all public mental health beds. Included in that 30 percent are patients who have 1) been in mental facilities all their lives, 2) those who have been admitted off and on throughout their lives and who cannot cope with added stresses of old age, and 3) those elderly patients who have become ill for the first time. Another 10 percent of our elderly population seeks care for physical and mental disorders on an outpatient basis from community clinics. Several million more elderly people live under economic and environmental conditions that contribute to emotional breakdown. Although the elderly now account for only 12.5 percent of our total population, approximately 20 percent (Butler, 1989) of all suicides in this country are committed by elderly individuals (although these figures vary from 20 to 35 percent depending on the study).

Of the elderly patients confined to mental health institutions, most suffer from senile brain atrophy or brain changes that occur due to arteriosclerosis. *Cerebral arteriosclerosis* is a condition marked by a thickening and hardening of the arteries of the brain. When this occurs, less blood and oxygen reach the brain and the patient experiences periods of confusion and varied levels of consciousness. These patients may also be forgetful and complain of headaches, dizziness, and weakness. They seem to have little emotional control and are often irritable and argumentative with family members, other patients, and staff. They may wander about aimlessly, having a noticeable shuffling gait and a tendency to lean backward as they try to maintain their balance.

The cause of senile brain atrophy is unknown, but in the course of the disease, calcium deposits appear in brain tissues. The size and weight of the brain decreases and the amount of cerebrospinal fluid increases. The patient becomes progressively more and more confused. The patient has trouble remembering recent events, but can recall in detail experiences of the past. Emotional instability is common, and tears or rage come quickly with little justification.

Another major problem for the elderly, and not so elderly, has been the increase in the number of cases of Alzheimer's disease and Alzheimer's-type dementias (called Dementia of the Alzheimer Type in *DSM-IV*). Although there is some indication that genetic factors may be involved, research is still lacking in terms of a definitive explanation for the cause of Alzheimer's disease, and treatment is equally lacking. This disease is characterized primarily by a gradual and progressive loss of cognitive or thinking and problem-solving ability, loss of memory, poor judgment, disorientation, and behavior and personality changes. Memory impairment is usually noticed first; the more obvious cognitive interruptions do not show up until the middle stages of the disease. In the late stage of the disease, individuals become mute and inattentive and cannot care for themselves. Death usually occurs within about 5 years of onset.

Elderly patients may also experience any of a number of psychiatric disorders. Depression is common and neurotic and paranoid reactions occur rather frequently. All forms of therapy are used in treating these disorders, and elderly patients respond to therapy in about the same manner as any other age group.

Staff members working with elderly patients must be careful to distinguish among individual mannerisms, temporarily stressful situations, and true psychotic or neurotic disorders. Is Mr. Jones, who walks up and down the hall talking to himself, confused because of a psychiatric disorder, disoriented because he was suddenly moved to unfamiliar surroundings in the middle of the night, still oversedated from his sleeping pill, or just a person who has always walked around mumbling to himself as he thought things over? Various physical factors such as infection, dehydration, hunger, traumatic injuries (e.g., broken bones) may cause the elderly patient to become temporarily confused. Restraining such patients often makes matters worse. Staff members must try to discover and understand the cause of behavior and help the patient to control it with as little loss of freedom and dignity as possible.

Extreme caution should be used when ordering or administering medications to elderly patients. Often a smaller amount of a given drug is indicated due to such factors as increased sensitivity to medications, decreased body weight, impaired circulation, and liver dysfunction. The likelihood of adverse drug reaction or overmedication (especially with barbiturates) is increased because kidney function is decreased and, therefore, drugs are not excreted from the system as quickly as in a younger person.

BASIC PRINCIPLES OF CARE

Working with elderly patients requires that certain basic principles of care be followed. Staff members should allow them to maintain as much independence as they can safely handle. Feelings of frustration that contribute to fears, anxieties, restlessness, and agitation are much like the frustration experienced by teenagers. Teenagers long for independence from adult authority, yet they are afraid to give up the security of having someone on whom to rely. Elderly patients, although wanting to maintain their independence, also long for the security of depending on others. Elderly persons may also be compared with toddlers in that both groups cannot quite accomplish all the functions necessary to allow complete freedom. A toddler can get her shoes on, but cannot tie the laces. An elderly person may have the same problem due to arthritic changes that make it difficult to bend over and to use the hands. Both situations cause feelings of frustration and possibly angry outbursts at anyone nearby.

Despite some similarities, elderly patients must not be treated as if they were children. This mistake is often made by well-meaning family members and friends. When bossed around in an authoritarian, condescending, or parent-to-child manner, their response may become obstinate and contrary. One of the authors was recently asked to evaluate an 87-year-old male nursing home patient. The staff reported that he had become combative and had attacked not only several staff members but another elderly patient as well. In the process of doing the evaluation, interviews with the family revealed that one of the male nursing aides had been joking with the patient, saying "Wanna fight? C'mon, put 'em up" and raising his hands into a fighting stance. This was interpreted by the patient and the family as taunting the patient, although the staff member meant no harm and thought he was "just joking around." The patient did have significant cognitive decline and lacked the ability to distinguish among such socially subtle distinctions as taunting and joking. The result was to further anger and frustrate the patient, who responded by attacking anyone who came near. Interviews also made it clear that the reason he had attacked the other patient was that he was trying to enter what he thought was his room and she was preventing him from entering the room because it was, in fact, her room.

Correct names should be used with elderly patients. Despite what many people believe, few of the elderly enjoy being called "Granny" or "Gramps" except by family members. Names are important to people and being addressed correctly conveys respect. Most elderly patients especially dislike being given pet names by staff members. An individual struggling to maintain self-identity and respect has no wish to become a mascot.

The feeling of being accepted is needed by the elderly as much as by younger persons. Personal habits such as dressing in a certain sequence or always drinking coffee from a saucer should be permitted. However, staff members should try to correct unsanitary or self-defeating habits by encouraging more appropriate behaviors and by restructuring the environment to eliminate the need for some of the inappropriate behavior. For example, if Mr. Green insists on taking a short walk despite the fact that he can hardly balance himself, a staff member might try to find an easily accessible place, provide him with a cane or walker, and walk with him. If he is clearly not able to walk very far, he might agree to a shorter walk if the staff member will get a picture book of world travels to show and discuss with him.

Loneliness is a major problem for older people, even those who are hospitalized. They greatly need someone they can trust and who will be supportive. Sometimes a simple pat on the arm, a gentle hug, or a back rub can communicate a sense of warmth and affection. Most elderly patients need this type of human closeness and should not be rejected when they reach out to a staff member for comfort.

Elderly patients need to be encouraged to talk about their feelings, fears, and worries. If they want to talk about old memories, they should be permitted to do so. Sometimes elderly patients have difficulty remembering recent events due to organic brain changes, but more often they dwell in the past as a means of dealing with the painfulness of the present. They may also be attempting to understand their present situation by reviewing past events in their lives. However, if elderly patients continually "live" in the past, staff members should attempt to focus their attention on daily events.

Patients and their families should be encouraged to maintain close communication. Fortunately, the pattern of hospitalizing mentally ill patients in their own community instead of sending them to large, distant state hospitals is well established. This fosters a continuing relationship with family and friends and helps the rehabilitation process. Many elderly patients do not need to be hospitalized if they can participate in day-care programs and return to their homes at night. Thus, many communities have day-care treatment centers for elderly persons.

Older individuals need to be encouraged to participate in activities that bring them in contact with other people. Staff members should help patients choose activities that they not only enjoy but that bring satisfaction and a sense of purpose while helping to fill the long hours of the day. They must practice their socialization skills in order to keep them. Socialization is also important because it helps patients to maintain a satisfactory orientation to their environment. They learn names and places and make friends. A few other things can also be done to help keep patients oriented. Placing a large clock in the room and a cube calendar that can have the date changed each day is helpful. Patients are more aware of the year, month, day, and time if such devices are available. To help with orientation to place, patients may be taken for walks or wheelchair rides or placed by windows so that the front, side, or back of buildings can be pointed out.

Older patients do not like to be rushed. They rise early and their days are long, so they should not be pushed. They also fare much better in a calm, consistent environment that functions at a moderately slow pace and follows a well-established routine.

The physical needs of the elderly are of primary importance and the staff should ensure that these needs are met. Most will readily report physical problems to staff members, but patients who are confused must be carefully observed. They may be unable to report problems accurately.

It is imperative for elderly patients to stay active and to participate in physician-approved exercise programs. Physical activity promotes good health by increasing circulation, stimulating appetite, helping regulate bowel function, and preventing the complications of inactivity such as joint immobility, muscle stiffness, bed sores, and pneumonia. Fresh air is good for the elderly and, if dressed warmly, being outside on cold winter days is not harmful.

Staff members should be constantly alert for potential hazards in the environment. Those having problems with dizziness should be assisted when walking, climbing stairs, or getting in or out of the tub. To minimize stumbling by those with impaired vision, furniture should not be rearranged. Floors should not be slippery and carpets and tiles should be kept in good repair. Throw rugs should never be used because they slide easily and may cause a fall. If elderly patients are confused or groggy they should not be allowed to smoke alone. A staff member should sit with them and utilize that time to interact with the patient.

Staff members should be aware that patients may need help with personal hygiene, especially if they are confused or forgetful. The degree of help needed will vary. Some patients will need total care, and others will need only minor assistance such as fastening a dress with buttons up the back or tying shoelaces. Patients should be allowed to do all they can for themselves even when it would be much quicker and simpler for a staff member to assist or do the task themselves.

It is usually not necessary for elderly patients to take a complete bath every day. The face, underarms, and perineum do need daily washing. Because the skin has a tendency to be dry, frequent washing will increase dryness. Soap must be thoroughly rinsed off to avoid itching and skin irritation. Elderly patients may enjoy showers because it is hard to get into and out of a tub and they are often afraid of falling. If a patient tires easily or is unstable, a chair can be placed in the shower stall so that he or she can shower in a sitting position. Remember, elderly patients are usually very modest, and their right to personal privacy and dignity should be respected whenever possible.

A well-balanced diet is essential to health; however, physical changes may lead to problems in this area. Ill-fitting dentures and tough, undercooked meats and foods may make chewing difficult if not impossible. Dentures must be worn consistently to avoid a misfit. Conversely, any time a patient consistently does not wear dentures, it usually means they hurt and are not properly fitted. Most elderly patients do not like to eat alone and appetite may decrease as activity level decreases. Constipation may cause discomfort and lead to a poor appetite. Plenty of fluids, fruits, and vegetables should be included in the diet to aid digestion. If a patient is used to taking a mild laxative on a routine basis, there is probably no harm in allowing this practice to continue. In the event of a problem, the patient's physician should be consulted. Elderly individuals often eat slowly and need to be allowed to finish their meals at a leisurely pace. Most seem to prefer small meals served frequently rather than three big meals a day.

Staff members must be alert to behavioral changes that indicate physical problems. If Mr. Jones does not answer when his name is called, he may not be acting stubbornly but may actually have a hearing problem due to a buildup of ear wax. A patient who stumbles over objects may need glasses. A male patient who urinates frequently may have an enlarged prostate. Bunions, corns, ingrown toenails, or ill-fitting shoes may be the real reason a patient refuses to go outside for a walk.

If patients do not sleep well at night, their sleeping patterns during the day should be observed. If they have been taking a daytime nap, the length of that nap might be shortened, bedtime delayed, activities increased, and relaxation methods such as a warm bath or warm milk used just before bedtime. If sleeping pills are used, the patient may be groggy and sleepy during the day and awaken just in time to go to bed again. This pattern is not uncommon and should be considered if a patient has difficulty sleeping.

Working with the elderly is not easy, and staff members who do this work need a great deal of patience. In not too many years, today's staff members will be elderly patients themselves. It is not a matter of if, but a matter of when. They might strive to be the kind of staff member they would like to have when they become the patients.

▼ KEY POINTS ▼

Elderly Patients

1. Americans have become engrossed with the idea of youthfulness, and billions of dollars are spent each year on beauty aids, cosmetic surgery, and other "miracle" treatments.

2. The elderly often feel they are no longer valued members of our society.

3. By the year 2000, it is predicted that more than half of our country's population will be over age 55 with one-third being 65 years of age or older.

continued on page 430

Key Points continued

4. Because many persons in Western cultures equate their worth as humans with what they contribute to society as workers, many elderly feel that to retire is to become worthless.

5. The sometimes drastic reduction in income associated with retirement also contributes to the loss of self-esteem.

6. Activities for the elderly are often restricted by a loss of hearing, poor eyesight, and other physical ailments.

7. A recent survey indicates that people live only an average of 60 months past retirement, possibly due to an overall diminished interest in living.

8. All people, regardless of age, need to love and be loved, to have sufficient economic resources, to feel a sense of achievement, and to receive recognition from others.

9. Emotional adjustment to old age is usually a continuation of lifelong adjustment patterns; the aging process often exaggerates basic personality traits and behaviors as the elderly person experiences the stress of losing authority, independence, and usefulness.

10. For the mentally healthy, the final years of life are years in which the elderly have an opportunity to acknowledge their contributions to themselves, their families, and their society (Erikson's eighth stage of development).

11. Elderly people who have not been successful and who do not feel reasonably fulfilled often experience neurotic or psychotic disorders or significant behavioral disorganization.

12. Available data suggest that only 5 percent of the elderly need custodial care and that only 1 percent are found in mental hospitals.

13. The elderly now account for only 12.5 percent of our total population; however, 20 to 35 percent of all suicides in this country are committed by elderly individuals.

14. Of the elderly patients confined to mental health institutions, most suffer from senile brain atrophy or brain changes that occur due to arteriosclerosis.

15. Alzheimer's disease and Alzheimer's dementias have proved to be another major problem for the elderly.

Key Points continued

16. Elderly patients may also experience any of a number of psychiatric disorders including depression and paranoid reactions.

17. Staff members working with elderly patients must be careful to distinguish between individual mannerisms, temporarily stressful situations, and true psychotic or neurotic disorders.

18. Due to increased sensitivity to medications, extreme caution should be used when ordering or administering medications to elderly patients.

Principles of Geriatric Care

19. Working with elderly patients requires that certain basic principles of care be followed. A primary principle is that elderly patients should be allowed to maintain as much independence as they can safely handle.

Other basic principles include:

20. Do not treat elderly patients as if they were children.

21. When addressing an elderly person, use correct names to convey respect.

22. The feeling of being accepted is needed as much by the elderly as by younger persons.

23. The elderly need someone they can trust and who will be supportive.

24. Elderly patients need to be encouraged to talk about their feelings, fears, and worries.

25. Elderly patients and their families should be encouraged to maintain close communication.

26. Encourage the elderly patient to participate in activities that bring them in contact with other people.

27. Do not rush older patients; they require a calm, consistent environment that functions at a moderately slow pace and follows a well-established routine.

28. The physical needs of elderly patients are of primary importance.

29. It is very important that the elderly patient stay active and participate in physician-approved exercise programs.

continued on page 432

Key Points continued

30. Be constantly alert for potential hazards in the elderly patient's environment.
31. Be aware that elderly patients may need help with personal hygiene, especially if they are confused or forgetful.
32. A well-balanced diet is essential to the health of the elderly; however, physical changes associated with age may lead to problems in this area.
33. Be alert to behavioral changes indicating physical problems in the elderly patient.
34. If an elderly patient does not sleep well at night, his or her sleeping pattern during the day should be observed.
35. Working with the elderly is not easy, and staff members must exercise a great deal of patience.

Annotated Bibliography

Agostinelli, B., Demers, K., Garrigan, D., and Waszynski, C.: Targeted interventions: Use of the mini-mental state exam. *Journal of Gerontology Nursing,* 1994, 20(8):15–23.

Discusses the use of the MMSE as a tool for global cognitive assessment of the elderly and assessment of their daily living skills.

Beck, C., Heacock, P., Mercer, S., Walton, C. G., and Shook, J.: Dressing for success: Promoting independence among cognitively impaired elderly. *Journal of Psychosocial Nursing and Mental Health Services,* 1991, 29(7):30–35.

Presents ideas on how to encourage cognitively impaired elderly patients to take more responsibility for personal care.

Bergman, R., Ehrenfeld, M., and Golander, H.: Stimulating research thinking: The case for mini research. *Journal of Psychosocial Nursing,* 1995, 33(7):34–39.

Discusses ways to improve patient care in gerontopsychiatric units.

Copenhaver, M.: Better late than never. *Journal of Psychosocial Nursing,* 1995, 33(7):17–22.

Discusses assessment techniques for differentiating between somatic complaints of normal aging versus somatic complaints associated with depression.

Curl, A.: Agitation and the older adult. *Journal of Psychosocial Nursing and Mental Health Services,* 1989, 27(12):12–14.

Focuses on agitation caused by delirium, dementia, parkinsonism, and depression and the appropriate management of these behaviors by nursing staff.

Dellasega, C.: Meeting the mental health needs of elderly clients. *Journal of Psychosocial Nursing and Mental Health Services,* 1991, 29(2):10–14.

Preliminary investigation exploring the availability of mental health resources for the elderly on the local level with emphasis on outpatient services available and long-term care facilities.

Erbs-Palmer, V. K., and Anthony, W.: Incorporating psychiatric rehabilitation principles into mental health nursing. *Journal of Psychosocial Nursing,* 1995, 8(3):36–44.

Discusses the implementation of consumer and family involvement as a core value in nursing practice.

Kroessler, D.: Personality disorders in the elderly. *Hospital and Community Psychiatry,* 1990, 41(12):1325–1329.

A review of the literature on the prevalence of personality disorders in the elderly.

Masters, J. C., and O'Grady, M.: Normal pressure hydrocephalus: A potentially reversible form of dementia. *Journal of Psychosocial Nursing and Mental Health Services,* 1992, 30(6):25–28.

Discusses the symptoms, diagnosis, etiology, treatment, and nursing care for normal pressure hydrocephalus (NPH), a form of dementia that has proved to be reversible.

Puntil, C.: Integrating three approaches to counter resistance in a noncompliant elderly client. *Journal of Psychosocial Nursing and Mental Health Services,* 1991, 29(2):26–30.

Discusses how resistance is used by the elderly patient and how nurses can work through the resistance.

Strumpf, N. E.: Innovative gerontological practices as models for health care delivery. *Nursing and Health Care,* 15(10):522–527.

Discusses various models that have been implemented in an attempt to control the high cost of geriatric care and improve services.

Tappen, R. M.: The effect of skill training on functional abilities of nursing home residents with dementia. *Research in Nursing and Health,* 17:159–165.

Examines the effects of skill training on the ability to perform daily living activities on nursing home residents with dementia.

Tillman-Jones, T. K.: How to work with the elderly patients on a general psychiatric unit. *Journal of Psychosocial Nursing and Mental Health Services,* 1990, 28(5):27–31.

Focuses on the care of the elderly on a psychiatric unit with regard to assessment, planning, treatment, and evaluation.

Vaicunas, J., and Belser, R.: Later adulthood: Physical and cognitive development. In: Zanden, J. W. (ed.): *Human Development,* McGraw-Hill, New York, 1993, pp. 538–561.

Discusses the physical changes and biologic theories of aging as well as cognitive functioning in the process of aging.

Vaicunas, J., and Belser, R.: Later adulthood: Psychosocial development. In: Zanden, J. W. (ed.): *Human Development,* McGraw-Hill, New York, 1993, pp. 566–586.

Discusses psychosocial tasks and aspects of aging, including personality and patterns of aging as well as theories of adjustment.

Zerhusen, J. D., Boyle, K., and Wilson, W.: Out of the darkness: Group therapy for depressed elderly. *Journal of Psychosocial Nursing and Mental Health Services,* 1991, 29(9):16–21.

Research study examining the benefits of nurses facilitating cognitive group therapy with nursing home residents suffering from depression.

References

Caldwell, E.: *Geriatrics: A Study of Maturity.* Albany, N.Y.: Delmar Publishers, 1975.

Butler, R. N.: Psychosocial aspects of aging. In: Kaplan, H. I., and Saddock, B. J., (eds.): *Comprehensive Textbook of Psychiatry, Vol. 2* (ed. 5). Baltimore: Williams & Wilkins, 1989, pp. 2014–2019.

Post-Test

True or False. Circle your choice.

T   F   1. Most elderly patients hospitalized for psychiatric problems suffer from senile brain atrophy or brain changes that occur due to arteriosclerosis.

T   F   2. Calling the elderly "Granny" or "Gramps" tends to make them feel more at home.

T   F   3. It is necessary to encourage the elderly to hurry because they tend to be so slow.

T   F   4. Many elderly people feel that they are no longer valued members of our society.

T   F   5. Life situations often cause elderly individuals to suffer a significant loss of self-esteem and, therefore, to develop negative feelings about themselves.

T   F   6. Emotional adjustment changes drastically with increasing age.

T   F   7. The majority of elderly people are alert, competent, and functioning in their community.

T   F   8. Depression is a common psychiatric disorder seen in the elderly.

T   F   9. It is important for the elderly to maintain their independence whenever possible.

T   F   10. Whenever elderly patients begin acting like children, they should be treated as children.

T   F   11. Twenty to thirty-five percent of all suicides in this country are committed by elderly individuals.

Short Answer. Answer the following questions as briefly and specifically as possible.

1. What is a major factor contributing to the elderly individual's loss of self-worth and self-esteem?

_____

_____

Post-Test

(continued)

2. What are some of the main factors that should be considered before administering medications to elderly patients?

_____

_____

3. What is one of the main reasons why elderly patients have difficulty remembering recent events?

_____

_____

4. What are some basic things the mental health workers can do to keep the elderly patient well oriented?

_____

_____

5. Why is it necessary for the elderly patient to stay active?

_____

_____

Multiple Choice. Circle the letter you think represents the best answer.

1. People become old:
   a. At the same rate.
   b. When they reach age 65.
   c. When they reach age 75.
   d. At a very individual rate.

2. The basic attitude of Western culture toward the elderly is that:
   a. They should be held in esteem.
   b. They are of lesser importance.
   c. Their opinions should be sought.
   d. Their skills are valuable.

3. Changes in self-image are brought about by:
   a. Loss of vigor and vitality.
   b. Loss of independence.

Post-Test

(continued)

c. Loss of physical stamina.
d. All of the above.

4. The mental health worker can help increase patients' self-esteem by:
   a. Calmly accepting them and their behavior.
   b. Being critical of their behavior.
   c. Firmly stating what behavior is acceptable.
   d. Ignoring them until they behave in an acceptable way.

5. If an elderly patient complains that everyone is mumbling these days, which of the following is most likely to be true?
   a. He or she is just being cranky.
   b. He or she is probably becoming emotionally disturbed.
   c. His or her hearing is becoming less acute.
   d. None of the above.

6. Staff members must come to an understanding of their own feelings about the aged and aging because:
   a. They can be more therapeutic.
   b. Feelings are difficult to hide.
   c. Anxiety about aging is easily transmitted.
   d. All of the above.

7. A person's identity is reinforced when he or she wears:
   a. His or her own clothes.
   b. A hospital gown.
   c. A uniform.
   d. A friend's clothing.

8. The elderly person will probably eat better if:
   a. Food servings are large.
   b. Hard rolls are included.
   c. The foods are chewy.
   d. Food servings are small.

Post-Test

(continued)

9. A general precaution to remember when considering the safety of the elderly is:
   a. Confine the elderly individual to a small area.
   b. Keep their clothing less fitting and long.
   c. Have sufficient light.
   d. Use open heaters in the bathroom.

10. The most common accident to the elderly involves:
    a. Falls.
    b. Burns.
    c. Cuts.
    d. Bruises.

Crisis Intervention

OBJECTIVES: Student will be able to:

1. Define *crisis.*
2. Identify the goal of crisis intervention.
3. Identify ways a crisis may be precipitated.
4. Define *social crisis.*
5. Identify the four phases of a crisis.
6. Identify the steps in crisis intervention.

Mental health authorities define *crisis* as a state of psychological disequilibrium brought about by a conflict, problem, or life situation that an individual perceives as a threat to self, which cannot effectively be handled by using previously successful problem-solving and coping techniques. The crisis develops not because of the event itself, but because of the person's inability to cope with the event. When this situation occurs, individuals become increasingly anxious and tense and feel that their self-esteem and well-being are seriously threatened.

Without swift and effective intervention these feelings usually intensify rapidly and the individual may become behaviorally disorganized, have difficulty thinking in a rational manner, and experience feelings of anger, depression, helplessness, and guilt.

Patients in crisis are likely to repeat phrases such as: "I don't know what to do," "I feel so helpless," or "What's happening to me?" over and over again.

Therefore, crisis intervention is usually conducted in an outpatient setting on a short-term basis and utilizes problem-solving techniques to help patients resolve stress-provoking problems. The goal of this type of therapy is to help patients return to a level of functioning that is at least equal to their precrisis state. It is hoped that crisis therapy will also enable patients to learn new coping and adaptive behaviors, thus actually improving levels of mental health.

A crisis state may be precipitated by two types of events. Developmental or maturational crises are those that occur at foreseeable stages in the lives of most individuals. As discussed in earlier chapters, each stage of development has its developmental task. To carry out these tasks, certain traits and behaviors must be prominently strengthened while others must be restrained. Such changes often produce a great deal of stress, especially during the transition period between two developmental stages.

For example, many middle-aged couples become depressed when their long-awaited freedom from dependent children is replaced with greater emotional and financial responsibility for elderly parents. Learning to find workable solutions to this problem is one of the predictable developmental tasks of the middle years of life. This type of crisis can often be prevented by *anticipatory guidance,* an education process that alerts individuals and their families to behavioral changes they are likely to experience in current stages of development. This process allows the patient to foresee problem areas and to develop ways to adapt in a positive manner. Anticipatory guidance also helps individuals and their families to distinguish between normal experiences and unusual ones. The anxiety normally produced when an individual faces an unknown situation is thus reduced.

A second circumstance that may produce a crisis state is called a *situational event.* This kind of crisis is precipitated by an unexpected event that suddenly disrupts a person's life and threatens his or her emotional security. Some examples of events that may lead to situational crises include the loss of a loved one from death or divorce, loss of a job, a move to a new city or a new job, graduation from school, marriage, or an unwanted pregnancy.

Even a long-awaited promotion or career change may cause trouble because of added stress. Such events produce new situations with increased demands and challenges that the individual must meet.

A person may experience both types of stress-producing situations at the same time. Many middle-aged women trying to adjust to an empty nest syndrome find themselves also adjusting to the loss of a mate through divorce and the economic need to return to the workforce. It is understandable that persons experiencing multiple stressful events in close succession are likely to have difficulty coping in a positive manner.

Some authorities break situational crises into two subtypes: the specific unexpected situational events discussed above, and the social crises. A *social crisis* is defined as an unanticipated crisis that involves multiple losses, extensive environmental changes, or both. Examples include fires, floods, war, murder, and racial persecution. This type of crisis does not usually occur in everyday life, but when it does, stress levels become so high that the coping mechanisms of most everyone involved are seriously threatened.

Every individual reacts to a stressful event in a different way. Some seem to be able to handle an extraordinary amount of stress, whereas others find minor occurrences upsetting. Some degree of stress resulting from routine changes and challenges is unavoidable in day-to-day living. This type of stress is not necessarily bad, because it motivates us to complete our daily tasks, such as working or studying, in a satisfactory manner. Although these stresses usually affect only the individual, the individual in crisis is rarely the only person affected by a given situation. The individual's support system of significant others (family, special friends, neighbors) is invariably involved, and the support system should also be assumed to be in a state of crisis.

The development of a crisis seems to follow four different, overlapping phases (Table 23–1). The first phase is denial and usually lasts only for a few hours. *Denial* is a mental mechanism to temporarily defuse overwhelming anxiety. In mentally healthy persons, reality is quickly recognized, leading to an understanding of what is occurring. An example of denial is a wife's refusal to believe that the husband she kissed good-bye that morning has died in an automobile accident on the way to work. She may insist that the police and medical personnel have mistaken his identity. As she is given more details concerning the accident, the wife will begin to confront the reality of her situation.

In phase two, anxiety increases as the individual tries to continue daily activities while also searching for ways to handle the increased tension. The new widow somehow manages to make the funeral arrangements for her late husband and to get through the formalities.

The next stage is one of disorganization, when individuals in crisis seem to "go to pieces." They are unable to think clearly and neglect many of the activities of daily living. They are also preoccupied with the event. Persons in this stage are conscious of extreme anxiety, because coping mechanisms have failed, and there may even be fears of insanity. In this stage individuals may seek professional help to deal with the situation. The young widow at this stage may become unable to cope with household tasks such as cooking meals, preparing the children for school, and cleaning. She may neglect her personal appearance while dwelling on her husband's death and her inability to live without him. Decisions may become difficult or impossible for her to make.

With professional help the fourth and final stage should be one of reorganization and the development of new skills that allow individuals to function in a similar manner as before their crises. This gives them

Table 23–1. **The Four Overlapping Phases of a Crisis**

Phase 1: Denial

Lasts only a few hours.
Purpose is to temporarily defuse overwhelming anxiety.
In mentally healthy persons, reality is quickly recognized.

Phase 2: Anxiety

Individual tries to continue daily activities despite crisis.
Person searches for ways to handle increased tension.

Phase 3: Disorganization

Person "goes to pieces."
Person is unable to think clearly, neglects daily activities, is preoccupied
  with the event.
Individual is aware of extreme anxiety as coping mechanisms fail.
Person may fear he or she is going insane and seek professional help.

Phase 4: Reorganization and development of new skills

Individuals reorganize their lives according to the new realities.
Persons develop new skills that allow them to function as well as or better
  than before the crisis.
Persons resume daily activities.

the opportunity and ability to once again face the challenges of day-to-day living. If there is no improvement, anxiety will continue to increase until the patient experiences a state of panic and possibly generalized personality disorganization.

For the individual whose usual defense mechanisms are already functioning poorly, the extreme levels of stress and anxiety experienced during crisis are strong motivators. During this period persons are more likely to change their behavior in response to new problem-solving and coping techniques.

Because the acute stage of a crisis usually lasts approximately 4 to 6 weeks, patients who have not resolved the crisis or learned to cope successfully in that length of time may be referred to other professionals or to mental health agencies equipped to provide long-term therapies.

Aguilera and Messick (1978) state that effective resolution of a crisis situation is more likely to occur if the individual's perception of the precipitating event is realistic, if there are significant others in the patient's environment who are available and willing to help, and if positive coping mechanisms to deal with the stressful events in life have previously been developed and can be called upon. Resolution is also affected in a positive way by the therapist who is able to establish rapport quickly and who conveys to the patient a warm and caring attitude.

The first step in crisis intervention is to collect information about the nature of the crisis and the effect it is having on the patient and his or her family and friends. In the initial interview the mental health professional should identify the precipitating event and the patient's perception of that event, learn the patient's positive characteristics and coping mechanisms, and determine the strength of support the patient can expect from family and friends.

People usually seek help within 2 weeks of the precipitating event. Often the event may have occurred as recently as a day before the patient asks for help. In this stage of intervention, questions such as the following will help the mental health professional to obtain useful information:

What has happened that brought you here for help?

When did it happen?

Tell me how you feel.

How is this situation affecting your life?

How is it affecting those around you?

Have you ever faced a problem like this before?

When you are anxious or tense, what do you do to feel better?

Have you tried that this time?

What do you think might help you feel better?

Do you live with someone? Who?

Do you have a friend that you trust?

Do you have someone that you feel understands you?

Questions such as those above may help patients and their families put their thoughts and feelings in order at a time when they are likely to be disorganized. It may also be helpful to have patients give an account of their activities for the weeks preceding the intervention if they have difficulty identifying the event that precipitated the crisis. Talking about the situation should help lower the patients' state of tension, helping them to see the situation more clearly. At this point the nurse may find it helpful to reassure patients that seeking help is both a sign of strength and a step toward resolution of the problem. False reassurance should never be given. Instead, the nurse should express belief in the patients' ability to learn to cope, while encouraging them to help themselves in every way possible.

Planning is the second stage of the intervention process. All available data from the patient, his or her family, and any other professional sources should be reviewed and evaluated. A solution or solutions should be outlined and alternatives provided. The skills the patient will need to work through the problem should be identified and supportive community resources pointed out.

The third stage of crisis intervention is to implement the plan developed in stage two. First, the mental health professional should discuss his or her perception of the problem with the patient to see if their perceptions correspond, making corrections as needed. As both explore the precipitating event and the resulting crisis, the patient should be encouraged to verbalize his or her feelings about the situation.

Next, possible solutions to the problem may be discussed. Identify any of the patient's coping skills that may be useful, and explore the availability of supportive individuals in the person's environment. The mental health worker and patient may even role-play the new problem-solving techniques to allow the patient to become more comfortable with them in a controlled environment.

Sometimes the best approach to alleviating a crisis situation is to change the patient's physical or interpersonal environment. A middle-aged woman who faces the prospect of serious surgery and who also is responsible for her healthy but sometimes slightly confused elderly mother may have to make other living arrangements for the mother, despite the latter's strenuous objections. The mother may have to live temporarily with another son or daughter, or if this is not a feasible solution, the patient may need help in finding a home for senior citizens that provides the level of care her mother needs. If this type of care is too expensive for the daughter to finance alone, she will need to be referred to social agencies that can help her apply for funds to defray the additional cost.

As mentioned earlier, anticipatory guidance is also an effective way of dealing with many situational crises. Stages of grief have been identified for those who are seriously ill or dying, and these stages also apply to the feelings associated with the loss of a spouse through death or divorce, or diminished feelings of self-worth due to the loss of a job. The theorized stages, phases, or tasks of grieving provide frameworks to better understand universal human responses yet acknowledge individuality. Elizabeth Kubler-Ross (1969) described the stages of grief as denial, anger, bargaining, depression, and acceptance. Bowlby's (1980) theory of grief describes three phases of normal grieving: protest, disorganization, and reorganization. Similar phases are described by Engel (1964). He identifies the tasks and phases of the grieving process as initial shock and disbelief, developing awareness, restitution, and resolving the loss.

Education concerning these stages may be a very effective way of helping patients deal with the situations and the emotions involved. In all crisis counseling it is extremely important to establish a rapport with patients and to provide a therapeutic climate in which patients feel comfortable in voicing their feelings and concerns.

The final stage of the crisis intervention process is evaluation. In this stage the nurse or mental health worker and the patient have the opportunity to compare the goals they set in the planning stage with the actual behavioral changes in the patient's lifestyle. In the evaluation process, other unmet needs may be identified and appropriate patient actions or referrals to other helping agencies can be initiated.

It should be kept in mind that the goal of successful crisis intervention is at least to return patients to their precrisis level of functioning, hopefully with improved adaptive capabilities and within a relatively short time. Such short-term therapy in an outpatient setting allows community mental health workers to reach a greater number of patients more quickly and in this manner to prevent more severe mental problems that might require long-term hospitalizations.

▼ KEY POINTS ▼

Crisis Intervention

1. Mental health authorities define *crisis* as a state of psychological disequilibrium brought about by a conflict, problem, or life situation that the individual perceives as a threat and is unable to handle using previously successful techniques.

2. Patients experiencing crises become increasingly anxious and tense and feel that their self-esteem and well-being are seriously threatened. Without intervention the individual may become behaviorally disorganized.

3. Patients in crisis tend to repeat phrases such as: "I don't know what to do," "I feel helpless," or "What's happening to me?"

4. A crisis state may be precipitated by foreseeable stages that occur in the lives of most individuals, or by situational events. Both types of stress may be experienced at the same time.

continued on page 446

Key Points continued

5. Some authorities break situational crises into two subtypes: specific unexpected situational events and social crises.

6. Every individual reacts to a stressful event in a different way. Some seem to be able to handle an extraordinary amount of stress, whereas others find minor occurrences upsetting.

7. The individual in crisis is rarely the only person affected by a given situation. The individual's support system of significant others should also be assumed to be in a state of crises.

8. The development of a crisis seems to follow four different overlapping phases: denial, increased anxiety, mental disorganization, and reorganization with professional help in developing new skills.

9. For the individual whose unusual defense mechanisms are already functioning poorly, the extreme levels of stress and anxiety experienced during crisis are strong motivators for treatment.

10. The acute stage of crisis usually lasts approximately 4 to 6 weeks. Patients who have not resolved the crisis or have not learned to cope successfully in that time may require long-term therapies.

11. Resolution of a crisis is more likely to occur if:
    a. the individual's perception of the event is realistic.
    b. there are significant others in the patient's environment who are willing to help.
    c. positive coping mechanisms can be called upon.

12. People usually seek help within 2 weeks of the precipitating event.

13. Asking patients questions may help them and their families put their thoughts and feelings in order at a time when they are likely to be disorganized.

14. Talking about the situation should help lower the patient's state of tension and see the situation more clearly.

15. False reassurance should never be given. Instead, express belief in the patients' ability to learn to cope, while encouraging patients to help themselves in every way possible.

16. Planning is the second stage of the intervention process. A solution or solutions should be outlined and alternatives provided. The skills the patient will need to work through the problem should be identified and supportive community resources pointed out.

Key Points continued

17. The third stage of crisis intervention is to implement the plan developed in stage two. Explore the precipitating event and the resulting crisis. Encourage patients to verbalize their feelings about the situation.

18. Discuss possible solutions to the problem, identify the patient's coping skills and the availability of supportive individuals in the person's environment, and consider temporarily changing the patient's physical or interpersonal environment.

19. Establishing a rapport, providing a therapeutic climate, offering anticipatory guidance, and educating the patient on the stages are all effective ways of dealing with many situational crises.

20. The final stage of crisis intervention process is evaluation. Compare the goals set in the planning stage with the actual behavioral changes in the patient's lifestyle.

21. The goal of successful crisis intervention is at least to return patients to their precrisis level of functioning, hopefully with improved adaptive capabilities and within a relatively short time.

Annotated Bibliography

Cowles, K. V., and Rodgers, B. L.: When a loved one has AIDS: Care for the significant other. *Journal of Psychosocial Nursing and Mental Health Services,* 1991, 29(4):6–12.

Addresses the needs of family members, friends, and partners upon learning a loved one has AIDS. These needs include support and reassurance, assistance in adjusting to personal relationship changes, and help in becoming involved in some form of AIDS-related work.

Eppard, J., and Anderson, J.: Emergency psychiatric assessment: The nurse, psychiatrist, and counselor roles during the process. *Journal of Psychosocial Nursing,* 1995, 33(10):17–23.

Discusses the increasing importance of psychiatric nurses' functioning interdependently.

Lewin, L.: Interviewing the young child sexual abuse victim. *Journal of Psychosocial Nursing,* 1995, 33(7):5–10.

Discusses practical suggestions for interviewing children of sexual abuse.

McArther, M. J.: Reality therapy with rape victims. *Archives of Psychiatric Nursing,* 1990, 4(6):360–365.

Discusses the use of reality therapy groups with rape victims to provide a supportive arena where the victim can tell her story, diminish her desire to withdraw from others, and recognize control over her behavior.

Musto, S. M.: Trauma junkie: Taking charge of my survival. *Journal of Psychosocial Nursing,* 1995, 33(7):11–13.

Discusses the importance of nurses' awareness of their individual responses to violent behavior, which may help in their survival of a critical incident.

Rew, L., Agor, W., Emery, M., and Harper, S.: Intuitive skills in crisis management. *Nursing Connections,* 1991, 4(2):3–12.

Discusses the nurse's use of analytic reasoning and intuition to manage the complex, rapidly changing and often unpredictable circumstances surrounding crisis.

Shelby, J. S., and Tredinnick, M. G.: Crisis intervention with survivors of natural disaster: Lessons from Hurricane Andrew. *Journal of Counseling & Development,* 1995, 73:491–497.

The authors provide pragmatic interventions, focusing particularly on children's issues with the inclusion of multicultural issues.

Smith, S. B.: Restraints: Retraumatization for rape victims? *Journal of Psychosocial Nursing,* 1995, 33(7):23–27.

Discusses the common negative experiences associated with traumatized individuals who are restrained while in a hospital setting.

Walker, V., and Gatzert-Snyder, S.: When disaster strikes: The concerns of staff nurses. *Journal of Psychosocial Nursing and Mental Health Services,* 1991, 29(6):9–13.

Discusses how the calamity of an earthquake affected patient care delivery, and presents what nurses need to continue providing safe and efficient care in the midst of such adversity.

References

Aguilera, D. C., and Messick, M.: *Crisis Intervention: Theory and Methodology* (ed. 3). St. Louis: C. V. Mosby, 1978.

Bowlby, J.: *Loss, Sadness and Depression—Attachment and Loss,* Vol. 3. New York: Basic Books, 1980.

Engel, G.: Grief and grieving. *American Journal of Nursing,* September, 1964, 64(9):93–98.

Kubler-Ross, E.: *On Death and Dying.* New York: Macmillan, 1969.

Post-Test

Short Answer. Answer the following as briefly and specifically as possible.

1. State the goal of crisis intervention therapy.

_____

_____

_____

2. List and describe the four overlapping phases in the development of a crisis.

_____

_____

_____

_____

3. Define *crisis*.

_____

_____

_____

4. Define *social crisis*.

_____

_____

_____

5. List the four steps in crisis intervention.

_____

_____

_____

_____

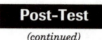

Post-Test

(continued)

Multiple Choice. Circle the letter or number you think represents the best answer.

1. A crisis state may be precipitated by which of the following events?
   a. Developmental and maturational stages.
   b. Transition period between two developmental stages.
   c. Unanticipated external event.
   d. b and c.
   e. a, b, and c.

2. Which of the following situations could precipitate a crisis?
   a. Marriage.
   b. Career change.
   c. Pregnancy.
   d. Job promotion.
      (1) a and b.
      (2) b and c.
      (3) a, b, and c.
      (4) All of the above.

3. Which of the following are manifestations of a person in crisis?
   a. Anxiety and tension.
   b. Increased feelings of self-esteem.
   c. Feelings of anger and depression.
   d. Behaviorally disorganized.
      (1) a and b.
      (2) b only.
      (3) a, c, and d.
      (4) All of the above.

4. Which of the following is not a recognized phase in the development of a crisis?
   a. Disorganization.
   b. Reorganization.
   c. Denial.
   d. Anger.

5. The acute stage of a crisis usually lasts approximately:
   a. 4 to 6 weeks.
   b. 6 to 8 hours.

Post-Test

(continued)

    c. 3 to 4 days.
    d. 4 to 6 days.

6. The initial step in crisis intervention is to:
    a. Try to resolve the problem.
    b. Collect information.
    c. Identify the strength of support.
    d. Identify the patient's positive characteristics.

7. The final stage of the crisis intervention process is:
    a. Evaluation.
    b. Anticipatory guidance.
    c. Implementing the plan of action.
    d. Exploring possible solutions.

8. Which of the following would not be considered a social crisis?
    a. Flood.
    b. War.
    c. Racial persecution.
    d. Loss of job.

True or False. Circle your choice.

T   F   1. Sometimes the best approach to alleviating a crisis situation is to actually change the patient's physical or interpersonal environment.

T   F   2. It is all right to give false assurance to patients if it helps them get through the crisis.

T   F   3. Most of the time it is necessary to hospitalize a person in a crisis situation.

T   F   4. The first phase in the development of a crisis is denial.

T   F   5. Anticipatory guidance is an effective way of dealing with many situational crises.

T   F   6. A certain amount of stress in life is unavoidable.

Answer Keys

Chapter 1

Attitude Inventory

1. F	11. T	21. F	31. F	41. T
2. F	12. F	22. F	32. F	
3. T	13. F	23. F	33. T	
4. F	14. F	24. F	34. F	
5. T	15. F	25. T	35. F	
6. F	16. F	26. T	36. F	
7. T	17. F	27. F	37. F	
8. F	18. T	28. T	38. F	
9. F	19. T	29. T	39. F	
10. F	20. F	30. F	40. F	

True or False

1. T	6. T
2. T	7. F
3. F	8. F
4. T	9. F
5. F	10. F

Fill in the Blanks

1. f, d
2. e
3. c
4. a
5. g

Multiple Choice

1. (3)
2. (2)
3. (4)
4. (4)
5. (3)

Chapter 2

Fill in the Blanks

1. b
2. a
3. d
4. c
5. e

True or False

1. F   6. F
2. T   7. F
3. T
4. F
5. F

Multiple Choice

1. b   6. b   11. b   16. d
2. c   7. a   12. (5)   17. c
3. b   8. d   13. b   18. (4)
4. (4)   9. c   14. c   19. c
5. a   10. d   15. (5)   20. a, b, c

Chapter 3

Matching

1. g
2. c
3. e
4. a
5. i
6. d
7. b
8. f

True or False

1. T
2. F
3. T
4. F
5. F
6. T

Fill in the Blanks

1. c
2. a
3. b, f
4. e
5. g

Multiple Choice

1. (4)   6. (3)   11. c   16. (2)
2. (3)   7. c   12. d   17. (4)
3. d   8. (5)   13. a   18. d
4. c   9. e   14. c
5. a   10. e   15. c

Chapter 4

True or False

1. F	6. T	11. T
2. T	7. T	12. F
3. F	8. F	13. F
4. F	9. T	14. T
5. T	10. T	

Matching

1. d
2. c
3. a
4. f
5. e

Short Answer

1. Willful neglect, abuse, harassment, or failure to attend adequately to a patient.
2. In a voluntary admission the patient admits himself. Involuntary admission involves legal action in which it is determined by a judge or a doctor (depending on state law) that a person is to be admitted.
3. Tell the patient you do not know the answer but will attempt to find out and tell him.
4. To protect the patient from harming himself or others.
5. A negligent act.

Chapters 5–7

Matching

1. d	6. i
2. a	7. b
3. h	8. c
4. e	9. f
5. f	

True or False

1. F	6. F	11. F
2. F	7. F	12. T
3. T	8. T	13. F
4. T	9. F	
5. F	10. F	

Short Answer

1. Persistent and irrational fear of some object, place, or condition.
2. Rigid; perfectionistic; often obstinate.

3. Tendency to be self-indulging; poor self-concept; exaggerated dependency needs.

4. Accept the patient.

5. In organic psychosis, pathology can be demonstrated; functional psychosis is caused by psychological stress.

6. Sexual disorders (paraphilia) involve sexual activity and arousal patterns that are not common to the general public; sexual dysfunctions involve problems with carrying through the usual sexual response cycle from attraction, to desire, to arousal, to intercourse, to orgasm.

Multiple Choice

1. a	6. c	11. (4)	16. c	21. b
2. b	7. d	12. d	17. b	22. a
3. d	8. a	13. d	18. b	
4. d	9. a	14. e	19. (3)	
5. b	10. c	15. c	20. d	

Chapter 8

True or False

1. T	6. T
2. T	7. F
3. T	8. T
4. F	9. F
5. T	10. T

Multiple Choice

1. d	6. b	11. (4)
2. d	7. d	12. d
3. d	8. (5)	13. d
4. d	9. b	
5. (3)	10. c	

Chapter 9

Matching

1. g
2. d
3. a
4. f
5. e
6. b
7. c

True or False

1. F
2. F
3. T
4. F
5. T
6. T
7. F
8. F
9. F
10. F
11. T
12. T
13. F
14. T
15. F

Multiple Choice

1. c
2. b
3. d
4. (2)
5. (1)
6. (2)
7. (1)
8. d
9. b
10. c
11. a
12. d
13. b
14. c

Chapter 10

Matching I

1. c
2. a
3. e
4. b
5. f

Matching II

1. e
2. d
3. f
4. e
5. b
6. a
7. c
8. d
9. a

True or False

1. F
2. T
3. F
4. T
5. F
6. F

Short Answer

1. Help calm the patient, control severe agitation, and decrease hallucinations.

2. Increase fluid intake to help prevent dry mouth, and caution the patient to decrease fatty foods and increase intake of salads because of excessive weight gain and constipation problems.

3. Tricyclic compounds and MAO inhibitors.

4. Dry mouth, fatigue, weakness, blurring vision, constipation, parkinsonian syndrome, and increased perspiration.

Multiple Choice

1. (4)   5. c
2. (5)   6. (5)
3. d   7. (3)
4. (2)

Chapter 11

True or False

1. F
2. F
3. T
4. F
5. T
6. F

Short Answer

1. Helps the patient to forget painful life experiences; perceived by the patient as a form of punishment.
2. Electroconvulsive therapy may place a great deal of strain on the patient's heart.
3. Depressed patients.
4. To prevent the patient from aspirating during the treatment.

Multiple Choice

1. a
2. d
3. (2)
4. a
5. (3)

Chapter 12

True or False

1. T
2. T
3. F
4. T
5. F
6. T
7. T

Short Answer

1. a. A patient must want to get better.
   b. Must come to a better understanding of what is causing the problems and learn methods of dealing with them more effectively.
   c. Have an environment that is possible for change.
2. An environment in which it is possible for change to take place.
3. Help patients gain insight and/or understanding into their problems so they can learn to deal with them more effectively.
4. Seven of the following: probability overestimation; all-or-none thinking; fortune-telling; disqualifying the positive; catastrophizing; magnification and minimization; emotional reasoning; phonyism; overgeneralization; selective abstraction; should/must/ought statements; personalization.

Multiple Choice

1. c
2. (1)
3. (4)
4. b
5. c
6. (3)
7. (3)

Chapter 13

True or False

1. T	6. F
2. F	7. T
3. T	8. F
4. T	9. T
5. T	

Multiple Choice

1. (3)
2. (6)
3. b
4. d
5. d

Short Answer

1. Confront him with the behavior.
2. Plan a program of activities that will not permit the patients so much free time that they become bored.
3. Feels threatened and unable to do anything else.
4. Patients are usually calmer when they don't have an audience.

Chapter 14

True or False

1. T	6. F
2. F	7. F
3. F	8. T
4. T	9. T
5. F	10. F

Multiple Choice

1. (4)	7. (3)
2. a	8. b
3. (3)	9. b
4. (3)	10. c
5. (2)	11. e
6. a	

Chapter 15

True or False

1. T
2. F
3. T
4. T
5. T
6. F
7. T

Multiple Choice

1. c
2. c
3. c
4. c
5. c
6. e

Chapter 16

True or False

1. T	6. F
2. T	7. F
3. F	8. T
4. F	9. T
5. T	10. F

Multiple Choice

1. d
2. (1)
3. b
4. d
5. c
6. c

Chapter 17

Short Answer

1. 10 to 20.

2. Persons who have previously attempted suicide, the terminally ill, the elderly, the alcoholic, the severely emotionally ill, and people who associate with persons who have made suicide attempts.

3. The need for help and the recognition that something is wrong and a change is necessary for survival.

4. One's acute awareness and alertness.

5. Any three of the following:
   a. Persons who continuously talk about suicide.
   b. Persons who show the vegetative signs of depression.
   c. Persons who have extreme difficulty sleeping.
   d. Persons who dwell on sad thoughts.

True or False

1. T	6. T	11. F
2. F	7. T	12. T
3. F	8. F	13. F
4. T	9. F	14. T
5. T	10. F	15. T

Matching

1. a, b
2. c
3. d
4. e
5. a
6. e

Multiple Choice

1. c
2. (4)
3. (3)
4. (3)
5. (4)

Chapter 18

True or False

1. F	4. F
2. F	5. T
3. T	6. T

Multiple Choice

1. b
2. b
3. (2)

Short Answer

1. Two of the following: schizophrenia, senile dementia, manic-depressive psychosis.

2. May first exhibit loud talk, rapid pacing, grandiose ideas.

3. Delusions, illusions, and hallucinations.

4. An *illusion* is a false interpretation or misinterpretation of a real sensory impression.

5. A *hallucination* is an idea or perception that does not exist in reality.

Chapter 19

Multiple Choice

1. (5)	6. b
2. (2)	7. b
3. e	8. b
4. (5)	
5. (1)	

True or False

1. F
2. T
3. T
4. F
5. F

Short Answer

1. J = Judgment
   O = Orientation
   C = Confabulation
   A = Affect
   M = Memory
2. Be as brief as possible.
3. Five of the following:
   a. Wear large name tags.
   b. Put patients' names on their room doors.
   c. Put up large calendars with big numbers.
   d. Use big clocks and place several around patient areas.
   e. Show patients around the unit and help them only as much as they need it; do not be overly helpful because this increases dependency.
   f. Let patients bring favorite and familiar things from home; this will help their new room to become "theirs."
4. The patient may not remember what he said or did and thus feels that he is being unfairly punished.
5. Routine and structure.

Chapter 20

Multiple Choice

1. d
2. c
3. d
4. c
5. d
6. a

Short Answer

1. Make sure the patient is stabilized; establish trust; promote improved nutrition; promote effective coping; promote improved perceptions of body image; and promote feelings of self-worth.
2. Promote effective coping; identify binge triggers; promote guilt reduction; and involve the patient in discharge planning.

3. Nurses need to display nonjudgmental acceptance; teach good nutrition; establish realistic nutritional goals; encourage social interaction; and promote a sense of well-being.

True or False

1. T
2. F
3. F
4. F
5. T
6. F

Chapter 21

True or False

1. T	6. F
2. T	7. T
3. F	8. F
4. T	9. T
5. T	10. T

Short Answer

1. When they have lost control of their drinking to the extent that interpersonal, family, and community relationships have become seriously threatened or disturbed.
2. Tend to be pale, skinny, and poorly nourished; may have dilated blood vessels in their faces and a bulblike, fleshy nose.
3. The process of being able to accept the fact that one is an alcoholic.
4. a. Depresses bone marrow and thus the production of RBCs.
   b. Causes brain tissue changes.
   c. Scar tissue formations in the liver (cirrhosis).
5. Marked by frequent "benders" and usually daily intake of alcohol in response to the physical "craving."
6. Through recognition of the alcoholic status by someone in the general hospital when admitted for some other reason.

Multiple Choice

1. d	6. a	11. a
2. (1)	7. d	12. b
3. b	8. a	
4. d	9. c	
5. b	10. c	

Chapter 22

True or False

1. T	6. F	11. T
2. F	7. T	
3. F	8. T	
4. T	9. T	
5. T	10. F	

Short Answer

1. Retirement.
2. Factors such as increased sensitivity to medications, decreased body weight, impaired circulation, and liver dysfunction.
3. Organic brain damage.
4. Placing a large clock and a cube calendar in the room.
5. Activity promotes good health by increasing circulation, stimulating appetite, helping regulate bowel function, and preventing the complications of inactivity such as joint immobility, bed sores, and pneumonia.

Multiple Choice

1. d	6. d
2. b	7. a
3. d	8. d
4. a	9. c
5. c	10. a

Chapter 23

Short Answer:

1. The goal of crisis intervention therapy is to help clients return to a level of functioning that is at least equal to their precrisis state.

2. a. The first phase is denial and usually lasts for only a few hours. Denial is a mechanism used by the mind to temporarily defuse overwhelming anxiety.
   b. In phase two, anxiety increases and the individual tries to continue his daily activities while attempting to find a way to handle the increased tension.
   c. The third state is one of disorganization, where the individual in crisis just seems to "go to pieces."
   d. The fourth stage is one of reorganization and the development of new skills that allow the individual to function at a precrisis level.

3. Mental health authorities define *crisis* as a state of psychological disequilibrium brought about by conflict, problems, or life situations that an individual perceives as a threat to self and cannot effectively handle by using previously successful problem-solving and coping techniques.

4. A *social crisis* is defined as an unanticipated crisis that involves multiple losses and/or extensive environmental changes, such as fires, floods, war, murder, and racial persecution.

5. Collecting information, planning, intervention, and evaluation.

Multiple Choice

1. e
2. (4)
3. (3)
4. d
5. a
6. b
7. a
8. d

True or False

1. T
2. F
3. F
4. T
5. T
6. T

A Patient's Bill of Rights

1. The patient has the right to considerate and respectful care.

2. The patient has the right to and is encouraged to obtain from physicians and other direct caregivers relevant, current, and understandable information concerning diagnosis, treatment, and prognosis.

   Except in emergencies when the patient lacks decision-making capacity and the need for treatment is urgent, the patient is entitled to the opportunity to discuss and request information related to the specific procedures and/or treatments, the risks involved, the possible length of recuperation, and the medically reasonable alternatives and their accompanying risks and benefits.

   Patients have the right to know the identity of physicians, nurses, and others involved in their care, as well as when those involved are students, residents, or other trainees. The patient also has the right to know the immediate and long-term financial implications of treatment choices, insofar as they are known.

3. The patient has the right to make decisions about the plan of care prior to and during the course of treatment and to refuse a recommended treatment or plan of care to the extent permitted by law and hospital policy and to be informed of the medical consequences of this action. In case of such refusal, the patient is entitled to other appropriate care and services that the hospital provides or transfer to another hospital. The hospital should notify patients of any policy that might affect patient choice within the institution.

These rights can be exercised on the patient's behalf by a designated surrogate or proxy decision maker if the patient lacks decision-making capacity, is legally incompetent, or is a minor.

Reprinted with permission of the American Hospital Association, copyright 1992.

4. The patient has the right to have an advance directive (such as a living will, health care proxy, or durable power of attorney for health care) concerning treatment or designating a surrogate decision maker with the expectation that the hospital will honor the intent of that directive to the extent permitted by law and hospital policy.

   Health care institutions must advise patients of their rights under state law and hospital policy to make informed medical choices, ask if the patient has an advance directive, and include that information in patient records. The patient has the right to timely information about hospital policy that may limit its ability to implement fully a legally valid advance directive.

5. The patient has the right to every consideration of privacy. Case discussion, consultation, examination, and treatment should be conducted so as to protect each patient's privacy.

6. The patient has the right to expect that all communications and records pertaining to his/her care will be treated as confidential by the hospital, except in cases such as suspected abuse and public health hazards when reporting is permitted or required by law. The patient has the right to expect that the hospital will emphasize the confidentiality of this information when it releases it to any other parties entitled to review information in these records.

7. The patient has the right to review the records pertaining to his/her medical care and to have the information explained or interpreted as necessary, except when restricted by law.

8. The patient has the right to expect that, within its capacity and policies, a hospital will make reasonable response to the request of a patient for appropriate and medically indicated care and services. The hospital must provide evaluation, service, and/or referral as indicated by the urgency of the case. When medically appropriate and legally permissible, or when a patient has so requested, a patient may be transferred to another facility. The institution to which the patient is to be transferred must first have accepted the patient for transfer. The patient must also have the benefit of complete information and explanation concerning the need for, risks, benefits, and alternatives to such a transfer.

9. The patient has the right to ask and be informed of the existence of business relationships among the hospital, educational institutions, other health care providers, or payers that may influence the patient's treatment and care.

10. The patient has the right to consent to or decline to participate in proposed research studies or human experimentation affecting care and treatment or requiring direct patient involvement, and to have those studies fully explained prior to consent. A patient who declines to participate in research or experimentation is entitled to the most effective care that the hospital can otherwise provide.

11. The patient has the right to expect reasonable continuity of care when appropriate and to be informed by physicians and other caregivers of available and realistic patient care options when hospital care is no longer appropriate.

12. The patient has the right to be informed of hospital policies and practices that relate to patient care, treatment, and responsibilities. The patient has the right to be informed of available resources for resolving disputes, grievances, and conflicts, such as ethics committees, patient representatives, or other mechanisms available in the institution. The patient has the right to be informed of the hospital's charges for services and available payment methods.

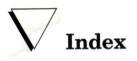

Index

Page numbers followed by "f" indicate figures; pages numbers followed by "t" indicate tables.